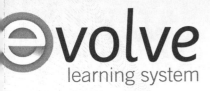

evolve
learning system

To access your free Evolve Resources, visit:

http://evolve.elsevier.com/Cairo

Register today and gain access to:

Instructor Only

- Test Bank
- Image Collection
- Instructor's Manual
- PowerPoint® Presentations

Student and Instructor

- Suggested Answers to Clinical Rounds
- Answers to Assessment Questions
- Answers Key to Workbook for Mosby's Respiratory Care Equipment
- Additional General-Use Ventilators
- Additional Transport, Home-Care and Alternative Ventilators
- Infectious Disease PowerPoint® Presentation
- Credits
- Weblinks

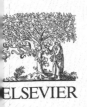

ELSEVIER

Workbook for Mosby's Respiratory Care Equipment

Eighth Edition

Sindee Kalminson Karpel, MPA, RRT
Clinical Coordinator
Respiratory Care and Cardiovascular Technology Programs
Edison State College
Fort Myers, Florida

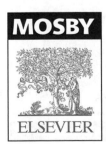

11830 Westline Industrial Drive
St. Louis, Missouri 63146

WORKBOOK FOR MOSBY'S RESPIRATORY CARE EQUIPMENT   ISBN: 978-0-323-05177-4

Notice

ISBN 13: 978-0-323-05177-4
ISBN 10: 0-323-05177-4

Publisher: Jeanne Wilke
Managing Editor: Billi Sharp
Senior Developmental Editor: Mindy Hutchinson
Publishing Services Manager: Julie Eddy
Project Manager: Marquita Parker
Designer: Paula Catalano

Printed in United States of America

Last digit is the print number: 9   8   7   6   5   4   3   2   1

To all my students, past, present, and future.
To my family for their unwavering support.

"Teachers open the door, but you must enter by yourself."
Chinese Proverb

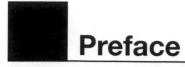

Preface

The primary purpose of this workbook is to help the respiratory care student in the comprehension and learning of the material presented in the eighth edition of *Mosby's Respiratory Care Equipment*, by James Cairo and Susan Pilbeam.

Reading and studying from a textbook like this requires active involvement, because comprehension of this type does not occur automatically. In order for you to get as much out of your study time as possible, your reading must be a conscious, organized, active undertaking. An active reading session is made up of four separate stages: (1) previewing, (2) reading to organize, (3) reading to find significant facts, and (4) summarizing. The purpose of this workbook is to focus the reader on the learning objectives of the textbook. Remember, the chapter learning objectives indicate what the author intends for the reader to know after finishing the chapter. Try as much as possible to use your own words to answer the questions. This will help with summarizing what you have learned.

At the end of each chapter there are NBRC-type questions. These may be used as a self assessment or by your instructor as an assignment. In addition, use the crossword puzzles to help test your knowledge of the chapter key terms.

Think of this workbook as a scaffold to assist you in building the foundation of your professional knowledge.

Sindee K. Karpel, MPA, RRT

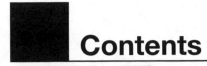

Contents

Basic Physics for the Respiratory Therapist

Upon completion of this chapter, you will be able to:
1. Differentiate between kinetic and potential energy.
2. Compare the physical and chemical properties of the three primary states of matter.
3. Explain why large amounts of energy are required to accomplish the changes associated with solid-liquid and liquid-gas phase transitions.
4. Convert temperature measurements from the Kelvin, Celsius, and Fahrenheit temperature scales.
5. Define pressure and describe two devices that are commonly used to measure it.
6. List various pressure equivalents for 1 atm.
7. Calculate the density and specific gravity of liquids and gases.
8. Explain how changes in pressure, volume, temperature, and mass affect the behavior of an ideal gas.
9. Calculate the partial pressure of oxygen in a room air sample of gas obtained at 1 atm.
10. List the physical variables that influence the flow of a gas through a tube.
11. Explain how the pressure, velocity, and flow of a gas change as it moves from part of a tube with a large radius to another part with a small radius.
12. Describe the Venturi and Coanda effects and how both can be used in the design of respiratory care equipment.
13. State Ohm's law and relate how changes in voltage and resistance affect current flow in a direct-current series circuit.
14. Describe three strategies that can be used to protect patients from electrical hazards.

"In physics, you don't have to go around making trouble for yourself — nature does it for you"
Frank Wilczek

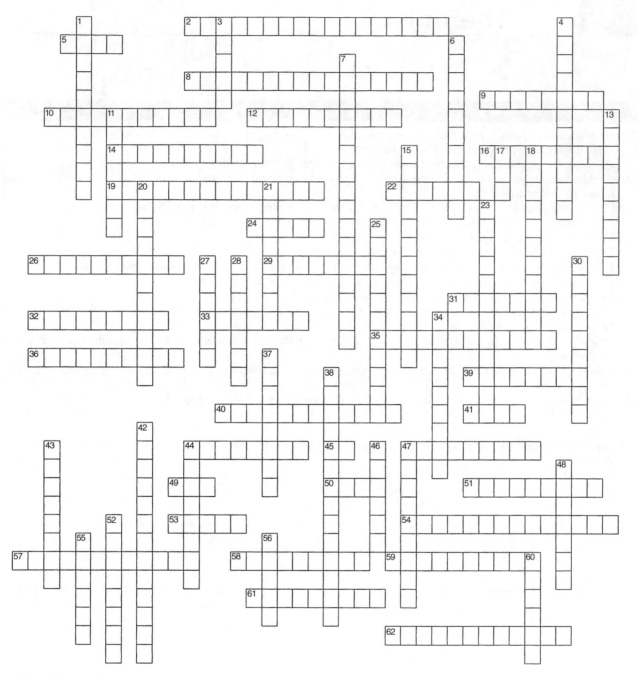

CROSSWORD PUZZLE 1-1
Created using Crossword Weaver, www.CrosswordWeaver.com.

Use the clues to complete the crossword puzzle.

Across

2. An amorphous solid, like margarine (*two words*).
5. A unit of power, equivalent to work done at the rate of 1 J/s.
8. A particular arrangement of multiple resistors in an electrical circuit (*two words*).

9. The type of humidity that is a ratio of actual to potential water vapor content.
10. Physical intermolecular forces that cause molecules to be attracted to each other (*three words*).
12. Animal power.

Chapter **1** **Basic Physics for the Respiratory Therapist**

14. Whose principle explains buoyancy?
16. The type of energy a body possesses by virtue of its position.
19. One of the fields of classical physics.
22. A field of study that deals with the electromagnetic radiation of wavelengths that are shorter than radio waves but longer than x-rays.
24. Another name for a liquid.
26. A common type of electrical thermometer.
29. The forces that cause the meniscus of a fluid to be convex.
31. The energy a body possesses by virtue of its motion.
32. The branch of physics dealing with the motion of material bodies and the phenomena of the action of forces on them.
33. A simple substance that cannot be broken down into any other substance by chemical means.
35. The temperature at which solids begin to turn into liquids (*two words*).
36. A device that determines the density of a liquid by comparing its weight with that of an equal volume of water.
39. Equal to 1000 W of electrical power.
40. The concept that all matter is made of submicroscopic atoms that are made of protons, electrons, and neutrons (*two words*).
41. The smallest division of an element composed of protons, electrons, and neutrons.
44. The pressure at which a material cannot exist as a gas.
45. An internationally accepted scientific system of units (*abbreviation*).
47. Glass and margarine are this type of solid.
49. The ability of electric energy to perform work (*abbreviation*).
50. The unit of electrical potential.
51. The branch of physics dealing with magnets.
53. A unit of energy equivalent to 1 W-second.
54. Materials with conductivity characteristics that are intermediate between conductors and insulators.
57. A change of state from gas to liquid is known as __ _____.
58. Whose number is 6.02×10^{23} (10 to the 23rd power)?
59. An imperceptible electrical current that is allowed to bypass the skin and follow a direct, low-resistance pathway into the body.
61. An instrument that measures the differences in potential between different points of an electric circuit.
62. The process whereby matter in its liquid form is changed into its gaseous form.

Down
1. The temperature scale in which the boiling point of water is 212 degrees.

3. A source of energy.
4. Direct transition of a substance from a solid to its gaseous state.
6. When applied externally to the skin, an electrical current of 1 mA or greater will deliver a _____ _____.
7. The actual content of water in a measured volume of air (*two words*).
11. The potential energy stored in a compressed spring.
13. In the equation PV/T = nR, *R* is whose universal gas constant?
15. The interaction of equal and opposite electrical charges.
17. A unit of measurement of electrical resistance.
18. The process by which liquids change into the vapor state.
20. The form of energy that can be produced by heat or generated by a voltaic cell or chemical activity.
21. A _____ is made up of two or more covalently bonded atoms.
23. The temperature at which a liquid begins to turn to a gas (*two words*).
25. An instrument for measuring temperature.
27. The standard unit of measurement of electric current.
28. An instrument for measuring the strength of an electric current in terms of amperes.
30. A nonconducting substance that is a barrier to heat or electricity passage.
34. The process of moving molecules from an area of high concentration to an area of lower concentration.
37. What type of potential energy is stored in coal, gas, or oil?
38. A concave meniscus is caused by _____ _____ (*two words*).
42. The potential energy an object can gain by falling.
43. The point at which a liquid becomes a solid.
44. A substance composed of two or more elements that are chemically combined in definite proportions; that may not be separated by physical means.
46. The amount of heat needed for a substance to change its state of matter.
47. The science of sounds.
48. A substance composed of ingredients that are not chemically combined.
52. A _____ limits current.
55. A Système International d'Unités (SI) unit of force that would impart 1 m/s acceleration to 1 kg of mass.
56. The type of pressure exerted during the transition state between a liquid and a gas.
60. An absolute temperature scale calculated in centigrade units from the point at which molecular activity apparently ceases.

ACHIEVING THE OBJECTIVES

1. Differentiate between kinetic and potential energy.

1A. Define kinetic energy.

_____

_____

1B. Define potential energy.

_____

_____

1C. List five common examples of kinetic energy.

_____

_____

_____

_____

1D. List five common examples of potential energy.

_____

_____

_____

_____

1E. As mass increases, potential energy and kinetic energy will

_____

_____

1F. As velocity increases, kinetic energy will

_____

_____

Think About This

When a car is going downhill, why does the driver have to apply more pressure on the brakes to stop the car than if the car was moving on a level street?

Helpful Web Sites

- University of Oregon, Virtual Laboratory, "Potential Energy" — http://jersey.uoregon.edu
- The Physics Classroom Tutorial, "Potential Energy Examples" — http://www.glenbrook.k12.il.us
- The Physics Classroom Tutorial, "Kinetic Energy Examples" — http://www.glenbrook.k12.il.us

2. Compare the physical and chemical properties of the three primary states of matter.

2A. List the three primary states of matter in order of greatest potential energy to least potential energy.

_____

_____

2B. List the three primary states of matter in order of greatest kinetic energy to least kinetic energy.

_____

_____

2C. The state of matter that possesses the weakest cohesive forces between constituent particles is

_____.

2D. Why are gases and liquids described as fluids?

_____

_____

2E. The two states of matter that have no definite shape are _____.

2F. A state of matter that has no defined shape or volume and has no cohesive forces between constituent particles is a

_____.

2G. A state of matter that has weak intermolecular forces between constituent particles and is essentially incomprehensible is

_____.

2H. The two states of matter that have definite volume and cannot be compressed are

_____.

2I. The one state of matter that has a definite shape and volume and cannot be compressed is a

_____.

2J. The one state of matter that has no definite shape and volume and can be compressed is a

_____.

Think About This

Why won't gas stay in a cup?

Helpful Web Sites

- National Aeronautics and Space Administration (NASA), "States of Matter" — http://exploration.grc.nasa.gov/education/rocket/state.html
- Purdue University, Department of Chemistry, "States of Matter" with illustrations and explanations — http://www.chem.purdue.edu

3. Explain why large amounts of energy are required to accomplish the changes associated with solid-liquid and liquid-gas phase transitions.

3A. Fill in the blanks in the following table.

Start from:	Change to:	Name(s)
Solid	Liquid	
Liquid	Solid	
Liquid	Gas	
Gas	Liquid	
Solid	Gas	

3B. The amount of heat that must be added to effect the change from a solid to liquid is called the

_____

_____.

3C. What effect does heat have on molecules?

_____

_____

3D. How does the application of heat to a liquid enhance the process of evaporation?

_____

_____

_____

3E. Explain why the boiling point of water is lower at the Mount Washington Observatory in New Hampshire.

_____

_____

_____

3F. The state of matter at which water exists at temperatures between 0°C and 100°C is

_____.

3G. What happens to water at temperatures above 374°C?

_____

_____

3H. Describe the difference between a gas and a vapor.

_____

_____

_____

_____

Think About This

Why is salt used to make ice cream?

Helpful Web Sites

■ Rader's Chem4Kids, "Changing States of Matter," — http://www.chem4kids.com

■ Birmingham Grid for Learning, "Changing Matter," shows how heat is necessary to the change of state from solid to liquid to gas — http://www.bgfl.org

4. Convert temperature measurements from the Kelvin, Celsius, and Fahrenheit temperature scales.

4A. Why is the Fahrenheit scale not a centigrade scale?

_____

_____

_____

4B. On which scale is absolute zero found?

_____

_____

4C. Convert 25°C to Kelvin.

_____

4D. Convert 150°K to Celsius.

_____

4E. Convert 92°F to Kelvin.

_____

4F. Convert 100°K to Fahrenheit.

_____

_____

Chapter **1** **Basic Physics for the Respiratory Therapist**

Think About This

Why shouldn't thermometers be placed directly in the sun to measure air temperature?

Helpful Web Sites

■ Visionlearning Web site, "Background of the Discovery of the Various Temperature Scales," Martha M. Day and Anthony Carpi — http://www.visionlearning.com

■ Fordham Preparatory School, Science Help Online Chemistry, "Lesson 2–9: Temperature Conversions," including practice quizzes and worksheets — http://www.fordhamprep.org

■ University of Alaska Fairbanks, Geophysical Institute, Alaska Science Forum: "Daniel Fahrenheit, Anders Celsius Left Their Marks; Article #1317," Ned Rozell — http://www.gi.alaska.edu

5. Define pressure and describe two devices that are commonly used to measure it.

5A. What is the definition of *gas pressure*?

_____

_____

5B. Why is the atmospheric pressure on Mount Washington less than that in New Orleans?

_____

_____

5C. Describe how a mercury barometer measures atmospheric pressure.

_____

_____

_____

_____

5D. Describe how an aneroid barometer measures atmospheric pressure.

_____

_____

_____

Think About This

Why will a potato chip bag packed and sealed in New Orleans burst open in Denver?

Helpful Web Sites

■ University of Toronto, Department of Physics, "The Mercury Barometer," David M. Harrison, information and video on how to use a mercury barometer — http://www.upscale.utoronto.ca

■ Potomac Elementary School, "Air Pressure: How to Measure the Air Around Us," Chad Williams — http://www.williamsclass.com

6. List various pressure equivalents for 1 atm.

6A. 1 atm = _____ psi.

6B. 1 atm = _____ mm Hg.

6C. 1 atm = _____ cm H_2O.

6D. 1 atm = _____ kPa.

Think About This

What is happening inside the highs and lows on a weather map?

Helpful Web Sites

■ Cornell University, Medical calculators — http://www-users.med.cornell.edu

■ National Oceanic and Atmospheric Administration (NOAA), National Weather Service, Southern Region Headquarters, Pressure Conversion Calculator — http://www.srh.noaa.gov

7. Calculate the density and specific gravity of liquids and gases.

7A. What is the formula for density?

_____

_____

7B. What are the units of expression for the density of a solid? _____

_____

7C. What are the units of expression for the density of a gas? _____

_____

7D. The volume in liters that 1 mole of gas occupies at standard temperature and pressure, dry (STPD) is

_____

_____.

7E. Given that the mass of oxygen (molecular weight) is 32 g, calculate the density of oxygen.

_____

_____

7F. Given that the mass of nitrogen is 28 g, calculate the density of nitrogen.

_____

_____

7G. Given that the mass of helium is 4 g, calculate the density of helium.

_____

_____

7H. What are the values for STPD?

_____

_____

Chapter **1** **Basic Physics for the Respiratory Therapist**

7I. A block of aluminum has a volume of 15.0 mL and weighs 40.5 g. What is its density?

_____

_____

7J. Note that 1.00 g of oxygen gas (O_2) has a volume of 670.2 mL. The same mass of carbon dioxide gas (CO_2) occupies 505.8 mL. What are the densities of the two gases?

_____

_____

7K. What is the reference substance used to calculate the specific gravity of a liquid?

_____

_____

7L. What is the difference between density and specific gravity?

_____

_____

7M. What does Avogadro's number represent?

_____

_____

7N. How is specific gravity calculated?

_____

_____

7O. If a liquid has a specific gravity of 1.21, is it lighter or heavier than water?

_____

_____

Think About This

What does the specific gravity of urine tell us about the function of the kidneys?

Helpful Web Sites

■ Wisconsin Online Resource Center, "Calculating Gas Density from Standard Molar Volume," available for purchase — http://www.wisc-online.com

■ General Chemistry Virtual Textbook: "Avogadro's number and the mole," Stephen Lower — http://www.chem1.com

■ Walter Fendt, "Buoyant Force in Liquids" — http://www.walter-fendt.de

■ Georgia State University, Department of Physics and Astronomy, "Examples of Surface Tension, Cohesion, and Adhesion" — http://hyperphysics.phy-astr.gsu.edu

8. Explain how changes in pressure, volume, temperature, and mass affect the behavior of an ideal gas.

Fill in the blanks in the following table:

	Law	Description	Formula
8A.	Boyle's law		
8B.		The volume of a given amount of gas held at a constant pressure increases proportionately with increases in the temperature of the gas.	
8C.			$P_1/T_1 = P_2/T_2$
8D.		Equal volumes of gas at the same pressure and temperature contain the same number of molecules.	
8E.			$PB = PO_2 + PN_2 + PCO_2 + P$ (trace gases)
8F.	Combined-gas law		
8G.		When a gas is confined in a space adjacent to a liquid, a certain number of gas molecules dissolve in the liquid phase.	
8H.	Graham's law		
8I.			$\dot{V}gas = A \times D \times \Delta P/T$

8J. Helium takes up 5.71 L at 0°C and 3.95 atm. What is the volume of the same amount of helium at 32°F and 800 mm Hg? What gas law did you use to calculate the answer?

_____

_____

_____

_____

8K. A 100-L sample of helium at 27°C is cooled at constant pressure to −55°C. Calculate the new volume of the helium. What gas law did you use in this situation?

_____

_____

_____

_____

8L. If you were to take a volleyball SCUBA (*self-contained underwater breathing apparatus*) diving with you, what would be its new volume if it started at the surface with a volume of 2.5 L, under a pressure of 760 mm Hg, and with a temperature of 22°C? On your dive, you take it to a place where the pressure is 2943 mm Hg and the temperature is 0.25°C. What gas law did you use in this situation?

_____

_____

_____

_____

_____

8M. Name the four factors that play roles in the diffusion of oxygen across the alveolar capillary membrane.

_____

_____

_____

_____

_____

Think About This
What happens to the volume of gas in a SCUBA diver's body cavities as the diver descends?

Helpful Web Sites
- World of Chemistry, "How Can the Ideal Gas Law be Applied in Dealing with How Gases Behave?," Ralph Logan — http://members.aol.com/profchm/idealgas.html
- The Woodrow Wilson Foundation Site, Chemistry Textbook, chapter on gases — http://www.woodrow.org/teachers/chemistry/links/chem1/Chapter12.html
- 1728 Software Systems, Chemistry Calculator Index — http://www.1728.com/indexche.htm

9. Calculate the partial pressure of oxygen in a room air sample of gas obtained at 1 atm.

9A. The air we breathe consists of what gases?

_____

_____

9B. List the gases contained in air and their percentage.

_____

_____

9C. How can total atmospheric pressure be calculated?

_____

_____

9D. What is the formula to calculate the partial pressure of a gas (in mm Hg) in a sample of room air?

_____

_____

9E. Calculate the partial pressure of oxygen in a room air sample of gas obtained at 1 atm.

_____

_____

9F. What formula is used to calculate the partial pressure of inspired oxygen?

_____

_____

9G. Mount Rainier's Columbia Crest (its current summit), in Washington state, is 14,411 feet above sea level. The barometric pressure is 459 mm Hg. Calculate the partial pressure of inspired oxygen at body temperature and saturation.

_____

_____

9H. A mixture of neon and argon gases exerts a total pressure of 2.39 atm. The partial pressure of the neon alone is 1.84 atm; what is the partial pressure of the argon?

_____

_____

Think About This
Why would an otherwise healthy visitor to Mesa Verde National Park, Colorado (6960 feet above sea level), be in the ranger station receiving supplemental oxygen for shortness of breath?

Helpful Web Site
- ChemTeam: Gas Laws, "Dalton's Law of Partial Pressures" — http://dbhs.wvusd.k12.ca.us/webdocs/GasLaw/Gas-Dalton.html

10. List the physical variables that influence the flow of a gas through a tube.
10A. Identify the three patterns of flow in Figure 1-1.

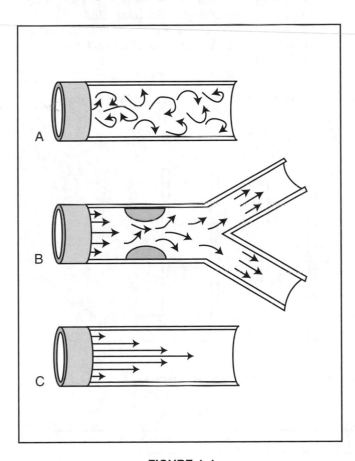

FIGURE 1-1

_____

_____

10B. Which of the flow pattern is normally associated with the movement of fluids through tubes with smooth surfaces and fixed radii?

_____

_____

10C. The pressure required to produce a given flow is influenced more by the density of the fluid than by its viscosity when which flow pattern is present?

_____

_____

10D. In the lung, where is flow predominantly laminar?

_____

_____

10E. In the lung, where is flow predominantly turbulent?

_____

_____

10F. In the lung, where is flow predominantly transitional?

_____

_____

Think About This
Why is laminar flow an important factor in flight?

Helpful Web Site
- Johns Hopkins School of Medicine's Interactive Respiratory Physiology Encyclopedia, "Air Flow" — http://oac.med.jhmi.edu/res_phys/Encyclopedia/AirFlow/AirFlow.html

11. Explain how the pressure, velocity, and flow of a gas change as it moves from part of a tube with a large radius to another part with a small radius.
11A. What two factors must be considered when describing gas movement through a tube?

_____

_____

11B. According to Poiseuille, what factors determine the resistance to flow?

_____

_____

11C. Calculate the resistance to flow if the viscosity = 1, length = 1, and radius = 1.

_____

_____

Chapter **1** **Basic Physics for the Respiratory Therapist**

11D. Calculate the resistance to flow if the viscosity = 1, length = 1, and radius = 0.5.

_____

_____

11E. Calculate the resistance to flow if the viscosity = 1, length = 1, and radius = 2.

_____

_____

11F. Calculate the resistance to flow if the viscosity = 2, length = 1, and radius = 1.

_____

_____

11G. Calculate the resistance to flow if the viscosity = 0.5, length = 1, and radius = 1.

_____

_____

11H. Calculate the resistance to flow if the viscosity = 1, length = 2, and radius = 1.

_____

_____

11I. Calculate the resistance to flow if the viscosity = 1, length = 0.5, and radius = 1.

_____

_____

11J. Using the previous seven calculations, determine which of the factors (viscosity, tube length, or tube radius) causes the greatest change in resistance to flow.

_____

_____

_____

_____

Think About This

What type of pulmonary problem will cause the radius of the airways to become smaller?

Helpful Web Site

■ Johns Hopkins School of Medicine Interactive Respiratory Physiology Encyclopedia, "Airway Resistance" — http://oac.med.jhmi.edu/res_phys/Encyclopedia/AirwayResistance/AirwayResistance.html

12. Describe the Venturi and Coanda effects and how both can be used in the design of respiratory care equipment.

12A. Explain why the fourth manometer in Figure 1-2 shows reduced pressure.

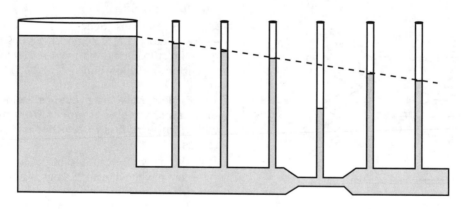

FIGURE 1-2
(Redrawn from Nave CR, Nave BC: *Physics for the health sciences*, ed 3, Philadelphia, 1985, WB Saunders.)

_____

_____

Questions 12B through 12D refer to Figure 1-3.

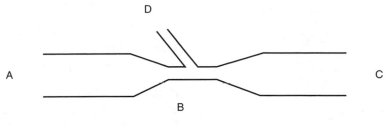

FIGURE 1-3

12B. As a gas moves from point *A* to point *C* in Figure 1-3, what happens to the speed of the gas as it flows through the constriction in the tube labeled *B*?

_____

_____

12C. As the gas passes through the constriction in the tube in Figure 1-3, what happens to the gas around point *D* in this figure?

_____

_____

12D. What happens to the speed of the gas as it emerges from the constriction in the tube in Figure 1-3 and flows toward point *C* in this figure?

_____

_____

Questions 12E through 12G refer to Figure 1-4.

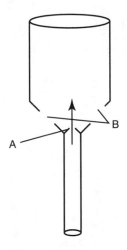

FIGURE 1-4

12E. What happens to the velocity of a gas as it flows through point *A* in Figure 1-4?

_____

_____

12F. What happens to the pressure as the gas flows through point *A* in Figure 1-4?

_____

_____

12G. What will happen to air just outside the "ports" labeled *B* in Figure 1-4 as a gas is going through the constriction labeled *A*?

_____

_____

12H. List three respiratory care devices that utilize the Venturi principle.

_____

_____

Chapter **1** **Basic Physics for the Respiratory Therapist**

12I. The Coanda effect will cause the water from the faucet to travel toward which direction — *A*, *B*, or *C* — after it touches the back of the spoon?

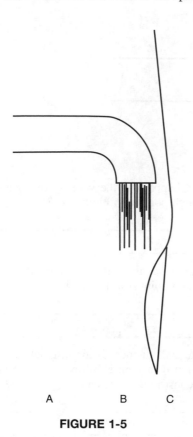

A   B   C

FIGURE 1-5

_____

_____

12J. What type of respiratory care device uses the Coanda effect?

_____

_____

Think About This

Which principle helps airplanes lift off the ground?

Helpful Web Sites

■ "Animated Demonstration of Bernoulli's Principle," M. Mitchell — http://home.earthlink.net/~mmc1919/venturi.html

■ *Drinking Water & Backflow Prevention* magazine, "Venturi Principle" — http://www.dwbp-online.com/venturi.htm

13. State Ohm's law and relate how changes in voltage and resistance affect current flow in a direct-current series circuit.

13A. Name the three factors involved in Ohm's law.

_____

_____

13B. What is the formula for Ohm's law?

_____

_____

13C. A 9-V battery supplies power to a pulse oximeter with a resistance of 18 Ω. How much current is flowing through the pulse oximeter? (See Figure 1-6.)

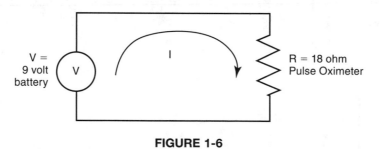

V = 9 volt battery   V   I   R = 18 ohm Pulse Oximeter

FIGURE 1-6

13D. Calculate the current for the schematic in Figure 1-7.

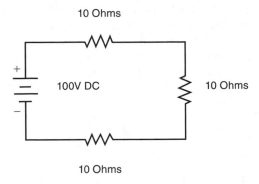

FIGURE 1-7

13E. Calculate the current for the schematic in Figure 1-8.

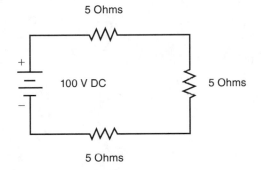

FIGURE 1-8

13F. Calculate the current for the schematic in Figure 1-9.

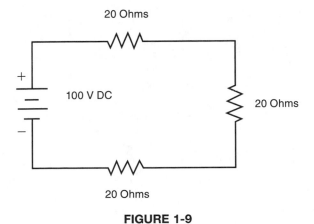

FIGURE 1-9

13G. What happens to the current flow in a direct-current series circuit when voltage remains constant and resistance increases?

_____

_____

13H. What happens to the current flow in a direct-current series circuit when resistance remains constant and the voltage is increased?

_____

_____

13I. Calculate the current in a direct-current parallel circuit when the voltage is 120 V and $R_1 = 30$, $R_2 = 60$, $R_3 = 30$, and $R_4 = 20\ \Omega$.

_____

_____

_____

_____

Think About This
Will a 1.5-V direct current (DC) circuit with one light bulb be brighter than a 3-V DC circuit with two light bulbs in series?

Helpful Web Sites
■ Science Joy Wagon, "Ohm's Law" — http://www.sciencejoywagon.com/physicszone
■ Science Joy Wagon, "The Parallel Circuit" — http://regentsprep.org/Regents/physics
■ Science Joy Wagon, "The Series Circuit" — http://regentsprep.org/Regents/physics

14. Describe three strategies that can be used to protect patients from electrical hazards.

14A. Describe how grounding offers protection from electrical hazards.

_____

_____

_____

_____

14B. How do ground-fault circuit interrupters protect against electrical hazards?

_____

_____

_____

_____

Chapter **1** **Basic Physics for the Respiratory Therapist**

14C. What is the purpose of regular inspection of respiratory equipment by a hospital's biomedical equipment department?

_____

_____

_____

_____

Think About This

Why is static electricity buildup hazardous in an operating room?

Helpful Web Sites

■ U.S. Department of Labor, Occupational Safety & Health Administration (OSHA) Hospital eTool: Healthcare Wide Hazards Module, "Electrical Hazards" — http://www.osha.gov/SLTC/etools/hospital/hazards/electrical/electrical.html

■ University of Southern Queensland, Self-Directed Learning 3: "Electricity and Electrical Safety" — http://www.usq.edu.au

NATIONAL BOARD FOR RESPIRATORY CARE (NBRC)–TYPE QUESTIONS

1. Another name for *supercooled liquids* is which of the following?
   A. *Elements*
   B. *Compounds*
   C. *Crystalline solids*
   D. *Amorphous solids*

2. The melting of ice demonstrates which of the following?
   A. An increase in potential energy
   B. An increase in kinetic energy
   C. The latent heat of fusion
   D. The process of sublimation

3. The opposite of evaporation is which of the following?
   A. Respiration
   B. Vaporization
   C. Condensation
   D. Sublimation

4. A sample of gas expands isothermally from 10.0 L to 30.0 L. If the initial pressure was 1140 mm Hg, what is the new pressure?
   A. 3420 mm Hg
   B. 380 mm Hg
   C. 127 mm Hg
   D. 760 mm Hg

5. A sample of gas initially occupies 3.0 cc at a pressure of 47.8 mm HG. The pressure is increased to 746 mm HG. What is the new volume?
   A. 0.192 cc
   B. 46.8 cc
   C. 0.0214 cc
   D. 5.21 cc

6. A gas system has an initial temperature of 142°C with the volume unknown. When the temperature changes to 46.20°K, the volume is found to be 1.58 L. What was the initial volume in liters?
   A. 2.05 L
   B. 4.9 L
   C. 10.8 L
   D. 14.2 L

7. Under the same conditions of temperature and pressure, a liquid differs from a gas because the particles of the liquid:
   A. Are in a constant straight-line motion
   B. Take the shape of the container they occupy
   C. Have no regular arrangement
   D. Have stronger forces of attraction between them

8. The volume of a given mass of an ideal gas at constant pressure is which of the following?
   A. Directly proportional to the Kelvin temperature
   B. Directly proportional to the Celsius temperature
   C. Inversely proportional to the Kelvin temperature
   D. Inversely proportional to the Celsius temperature

9. A mixture of helium and oxygen exerts a combined pressure of 6 atm, and the partial pressure of oxygen is 4 atm. What is the partial pressure of helium?
   A. 1520 mm Hg
   B. Not enough information
   C. 6600 mm Hg
   D. 7600 mm Hg

10. A cylinder contains helium and oxygen and exerts a total pressure of 7.00 atm. The cylinder has 42.8% helium. What is the partial pressure of oxygen in this cylinder?
    A. 435 mm Hg
    B. 2277 mm Hg
    C. 3043 mm Hg
    D. 4004 mm Hg

11. Calculate the total current through the circuit in Figure 1-10.

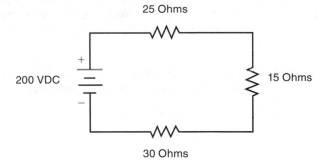

25 Ohms

200 VDC

15 Ohms

30 Ohms

FIGURE 1-10

    A. 0.35 A
    B. 2.86 A
    C. 3.50 A
    D. 28 A

12. According to Fick's first law of diffusion, flow of gas across a semipermeable membrane will be reduced when which of the following occurs?
    A. Surface area increases
    B. Wall thickness increases
    C. Wall thickness decreases
    D. Gas diffusivity increases

15

2 Manufacture, Storage, and Transport of Medical Gases

Upon completion of this chapter, you will be able to:

1. Describe the chemical and physical properties of the medical gases most often encountered in respiratory care.
2. Identify various types of medical gas cylinders (e.g., types 3, 3A, 3AA, and 3AL).
3. Identify the following cylinder markings: Department of Transportation (DOT) specifications, service pressure, hydrostatic testing dates, manufacturer's identification, ownership mark, serial number, and cylinder size.
4. List the color codes used to identify medical gas cylinders.
5. Discuss United States Pharmacopeia (USP) purity standards for medical gases.
6. Compare the operation of direct-acting cylinder valves with that of diaphragm-type cylinder valves.
7. Explain American Standards Association (ASA) indexing, the Pin Index Safety System (PISS), and the Diameter Index Safety System (DISS).
8. Identify and correct a problem with cylinder valve assembly.
9. Calculate the gas volume remaining in a compressed-gas cylinder and estimate the duration of gas flow based on the cylinder's gauge pressure.
10. Describe the components of a bulk liquid oxygen system and discuss National Fire Protection Association (NFPA) recommendations for the storage and use of liquid oxygen in bulk systems.
11. Discuss the operation of a portable liquid oxygen system and describe NFPA recommendations for these systems.
12. Calculate the duration of a portable liquid oxygen supply.
13. Identify three types of medical air compressors and describe the operational theory of each.
14. Summarize NFPA recommendations for medical air supply safety.
15. Compare continuous supply systems with alternating central supply systems.
16. Identify a DISS station outlet and a quick-connect station outlet.
17. Compare the operational theory of a membrane oxygenator with that of a molecular sieve oxygenator.

"Not all chemicals are bad. Without chemicals such as hydrogen and oxygen, for example, there would be no way to make water, a vital ingredient in beer."
Dave Barry

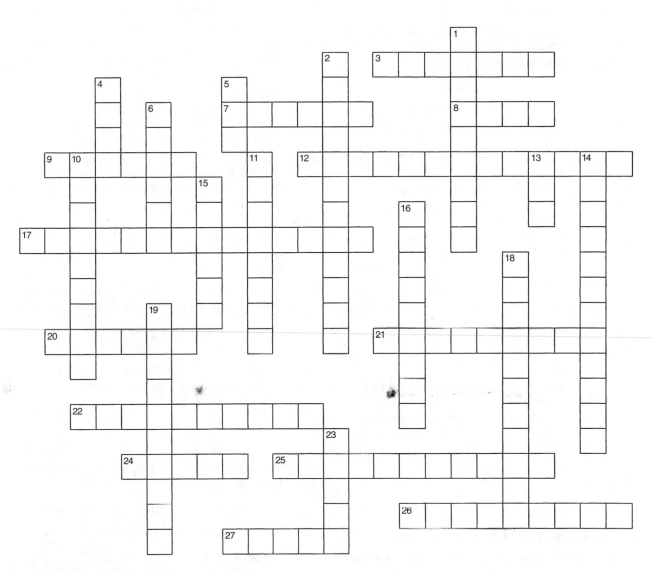

CROSSWORD PUZZLE 2–1
Created using Crossword Weaver, www.CrosswordWeaver.com.

Use the clues to complete the crossword puzzle.

Across

3. The type of plug that melts when the temperature rises.

7. _____-loaded devices are susceptible to leakage around the metal seal.

8. The indexing system used for small cylinders, sizes A to E (*abbreviation*).

9 The type of compressor that is typically used to power a mechanical ventilator.

12. A type of membrane that allows certain things to pass through it.

17. A constant or "tank factor" used to calculate the duration of a cylinder of gas (*two words*).

20. A type of compressor that uses a rotating vane.

21. The type of container in which liquid air is shipped.

22. The type of supply system that contains two sources of gas, one of which is a reserve source for emergencies.

24. _____ metal is a type of metal that melts when cylinder temperature rises.

25. The term _____ *effect* was introduced by Karl von Linde to describe the production of bulk liquid oxygen (*two words*).

26. A _____ disk is a thin metal disk that ruptures when the pressure is high.

27. A type of valve used in a supply system.

Down

1. A _____ valve uses a threaded stem.

2. A type of device that supplies oxygen by separating it from air.

4. The threaded safety system used at station outlets (*abbreviation*).

5. A method used to ensure that an oxygen concentrator functions properly (*abbreviation*).

6. _____-tube flowmeter.

10. A type of valve that is used to shut off oxygen supply to various patient rooms or a floor.

11. _____ separation is a method of producing oxygen for home care settings.

13. The indexing system used for large cylinders (*abbreviation*).

14. The process that turns air into a liquid.

15. A/an _____-acting valve contains two fiber washers.

16. A type of compressor that is typically used in small nebulizer compressors.

18. The type of supply system that usually consists of a primary bank and a secondary bank of cylinders.

19. _____ distillation is a method of producing bulk oxygen.

23. This type of station outlet connection uses a plunger.

ACHIEVING THE OBJECTIVES

1. Describe the chemical and physical properties of the medical gases most often encountered in respiratory care.

1A. The nonflammable substance that can exist as a liquid or a gas, is colorless, odorless, has a slightly acidic taste, and has a molecular weight of 44.01 and a boiling point of −78.4° C_____
_____.

1B. The nonflammable gas that has a molecular weight of 4.00, is tasteless, and has a critical temperature of −267.0° C is _____.

1C. _____ is a gas that is a powerful pulmonary vasodilator used to treat persistent pulmonary hypertension of the newborn.

1D. The nonflammable substance that can exist as a liquid or a gas, has a molecular weight of 44.01, and is used as an anesthetic is _____
_____.

1E. _____ is a colorless, odorless, tasteless flammable gas that binds easily to hemoglobin.

1F. The nonflammable gas or liquid that supports combustion, has a critical temperature of −118.4° C and is used to treat hypoxemia is _____
_____.

1G. The substance that can exist as either a gas or liquid, is nonflammable but supports combustion, as a gas has a specific gravity of 1, and is made up of 78% nitrogen is _____.

1H. _____ can be obtained as a by-product in the production of ammonia and lime and is purified by liquefaction and the fractional distillation process.

1I. Patients with severe airway obstruction may benefit from the use of what mixture of gases? _____
_____
_____

1J. Which gas is used as a standard calibration gas for blood gas analyzers, certain transcutaneous monitors, and capnographs?
_____
_____

1K. Which gas can be produced by the physical separation of atmospheric air in patients' homes?
_____
_____

Think About This

Why does inhaling helium make your voice sound strange?

Helpful Web Sites

■ Jefferson Lab, "The Periodic Table of Elements" — http://education.jlab.org/itselemental/index.html

■ Lenntech B.V., "Carbon Dioxide Information" — http://www.lenntech.com/carbon-dioxide.htm

■ Consumer Product Safety Commission, "Carbon Monoxide Questions and Answers" — http://www.cpsc.gov

■ Kansas University Medical Center, Respiratory Care Web Ed (Web education), "Therapeutic Delivery of Inhaled Nitric Oxide" — http://classes.kumc.edu/

- University of Bristol, School of Chemistry, "Nitrous Oxide — Laughing Gas" — http://www.chm.bris.ac.uk

2. Identify various types of medical gas cylinders (e.g., types 3, 3A, 3AA, and 3AL).

2A. What three types of metal are used to construct seamless compressed-gas cylinders?

_____

_____

2B. What agency issues regulations for all cylinders used to store and transport compressed gases?

_____

_____

2C. Type 3 cylinders are made of _____

_____.

2D. What type of cylinder is made from heat-treated, high-strength steel?

_____

_____

2E. What type of cylinder is constructed of specially prescribed seamless aluminum alloys?

_____

_____

2F. The filling pressure of a type 3AA "H" size cylinder is 2265 pound-force per square inch gauge (psig). What is the maximum amount of pressure this cylinder can hold?

_____

_____

Think About This

Why are compressed-gas cylinders capable of holding 10% more than their maximum filling pressure?

Helpful Web Site

- The Compressed Gas Association — http://www.cganet.com

3. Identify the following cylinder markings: Department of Transportation (DOT) specifications, service pressure, hydrostatic testing dates, manufacturer's identification, ownership mark, serial number, and cylinder size.

Questions 3A through 3I refer to Figure 2-1.

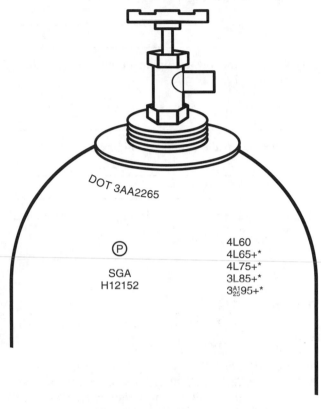

DOT 3AA2265

(P)

SGA
H12152

4L60
4L65+*
4L75+*
3L85+*
3$^{A1}_{25}$95+*

FIGURE 2-1

3A. From what type of metal is the cylinder in Figure 2-1 made?

_____

_____

3B. What is the service pressure for the cylinder in Figure 2-1?

_____

_____

3C. What year was the cylinder in Figure 2-1 last hydrostatically tested?

_____

_____

3D. What is the serial number for the cylinder in Figure 2-1?

_____

_____

3E. What is the manufacturer's mark on the cylinder in Figure 2-1?

_____

_____

3F. What is the year of the original hydrostatic test for the cylinder in Figure 2-1?

_____

_____

3G. What is the ownership mark on the cylinder in Figure 2-1?

_____

_____

3H. What size is the cylinder in Figure 2-1?

_____

_____

3I. Why should the cylinder in Figure 2-1 not be used at this time?

_____

_____

Think About This

What should be done with a cylinder that has lost its elasticity?

Helpful Web Site

■ CFC StarTec LLC, "DOT Cylinder Maintenance, Retest and Certification Requirements" — http://www.c-f-c.com/gaslink/docs/dot_cylinder.htm

4. List the color codes used to identify medical gas cylinders.

	Gas	Color (in the United States)
4A.	Oxygen	
4B.	Nitrogen	
4C.	Helium	
4D.	Ethylene	
4E.	Cyclopropane	
4F.	Air	
4G.	Nitrous oxide	
4H.	Nitric oxide	
4I.	Helium/oxygen	
4J.	Carbon dioxide	
4K.	Carbon dioxide/oxygen	

4L. What are the two major exceptions to the international cylinder color-coding system?

_____

_____

Think About This

Why are there two forms of identification for compressed-gas cylinders?

Helpful Web Site

■ European Union, "Compressed Gas Cylinder Colour Codes" — http://physchem.ox.ac.uk/MSDS/cylinders.html

5. Discuss United States Pharmacopeia (USP) purity standards for medical gases.

5A. What agency requires that compressed gases used for medical purposes meet certain minimum requirements for purity?

_____

_____

5B. Where is the purity of a gas indicated?

_____

_____

5C. Where are the purity standards for medical gases listed?

_____

_____

5D. Which gas has a purity standard of 97%?

_____

_____

5E. What is the purity standard for all medical gases except one?

_____

_____

Think About This

Why are medical gases regulated for purity?

Helpful Web Sites

■ United States Pharmacopeia, "About USP — An Overview" — http://www.usp.org/aboutUSP

■ National Formulary, "USP-NF — An Overview" — http://www.usp.org/USPNF

6. Compare the operation of direct-acting cylinder valves with diaphragm-type cylinder valves.

Identify the common elements in Figure 2-2:

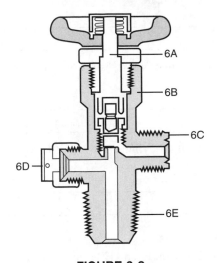

FIGURE 2-2

6A. _____

_____

6B. _____

_____

6C. _____

_____

6D. _____

_____

6E. _____

_____

Identify the common elements in Figure 2-3:

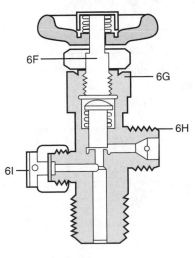

FIGURE 2-3

6F. _____

_____

6G. _____

_____

6H. _____

_____

6I. _____

_____

6J. _____

_____

6K. What is the difference between Figure 2-2 and Figure 2-3?

_____

_____

_____

_____

6L. Which type of cylinder valve can withstand pressures of more than 1500 psi?

_____

_____

6M. Which type of cylinder valve is preferred for use with flammable anesthetics? Why?

_____

_____

_____

_____

Think About This

What type of valves should be used on cylinders used for *s*elf-contained *u*nderwater *b*reathing *a*pparatus (SCUBA) diving?

Helpful Web Site

■ Oklahoma State University, "Compressed Gas Cylinder Safety" — http://www.pp.okstate.edu

7. Explain the American Standards Association (ASA) indexing, the Pin Index Safety System (PISS), and the Diameter Index Safety System (DISS).

7A. What is the purpose of cylinder safety systems?

_____

_____

7B. What safey system prevents an oxygen regulator from being placed on a large nitrous oxide cylinder?

_____

_____

7C. In which direction do non–life support gas cylinders thread?

_____

_____

7D. What safety system is used for small cylinders (size A to E)?

_____

_____

7E. How does the small-cylinder safety system differ from the large-cylinder safety system?

_____

_____

_____

_____

7F. Name the two safety systems that are used at station outlets.

_____

_____

Think About This

With all the safety systems preventing the interchange of regulating equipment, is it still possible to hook up an oxygen-delivery device (i.e., a nasal cannula) to compressed air?

Helpful Web Site

■ Agency for Healthcare Research and Quality, Web M&M (Morbidity & Mortality Rounds on the Web) "Case and Commentary" — http://www.webmm. ahrq.gov

8. Identify and correct a problem with a cylinder valve assembly.

8A. How would a respiratory therapist know whether there is a loose seal between a cylinder and a regulator?

_____

_____

_____

_____

8B. The respiratory therapist prepares an "E" size cylinder for transport. When the RT turns the cylinder, there is a loud hissing noise. What is the most likely cause of the leak?

_____

_____

8C. What are two causes of low gas flow from a cylinder?

_____

_____

8D. Why should a cylinder valve not be opened up all the way?

_____

_____

Think About This

What would happen to an "H" size cylinder if the valve assembly were to be broken off?

9. Calculate the gas volume remaining in a compressed-gas cylinder and estimate the duration of gas flow based on the cylinder's gauge pressure.

9A. Calculate the volume of gas in an "E" size cylinder with a pressure of 1500 psi.

_____

_____

9B. Calculate the volume of gas in an "H" size cylinder with a pressure of 1050 psi.

_____

_____

9C. Calculate the volume of gas in a "G" size cylinder with a pressure of 1800 psi.

_____

_____

9D. Calculate the duration of gas flow for an "E" size cylinder with a pressure of 2200 psi and a flow of 3 L/min to a nasal cannula.

_____

_____

9E. Calculate the duration of gas flow for a "G" size cylinder with a pressure of 1600 psi and a flow of 6 L/min to an oxygen mask.

_____

_____

9F. Calculate the duration of gas flow, in hours, for an "H" size cylinder with a pressure of 1000 psi and a flow of 10 L/min to an oxygen device.

_____

_____

9G. An "H" size cylinder of oxygen contains 2000 psi of pressure, with a set flow of 12 L/min. How many hours will it take for this cylinder to get to 800 psi of pressure?

_____

_____

_____

_____

9H. A patient will be transferred from one hospital to another 50 miles away. The patient is receiving oxygen to his tracheostomy tube at a flow of 8 L/min. Travel time should be 1 hour. Will an "E" size cylinder with 1200 psi of pressure be able to last the trip? (Support your answer with a mathematical calculation.)

_____

_____

_____

_____

9I. A patient is being moved to the radiology department for a computed tomography scan. The round-trip to radiology and the procedure will take 45 minutes. The patient is receiving oxygen via a nasal cannula at 2 L/min. The "E" size cylinder has 1000 psi of pressure. Is there enough gas in the cylinder for the procedure? (Support your answer with a mathematical calculation.)

_____

_____

_____

_____

9J. Calculate how much time it will take for an "H" size cylinder with 800 psi of pressure to get to 200 psi of pressure with an oxygen device set at a flow rate of 4 L/min.

_____

_____

Think About This

What other individuals need to calculate gas duration?

10. Describe the components of a bulk liquid oxygen system and discuss National Fire Protection Association (NFPA) recommendations for the storage and use of liquid oxygen in bulk systems.

Identify the components in Figure 2-4:

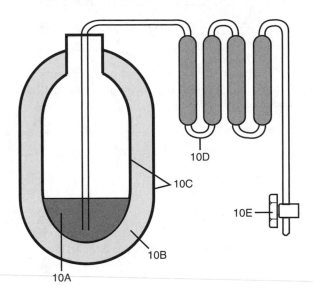

FIGURE 2-4

10A. _____

_____

10B. _____

_____

10C. _____

_____

10D. _____

10E. _____

_____

10F. In Figure 2-4, where does the oxygen gas exist?

_____

_____

10G. Why are bulk liquid oxygen systems used in hospitals and large health care facilities?

_____

_____

_____

Chapter **2** **Manufacture, Storage, and Transport of Medical Gases**

10H. What is the NFPA definition of a *bulk oxygen system*?

_____

_____

_____

_____

_____

10I. What is the purpose of the vaporizer on the bulk liquid oxygen system?

_____

_____

_____

Fill in the following table.

	Structure/person	Distance from bulk oxygen system
10J.	Place of public assembly	
10K.	Nearest nonambulatory patient	
10L.	Public sidewalk	
10M.	Property line	
10N.	Parked vehicle	
10O.	Wood-frame structure	

Think About This
Why shouldn't a child in a croup tent who is receiving oxygen play with a metal toy car?

Helpful Web Site
■ NFPA, "Review NFPA 99: Standard for Health Care Facilities, 2005 Edition" — http://www.nfpa.org

11. Discuss the operation of a portable liquid oxygen system and describe NFPA recommendations for these systems.

11A. What are the main components of a home liquid oxygen system?

_____

_____

11B. The capacity of a stationary home unit is _____

_____, whereas the capacity of a

portable unit is _____

of liquid oxygen.

11C. What is the approximate working pressure of a portable liquid oxygen system?

_____

_____

11D. What is the purpose of the pressure-relief valve?

_____

_____

11E. How are portable liquid oxygen units filled?

_____

_____

11F. According to the NFPA, what actions should be taken if liquid oxygen comes in contact with the skin?

_____

_____

_____

_____

_____

_____

_____

_____

Think About This
Why does fog appear when a liquid oxygen spill occurs?

Helpful Web Sites
■ HELiOS Personal Oxygen System — http://www.heliosoxygen.com
■ The Respiratory Group, Certificates and User Guides — http://www.respiratorygroup.com

12. Calculate the duration of a portable liquid oxygen supply.

12A. How long would a liquid oxygen supply weighing 8 lb last if a patient is receiving oxygen through a nasal cannula at 3 L/min?

_____

_____

_____

_____

12B. How long would a liquid oxygen supply weighing 12 lb last if a patient is receiving oxygen through a nasal cannula at 1.5 L/min?

_____

_____

_____

_____

12C. A portable liquid oxygen system weighs 1.5 lb when empty and 3.5 lb when full. How long will this system last when it is running at 1 L/min?

_____

_____

_____

_____

12D. How long will a portable liquid oxygen system containing 1.2 L of oxygen last when it is running at 2 L/min?

_____

_____

_____

_____

12E. Calculate the duration of a liquid oxygen supply if the liquid supply weighs 60 lb and is running at 3 L/min.

_____

_____

_____

_____

12F. Calculate the duration of a liquid oxygen supply when the empty container's weight is 6 lb, the full weight is 40 lb, and the oxygen flow is 5 L/min.

_____

_____

_____

_____

Think About This

What use does the National Aeronautics and Space Administration (NASA) have for liquid oxygen?

Helpful Web Site

■ "Portable Oxygen: A User's Perspective" — http://www.portableoxygen.org

13. Identify three types of medical air compressors and describe the operational theory of each.

Questions 13A through 13C refer to Figure 2-5.

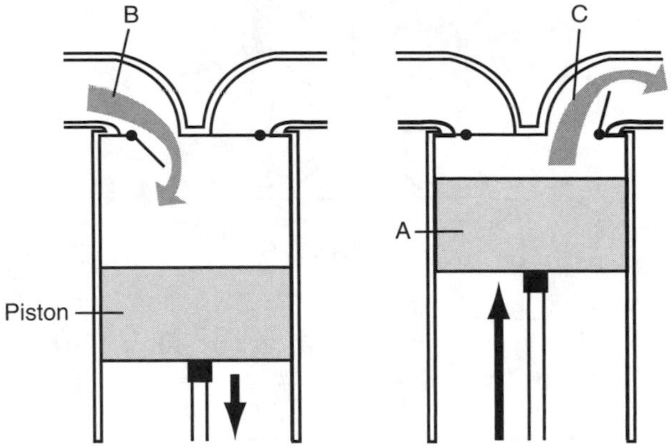

FIGURE 2-5

13A. What type of medical air compressor is shown in Figure 2-5?

_____

_____

13B. Label the components of Figure 2-5.

A. _____

B. _____

C. _____

13C. Describe the basic operation of the compressor in Figure 2-5.

_____

_____

_____

_____

_____

Questions 13D through 13F refer to Figure 2-6.

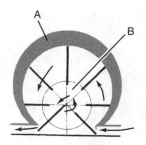

FIGURE 2-6

13D. What type of medical air compressor is shown in Figure 2-6?

_____

_____

13E. Label the components of Figure 2-6.

A. _____

B. _____

13F. Describe the basic operation of the compressor in Figure 2-6.

_____

_____

_____

_____

_____

_____

Questions 13G through 13I refer to Figure 2-7.

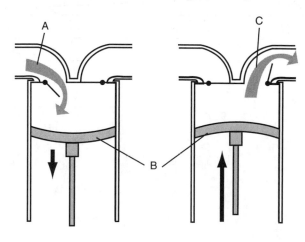

FIGURE 2-7

13G. What type of medical air compressor is shown in Figure 2-7?

_____

_____

13H. Label the components of Figure 2-7.

A. _____

B. _____

C. _____

13I. Describe the basic operation of the compressor in Figure 2-7.

_____

_____

_____

_____

13J. Which type/types of compressors is/are best suited to provide 50 psi of pressure to mechanical ventilators?

_____

_____

Think About This

What other applications do compressors have?

Helpful Web Sites

- Four Seasons Controlled Climates, *PilotLight* magazine, "Compressors: How They Work" — http://www.fscc-online.com
- Pressure Products Industries, Inc., "Diaphragm Compressors Explained" — http://www.pressureproductsindustries.com

14. Summarize NFPA recommendations for medical air supply safety.

14A. From what source must medical air come?

_____

_____

14B. What are the recommendations for where the air intake port should be located?

_____

_____

_____

_____

14C. What are the recommendations for the air taken into the system?

_____

_____

_____

14D. The minimum number of compressors recommended by the NFPA is _____.

14E. What dictates how many compressors a system should have?

_____

_____

14F. What determines the need for intake filters, aftercoolers for air dryers, and additional downstream regulators?

_____

_____

14G. What features must air storage tanks or receivers have?

_____

_____

Think About This
What are the everyday uses for compressed air?

Helpful Web Site
■ Anesthesia Patient Safety Foundation, Resource Center, "Medical Air," Ervin Moss, MD, and Thomas Nagle, MBA — http://www.apsf.org/resource_center/newsletter/1996/summer/apsfmedair.html

15. Compare continuous supply systems with alternating central supply systems.

15A. How many sources of gas supply does a continuous supply system have?

_____

_____

15B. What are the names for the gas sources in a continuous supply system?

_____

_____

15C. List four NFPA requirements for a continuous supply system.

_____

_____

_____

_____

15D. What would happen if the liquid source being used by a continuous supply system fails?

_____

_____

15E. Describe the gas sources for an alternating supply system.

_____

_____

_____

_____

_____

15F. What happens when one of the gas sources in an alternating supply system becomes depleted?

_____

_____

_____

_____

15G. When are switch signals activated in an alternating supply system?

_____

_____

15H. What type of central supply system is shown in Figure 2-8?

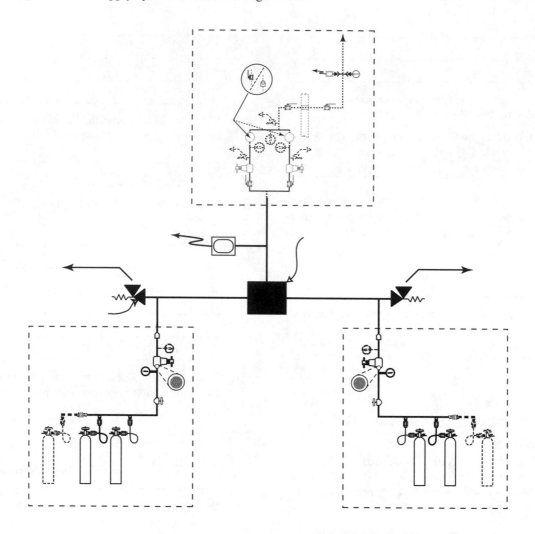

FIGURE 2-8
(From Kacmarek RM, Dimas S: *The essentials of respiratory care*, ed 4, St Louis, 2005, Mosby.)

Think About This
What type of contingency plans should a hospital have for its central oxygen supply system during extreme weather?

16. Identify a DISS station outlet and a quick-connect station outlet.

Questions 16A and 16B refer to Figure 2-9.

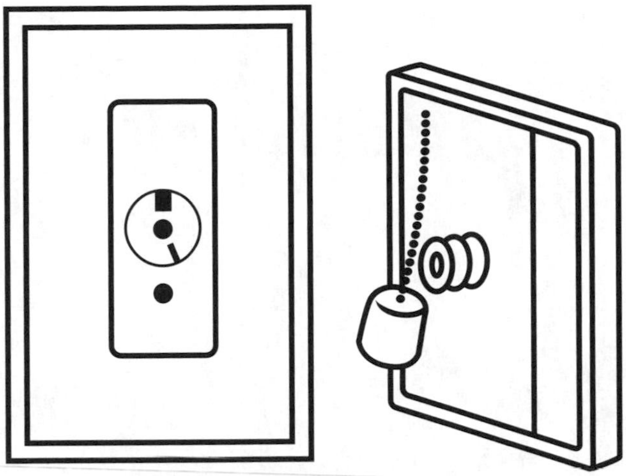

A   B

FIGURE 2-9

16A. Identify the type of station outlet in Figure 2-9*A*.

_____

_____

16B. Identify the type of station outlet in Figure 2-9*B*.

_____

_____

Think About This
What would happen if all existing intensive care unit oxygen station outlets were purged with nitrogen?

Helpful Web Site
■ Susquehanna Micro, Inc., homepage (Precision Medical Fittings) — http://www.susquemicro.com

17. Compare the operational theory of a membrane oxygenator with that of a molecular sieve oxygenator.

17A. Describe the characteristics of the semipermeable membrane used in oxygen concentrators.

_____

_____

_____

_____

17B. How does a semipermeable membrane separate atmospheric gases?

_____

_____

_____

_____

17C. What is the usual output from an oxygen concentrator that uses a semipermeable membrane?

_____

_____

17D. How does a semipermeable membrane oxygen concentrator provide a constant flow of atmospheric gas to the membrane?

_____

_____

17E. How is nitrogen removed from the atmospheric gas in a molecular sieve oxygen concentrator?

_____

_____

17F. How many molecular sieves are contained in an oxygen concentrator?

_____

_____

17G. What is the pressure swing adsorption (PSA) method?

_____

_____

_____

_____

17H. What is the typical output from a molecular sieve oxygen concentrator?

_____

_____

17I. The outlet pressure for a molecular sieve oxygen concentrator is _____

_____.

17J. Why can't regular oxygen flowmeters be used on molecular sieve oxygen concentrators?

_____

_____

_____

Think About This?

There are now portable oxygen concentrators that weigh less than 5 lb.

Helpful Web Sites

- National Lung Health Education Program, "Guide to Prescribing Home Oxygen," Thomas L. Petty, MD — http://www.nlhep.org/resources

- University of Oxford, Nuffield Department of Anaesthetics, World Anaesthesia Online, "The Oxygen Concentrator," Dr. Roger Eltringham, from *Update in Anaesthesia,* — http://www.nda.ox.ac.uk

NATIONAL BOARD FOR RESPIRATORY CARE (NBRC)–TYPE QUESTIONS

1. An "E" size cylinder, with 1500 psig of pressure and set at a flow rate of 3 L/min will last how long?
   A. 0.2 hour
   B. 2.3 hours
   C. 20.1 hours
   D. 26.2 hours

2. The duration of oxygen flow for an "H" size cylinder with 2000 psig of pressure running at 6 L/min will be which of the following?
   A. 1.6 hours
   B. 11.9 hours
   C. 17.4 hours
   D. 23.7 hours

3. A full liquid oxygen cylinder weighs 10 lb; when empty, it weighs 2.5 lb. How many liters of oxygen does this liquid cylinder contain when it is full?
   A. 2 L
   B. 3 L
   C. 4 L
   D. 5 L

4. If the net weight of liquid oxygen in a cylinder is 3 lb, how long will the liquid oxygen last if the oxygen flow is running at 1.5 L/min?
   A. 4 hours 29 minutes
   B. 11 hours 28 minutes
   C. 28 hours 40 minutes
   D. 34 hours 24 minutes

5. A respiratory therapist sets up an "E" size oxygen cylinder to transport a patient. When the cylinder is turned on, a loud whistling noise is heard from the cylinder. The most appropriate action is which of the following?
   A. Replace the regulator
   B. Check the plastic washer
   C. Loosen the regulator
   D. Check for cross-threading

6. Safety systems used at station outlets include which of the following?
   I. A.S.S.S.
   II. P.I.S.S.
   III. D.I.S.S.
   IV. Quick-connect
      A. I and III
      B. I and II

C. II and IV
D. III and IV

7. What is the gaseous capacity of a liquid oxygen cylinder that has 0.52 L when full?
   A. 172 L
   B. 30 L
   C. 447 L
   D. 452 L

8. A stationary liquid oxygen system contains 80 lb of oxygen when full. A home care patient is using it 8 hours each day, during sleep, at a rate of 3 L/min. At this usage, how many days will the liquid oxygen last?
   A. 6
   B. 8
   C. 19
   D. 27

9. Which of the following "E" size oxygen cylinders will run out of oxygen first?

Cylinder	Pressure (in psig)	Flow (in L/min)
A.	700	0.5
B.	900	1.5
C.	1100	2
D.	1600	3

10. The liquid capacity of a full stationary liquid oxygen system is 35 L, and the home care patient is using it 7 hours per night with a flow rate of 1.5 L/min. On the basis of this usage, the number of days that this liquid oxygen system will last is which of the following?
    A. 14 days
    B. 33 days
    C. 41 days
    D. 47 days

3

Administering Medical Gases

Upon completion of this chapter, you will be able to:
1. Compare the design and operation of single-stage and multistage regulators.
2. Identify the components of preset and adjustable regulators.
3. Explain the operational theory of a Thorpe tube flowmeter, a Bourdon flowmeter, and a flow restrictor.
4. Demonstrate a method for determining whether a flowmeter is pressure-compensated.
5. Compare low-flow and high-flow oxygen-delivery systems.
6. Name several commonly used low-flow oxygen-delivery systems.
7. Discuss the advantages and disadvantages of oxygen-conserving devices.
8. Explain the operational theory of air-entrainment devices.
9. Compare the operation of oxygen blenders with that of oxygen mixers and adders.
10. Describe the physiologic effects of hyperbaric oxygen therapy.
11. List the indications and contraindications of nitric oxide therapy.
12. Describe the appropriate use of mixed-gas (e.g., heliox, carbogen) therapy.

"What oxygen is to the lungs, such is hope to the meaning of life."
Emil Brunner

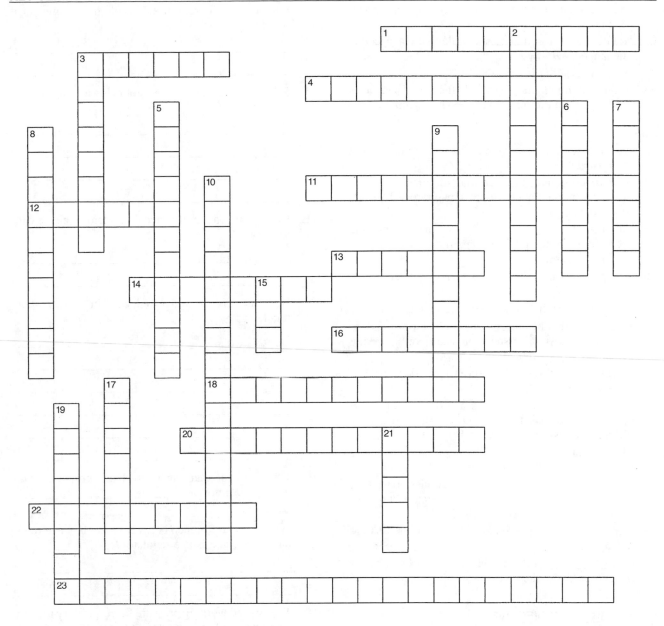

CROSSWORD PUZZLE 3-1
Created using Crossword Weaver, www.CrosswordWeaver.com.

Use the clues to complete the crossword puzzle.

Across

1. A walk-in hyperbaric chamber for two or more patients simultaneously.
3. A mixture of helium and oxygen used to treat patients with airway obstruction.
4. A regulator that allows the user to determine pressure limits.
11. A device that provides a variety of fractional inspired oxygen (F_IO_2) levels reliably (*two words*).

12. The most common type of flowmeter used in respiratory care.
13. A regulator that decreases the pressure from a gas supply system to a predetermined lower pressure.
14. A _____ performance device's F_IO_2 depends on the patient's inspiratory demand.
16. A type of nasal cannula that has a 20-mL reservoir.

18. A device consisting of two flowmeters, one to oxygen and one to air. It is the simplest oxygen proportioner (*two words*).
20. A flow restrictor that has a hole with a specific, unchanged size (*two words*).
22. A single hyperbaric chamber.
23. A type of flowmeter in which the needle valve is located before the indicator tube (*two words*).

Down

2. A system to deliver oxygen on demand to the patient (*two words*).
3. An oxygen-delivery device that supplies oxygen at flow rates higher than a patient's inspiratory demands (*two words*).
5. Pressure _____ flowmeters provide accurate estimates of flow, regardless of the downstream pressure.
6. A type of nasal cannula that has a reservoir of approximately 40 mL.
7. The flowmeter that is actually a reducing valve.
8. A regulator that has more than one level of pressure reduction between system pressure and working pressure (*two words*).
9. A regulator that lowers pressure to 50 psi in one step (*two words*).
10. A flow restrictor that utilizes a series of calibrated openings in a disk that can be adjusted to deliver different flows (*two words*).
15. The type of mask from which the partial rebreathing mask was derived (*abbreviation*).
17. An oxygen-delivery device that supplies oxygen at flow rates lower than a patient's inspiratory demands (*two words*).
19. A mixture of carbon dioxide and oxygen used to treat hiccups.
21. A _____ performance device's F_IO_2 does not depend on the patient's inspiratory demand.

ACHIEVING THE OBJECTIVES

1. Compare the design and operation of single-stage and multistage regulators.

1A. What divides the body of a single-stage regulator in half?

_____

_____

1B. How is excessively high pressure handled by a single-stage regulator?

_____

_____

1C. What are the two opposing forces that dictate flow into the high-pressure side of the single-stage regulator?

_____

_____

1D. What closes the valve stem in a single-stage regulator?

_____

_____

_____

_____

1E. How can a multistage regulator be easily identified?

_____

_____

1F. How is gas pressure reduced in a two-stage regulator?

_____

_____

_____

_____

_____

_____

1G. The regulator that can control gas pressures with more precision is a _____ _____.

1H. What is the difference between a single-stage regulator and a multistage regulator?

_____

_____

1I. The desired working pressure for respiratory therapy equipment is how many pounds per square inch?

_____

_____

1J. When incoming gas pressure is greater than the spring tension in the ambient chamber, what happens to the inlet valve?

_____

_____

Questions 1K and 1L refer to Figure 3-1.

1K. What type of regulator is shown in Figure 3-1?

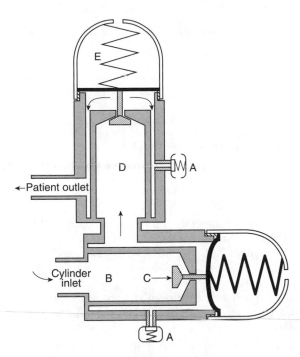

FIGURE 3-1

_____

_____

1L. Identify the components of Figure 3-1.

A. _____

B. _____

C. _____

D. _____

E. _____

Think About This

What commercial use does a gas regulator have?

Helpful Web Site

■ U.S. Food and Drug Administration (FDA), Center for Devices and Radiological Health, "FDA and NIOSH Public Health Notification: Oxygen Regulator Fires Resulting from Incorrect Use of CGA 870 Seals" — http://www.fda.gov

2. Identify the components of preset and adjustable regulators.

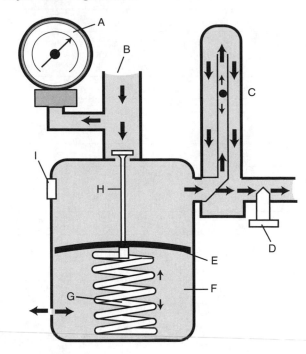

FIGURE 3-2

(Redrawn from Persing G: *Entry-level respiratory care review*, Philadelphia, 2005, WB Saunders.)

In questions 2A through 2I, label the components identified with letters in Figure 3-2.

2A. "A"

_____

_____

2B. "B"

_____

_____

2C. "C"

_____

_____

2D. "D"

_____

_____

2E. "E"

_____

_____

2F. "F"

_____

_____

2G. "G"

_____

_____

2H. "H"

_____

_____

2I. "I"

_____

_____

2J. The type of regulator shown in Figure 3-2 is a

_____

_____.

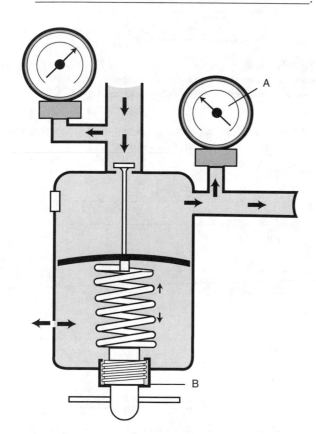

FIGURE 3-3
(Redrawn from Persing G: *Entry-level respiratory care review*, ed, F Known, Philadelphia, 2005, WB Saunders.)

In questions 2K and 2L, label the components identified with letters in Figure 3-3.

2K. "A" _____

_____

2L. "B" _____

_____

2M. The type of regulator shown in Figure 3-3 is a ___

_____.

Think About This
What is the typical pressure setting for an outdoor propane cooking tank?

Helpful Web Site
- U.S. Environmental Protection Agency, "Medical Devices; Anesthesiology Devices; Oxygen Pressure Regulators and Oxygen Conserving Devices" — http://www.epa.gov

3. Explain the operational theory of a Thorpe tube flowmeter, a Bourdon flowmeter, and a flow restrictor.
3A. Name the components of a Thorpe tube flowmeter.

_____

_____

_____

_____

3B. Adult flowmeters are usually calibrated in _____

_____, whereas neonatal and pediatric flowmeters are calibrated in _____.

3C. Why is the hollow tube of a Thorpe tube flowmeter wider at the top than at the bottom?

_____

_____

3D. What are the two opposing forces in the Thorpe tube flowmeter?

_____

_____

3E. If you put your finger over part of the outlet in flowmeter *B* in Figure 3-4, what would happen to the ball float and why?

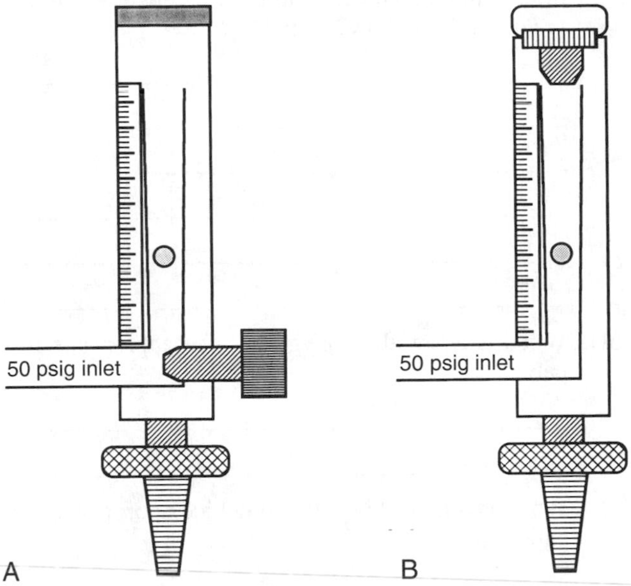

A   B

FIGURE 3-4

_____

_____

_____

3F. State the operational principle of the Bourdon flowmeter.

_____

_____

_____

3G. If the flow from a Bourdon flowmeter is set to 8 L/min and the outlet is totally occluded, what will the needle indicator reading be?

_____

_____

3H. How does a flow restrictor operate?

_____

_____

_____

_____

3I. Name the two types of flow restrictors.

_____

_____

3J. In the home care setting, where would flow restrictors be used most?

_____

_____

Think About This

How can flow restrictors save money in your home?

Helpful Web Site

■ RT Corner, "Gas Regulators and Flow Meters"—http://rtcorner.net/rt_regulators_flow_meters.htm

4. Demonstrate a method for determining whether a flowmeter is pressure-compensated or not pressure-compensated.

4A. Without plugging in the flowmeter, what two ways can you use to determine whether it is pressure-compensated or non–pressure-compensated?

_____

_____

_____

_____

_____

4B. What test can be performed to determine whether a Thorpe tube flowmeter is pressure-compensated or not?

_____

_____

4C. Which of the two Thorpe tube flowmeters in Figure 3-4 is not back-pressure–compensated? Why?

_____

_____

_____

_____

Think About This

Which type of Thorpe tube flowmeter would be most accurate to use in a hospital?

Helpful Web Sites

■ Kingwood College Respiratory Program: Gas Regulators and Flow Meters: Lecture by Elizabeth Kelley Buzbee A.A.S., R.R.T.-N.P.S., R.C.P__ http://wwwappskc.lonestar.edu/programs/respcare/resp.htm

5. Compare low-flow and high-flow oxygen-delivery systems.

5A. Why are low-flow devices also called *variable-performance devices*?

_____

_____

_____

_____

_____

5B. Name three factors that cause the F_IO_2 of a low-flow device to vary.

_____

_____

5C. Why are high-flow devices also called *fixed-performance devices*?

_____

_____

_____

_____

_____

_____

5D. How much can low-flow device F_IO_2 levels vary?

_____

_____

5E. What is the range for high-flow device F_IO_2 levels?

_____

_____

5F. A patient has been receiving supplemental oxygen via a low-flow device for 2 days. The patient's breathing becomes shallow. How would the F_IO_2 level when the patient is breathing with a normal tidal volume compare with the F_IO_2 level when the breathing is shallow? Why?

_____

_____

_____

_____

_____

_____

5G. A patient has been receiving supplemental oxygen via a high-flow device for 2 days. The patient's breathing becomes shallow. How would the F_IO_2 level when the patient is breathing with a normal tidal volume compare with the F_IO_2 level when the breathing is shallow? Why?

_____

_____

_____

_____

_____

_____

5H. When is a low-flow oxygen device appropriate for patient use?

_____

_____

5I. When is a high-flow oxygen device appropriate for patient use?

_____

_____

Think About This

When can a high-flow oxygen device become a low-flow device?

Helpful Web Site

■ University of Pennsylvania, Critical Care Medicine Tutorial: "How Do I administer Oxygen?," Patrick Neligan, — http://www.ccmtutorials.com/rs/oxygen/page13.htm

6. Name several commonly used low-flow oxygen delivery systems.

6A. Which low-flow oxygen-delivery device is most often used to treat hypoxemic patients who are breathing spontaneously?

_____

_____

6B. Name three common problems related to the use of the device from question 6A.

_____

_____

_____

_____

_____

6C. What is the theoretical oxygen concentration for use of the aforementioned low-flow oxygen device for adult patients? For pediatric patients?

_____

_____

_____

_____

6D. What F_IO_2 level can a simple mask deliver?

_____

_____

6E. Why is 5 L/min the minimum flow for a simple mask?

_____

_____

6F. List at least four disadvantages to the use of simple oxygen masks.

_____

_____

_____

_____

_____

6G. What is the structural difference between a simple mask and a partial rebreathing mask?

_____

_____

6H. What happens to the patient's anatomical dead space volume during exhalation with a partial rebreathing mask in use?

_____

_____

6I. Why does the anatomical dead space of a patient using a partial rebreathing mask have a high F_IO_2 level?

_____

_____

_____

_____

6J. What F_IO_2 range can a disposable partial rebreathing mask deliver?

_____

_____

6K. What is the structural difference between a partial rebreathing mask and a nonrebreathing mask?

_____

_____

_____

_____

_____

_____

6L. What F_IO_2 range can a disposable nonrebreathing mask deliver?

_____

_____

6M. How is the appropriate oxygen flow rate determined for a reservoir-type mask?

_____

_____

_____

_____

6N. Name the oxygen-conserving device that requires surgery for placement.

_____

_____

6O. Why can transtracheal oxygen (TTO) therapy make use of very low oxygen flow rates to achieve a desired level of oxygenation?

_____

_____

_____

_____

Think About This

How can you change a nonrebreathing mask into a partial rebreathing mask?

Helpful Web Sites

- Johns Hopkins Bayview Medical Center, "Healthy Directions: Transtracheal Oxygen Therapy" — http://www.hopkinsbayview.org
- University of Michigan, Oxygen Delivery Devices — http://www.respcare.med.umich.edu

7. Discuss the advantages and disadvantages of oxygen-conserving devices.

Complete the following chart.

Oxygen-conserving device	Advantages	Disadvantages
7A.	7B.	7C.
7D.	7E.	7F.
7G.	7H.	7I.

Questions 7J and 7K refer to Figure 3-5.

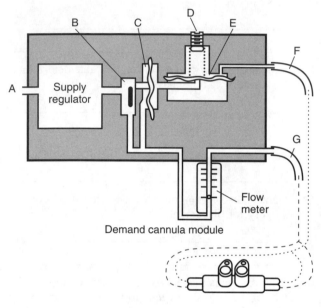

FIGURE 3-5
(Redrawn from Barnes TA: *Core textbook of respiratory care practice*, ed 2, St Louis, 1994, Mosby.)

7J. What is the inlet pressure (*A* in Figure 3-5) for the demand cannula module?

_____

_____

7K. Label the letters *B* through *G* in Figure 3-5, the demand cannula module.

B. _____

_____

C. _____

_____

D. _____

_____

E. _____

_____

F. _____

_____

G. _____

_____

Think About This

If you required home oxygen, which type of oxygen-conserving device would you want to have?

Helpful Web Sites

- National Lung Health Education Program, "Guide to Prescribing Home Oxygen," Thomas L. Petty, MD — http://www.nlhep.org
- American Association for Respiratory Care, "Oxygen-Conserving Techniques and Devices", R. McCoy, *Respir Care* 45:95–103, 2000 — http://www.aarc.org
- *Chest* journal, BL Tiep and MI Lewis: Oxygen conservation and oxygen-conserving devices in chronic lung disease: a review. *Chest* 92:263, 1987 — http://www.chestjournal.org

8. Explain the operational theory of air-entrainment devices.

8A. The three factors that dictate the concentration of oxygen delivered by an air-entrainment device are:

(1) _____

_____

(2) _____

_____

(3) _____

_____.

8B. How does the oxygen exiting the jet nozzle become diluted to a specific oxygen concentration?

_____

_____

_____

_____

8C. How do most commercially available air-entrainment masks vary oxygen concentration?

_____

_____

8D. What happens to the F_IO_2 when there is a partial obstruction of the gas flow downstream or partial obstruction of the entrainment ports?

_____

_____

_____

_____

8E. Calculate the air-to-oxygen ratio, using Figure 3-6, when the F_IO_2 of an air-entrainment device is 45%.

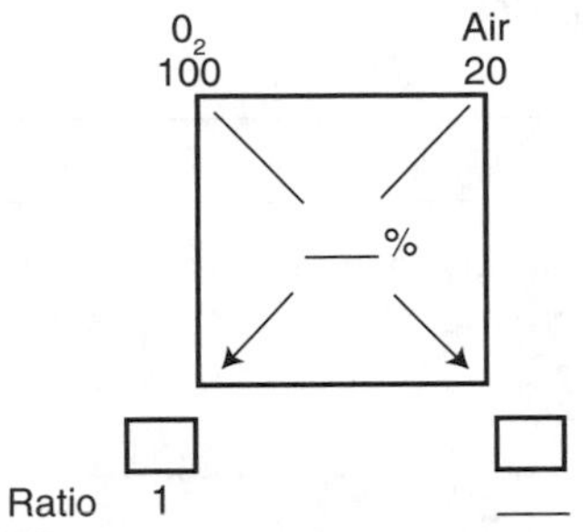

FIGURE 3-6

_____

8F. What are the total parts for 45%?

_____

_____

8G. Calculate the total flow for a 45% air-entrainment device when the oxygen flow is set to 10 L/min.

_____

_____

8H. What happens to the actual delivered F_IO_2 when a patient's inspiratory demand exceeds the total flow of an air-entrainment device?

_____

_____

_____

_____

8I. At what F_IO_2 range do air-entrainment masks function appropriately?

_____

_____

8J. Calculate the total flow for a 35% air-entrainment mask with a set oxgyen flow rate of 8 L/min.

_____

_____

8K. Accumulated moisure in the tubing of an air-entrainment large-volume nebulizer will cause what to happen to the delivered F_IO_2?

_____

_____

Think About This

What are some practical uses of the Venturi effect?

Helpful Web Sites

■ Salter Labs, "Percent-O_2-Lock Venturi System" — http://www.salterlabs.com

■ Keomed site — http://www.keomed.com

9. Compare the operation of oxygen blenders with that of oxygen mixers and adders.

9A. What are the components of a typical oxygen-adder system?

_____

_____

9B. With an oxygen-adder system, how can an F_IO_2 of 35% be achieved?

_____

_____

_____

_____

9C. What are the components of an oxygen blender?

_____

_____

_____

_____

_____

_____

9D. Why does an oxygen blender require a filter for the gases entering the blender housing?

_____

_____

_____

_____

9E. What device is most reliable for providing a variety of F_IO_2 levels for mechanical ventilators?

_____

_____

Think About This

What are the similarities and differences between an oxygen blender and the blender you used for food?

Helpful Web Sites

- Inspiration Healthcare Air/Oxygen Blender — http://www.inspiration-healthcare.co.uk
- Precision Medical Blender — http://www.precisionmedical.com

10. Describe the physiologic effects of hyperbaric oxygen therapy.

10A. What are the two problems that hyperbaric therapy was originally used to treat?

_____

_____

10B. List six other disorders that hyperbaric therapy is used to treat.

_____

_____

_____

10C. What happens to lung volumes during hyperbaric therapy?

_____

_____

_____

10D. Which gas law explains what happens to the alveolar and arterial partial pressures of oxygen during hyperbaric therapy?

_____

_____

10E. Calculate the PAO_2 during hyperbaric therapy when the barometic pressure (P_{bar}) equals 3 atm, F_IO_2 equals 1.00, $PaCO_2$ equals 45 mm HG, and water vapor pressure is 47 mm HG.

_____

_____

_____

_____

10F. Which gas law explains the changes in the PaO_2 that occur with exposure to hyperbaric therapy?

_____

_____

10G. Calculate the oxygen-carrying capacity of plasma when P_{bar} equals 3 atm, F_IO_2 equals 1.00, $PaCO_2$ equals 45 mm HG, and water vapor pressure is 47 mm HG.

_____

_____

_____

_____

10H. Calculate the oxygen-carrying capacity of plasma when P_{bar} equals 2.5 atm, F_IO_2 equals 1.0, $PaCO_2$ equals 40 mm HG, and water vapor pressure is 47 mm HG.

_____

_____

10I. What gas law would cause the temperature within a hyperbaric chamber to rise when pressure is exerted?

_____

_____

10J. How is temperature controlled within a hyperbaric chamber?

_____

_____

10K. Why is hyperbaric oxygen therapy useful in the treatment of skin grafts?

_____

_____

10L. Why is hyperbaric oxygen therapy used to treat anaerobic infections?

_____

_____

_____

_____

Think About This

What neurologic disorders may be treated with hyperbaric oxygen therapy?

Helpful Web Sites

- eMedicine from WebMD, "Hyperbaric Oxygen Therapy," Michael Neumeister, MD, FRCSC, FACS — http://www.emedicine.com
- University of Tennessee College of Veterinary Medicine, Veterinary Hyperbaric Medicine Society, "The Physiology of Hyperbaric Oxygen Therapy" — http://www.vet.utk.edu

11. List the indications and contraindications for nitric oxide therapy.

11A. What property does nitric oxide have that makes it useful in the treatment of various pulmonary disorders?

_____

_____

11B. List the indications for nitric oxide therapy.

_____

_____

_____

_____

11C. How is nitric oxide supplied?

_____

_____

11D. The by-products of nitric oxide and oxygen and water are:

_____

_____.

11E. The therapeutic dose of nitric oxide is between ___ _____ and _____

_____.

11F. What three gases are monitored during nitric oxide therapy?

_____

_____

Think About This

What physiologic and cellular processes does nitric oxide play a role in within the body?

Helpful Web Site

■ American Heart Association, *Circulation* journal, "Inhaled Nitric Oxide: A Selective Pulmonary Vasodilator: Current Uses and Therapeutic Potential," *Circulation* 109:3106–3111, 2004 — http://www.circ.ahajournals.org

12. Describe the appropriate use of mixed-gas (e.g., heliox, carbogen) therapy.

12A. How are heliox mixtures supplied?

_____

_____

12B. What property of heliox makes it useful in the treatment of certain respiratory problems?

_____

_____

12C. List five indications for heliox therapy.

(1) _____

_____

(2) _____

_____

(3) _____

_____

(4) _____

_____

(5) _____

_____

12D. Calculate the actual flow for an 80:20 heliox mixture being delivered to a patient via an oxygen flowmeter set at 10 L/min.

_____

_____

12E. The reservoir bag of a nonrebreathing mask needs to be maintained at 12 L/min to keep from collapsing. A 70:30 mixture of heliox is now connected to this mask. Calculate the set flow needed for actual heliox mixture to be 12 L/min.

_____

_____

_____

_____

12F. Calculate the actual flow for a 60:40 heliox mixture being delivered to a patient via an oxygen flowmeter set at 8 L/min.

_____

_____

12G. An insufficient amount of oxygen in the heliox mixture can result in:

_____

_____

43

12H. List four indications for carbogen.

(1) _____ (2) _____

(3) _____ (4) _____

12I. What are the clinical manifestations of carbon dioxide toxicity?

_____

_____

12J. How is carbogen supplied?

_____

_____

12K. What mask should be used to deliver carbogen?

_____

_____

12L. During carbogen therapy, what should the respiratory therapist be monitoring to help prevent carbon dioxide toxicity?

_____

_____

_____

_____

Think About This

How should a small-volume nebulizer be set up to deliver aerosolized medication with heliox?

Helpful Web Sites

■ *Respiratory Care* journal, Fink JB: Opportunities and risks of using heliox in your clinical practice, *Respir Care* 51:651–660, 2006 — http://www.rcjournal.com

■ Praxair, heliox overview — http://www.praxair.com

NATIONAL BOARD FOR RESPIRATORY CARE (NBRC)–TYPE QUESTIONS

1. Spring tension and gas pressure are the two opposing forces in which of the following?
   A. Bourdon gauge
   B. Kinetic tube
   C. Flowmeter
   D. Regulator

2. When a closed Thorpe tube flowmeter is attached to a 50-psi oxygen source, the indicator float jumps up then quickly falls to 0. This flowmeter is which of the following?
   A. Broken
   B. A Bourdon gauge flowmeter
   C. Compensated for back pressure
   D. Uncompensated for back pressure

3. Absorption atelectasis and oxygen toxicity may occur with which of the following?
   A. $F_IO_2 < 0.30$
   B. $F_IO_2 < 0.70$
   C. $F_IO_2 \geq 0.50$
   D. $F_IO_2 = 0.50$

4. A patient is receiving oxygen via a nasal cannula at 3 L/min. The patient's respiratory rate and tidal volume have decreased significantly. The F_IO_2 will do which of the following?
   A. Increase
   B. Stabilize
   C. Decrease
   D. Not change

5. A home care patient calls to inform the respiratory therapist that his *trans*tracheal *c*atheter (TTC) accidentally fell out last night and that he was unable to reinsert it. The respiratory therapist should tell the patient which of the following?
   A. Insert a dilating or stenting device
   B. Continue attempts to reinsert the catheter
   C. Use a nasal cannula and call his physician as soon as possible
   D. Use a nasal cannula until another TTC is delivered to the home

6. How much air will be entrained when a person is using a 35% air-entrainment adapter with 8 L/min oxygen?
   A. 35 L/min
   B. 40 L/min
   C. 45 L/min
   D. 55 L/min

7. If 35 L/min of humidified oxygen is added to 10 L/min of humidified air, what is the resultant F_IO_2?
   A. 0.82
   B. 0.74
   C. 0.40
   D. 0.38

8. A patient requires 15 L/min to prevent the reservoir bag on a nonrebreathing mask from collapsing. For an 80:20 heliox mixture, what is the correct flow rate to maintain the reservoir bag?
   A. 8 L/min
   B. 15 L/min
   C. 24 L/min
   D. 27 L/min

9. Which type of oxygen-delivery device should be used in the treatment of smoke inhalation?
   A. Nasal cannula at 6 L/min
   B. Simple mask at 10 L/min
   C. Nonrebreathing mask at 15 L/min
   D. Large-volume aerosol nebulizer at 0.60 setting

10. A home care patient reports no oxygen coming out of his pulse demand oxygen system. What are the probable causes?
    I. Flow set too low
    II. Improperly placed sensor
    III. Decreased or no power to the unit
    IV. Solenoid valve not properly opening
       A. I and IV only
       B. I and II only
       C. II and III only
       D. II and IV only

11. The work of breathing of a patient with limited lung reserves will increase with increased ambient pressure because of which of the following?
    A. Increased gas density
    B. Decreased gas volume
    C. Increased gas temperature
    D. Decreased oxygen solubility

Chapter 3 Administering Medical Gases

Humidity and Aerosol Therapy

LEARNING OBJECTIVES

Upon completion of this chapter, you will be able to:

1. Differentiate between the role of humidity and that of aerosol in respiratory care.
2. Describe the mechanisms of humidification.
3. Differentiate between humidity and aerosol.
4. Describe the natural physiologic humidification process throughout the respiratory tract.
5. Identify indications, contraindications, and hazards associated with humidity therapy.
6. Describe how various types of humidifiers work.
7. Compare and contrast low-flow and high-flow humidifiers.
8. Explain the importance of monitoring and maintaining humidity therapy.
9. Describe the physical characteristics of an aerosol.
10. Discuss factors that influence aerosol deposition.
11. Determine the optimal technique for administering aerosol: small-volume nebulizer, large-volume nebulizer, pressurized metered-dose inhaler, or dry powder inhaler.
12. Describe the therapeutic indications for aerosol therapy.
13. Explain how pneumatic, ultrasonic, and vibrating mesh aerosol generators work.
14. Discuss criteria for device selection.
15. Describe how each type of device should be set up, used, and maintained.
16. Identify special considerations for administering aerosol therapy.

"It's not the heat; it's the humidity."
Proverb

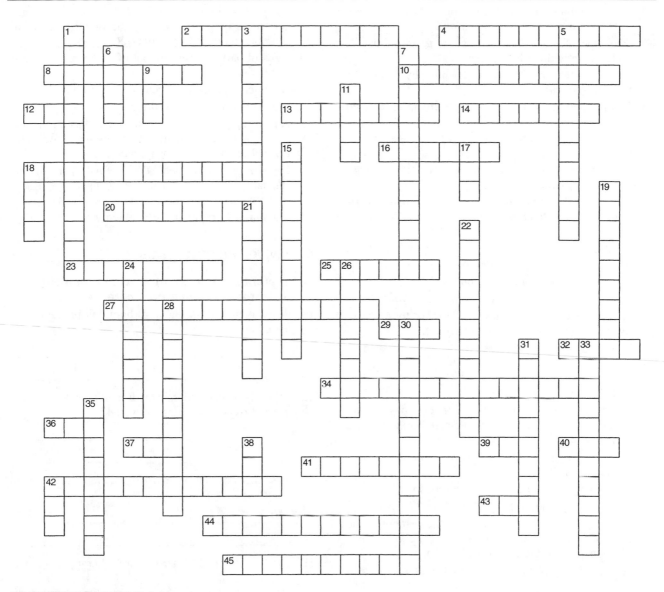

CROSSWORD PUZZLE 4-1
Created using Crossword Weaver, http://www.CrosswordWeaver.com.

Use the clues to complete the crossword puzzle.

Across

2. An index that describes a drug's toxic effect and its desired effect.
4. Measures humidity.
8. _____ humidity is the actual content or weight of water present in a given volume of gas.
10. The amount of drug inhaled (*two words*).
12. A propellant that does not have fluorocarbons (*abbreviation*).
13. A type of aerosol generator that creates aerosols for the upper airway.

14. A suspension of solid or liquid particles in a gas.
16. Any obstruction in an aerosol's path that breaks the aerosol into smaller particles.
18. A type of aerosol that consists of particles of similar size.
20. The type of movement that is the primary mechanism for the deposition of small particles.
23. Molecular water.
25. A valveless extension device that adds distance to the device referred to in **11 down**.

27. Aerosol particles of varying sizes.
29. Point at which inhaled gas reaches 100% saturation at body temperature (*abbreviation*).
32. The type of humidifier that passes gas flow over a water-saturated cloth or paper.
34. The product of inhaled mass multiplied by the answer to **7 down** (*two words*).
36. Small pneumatic device used to create medicated aerosols (*abbreviation*).
37. A statistical measure of the average aerosol droplet size (*abbreviation*).
39. An aerosol device for delivering a drug in powder form (*abbreviation*).
40. The variability of particle sizes in an aerosol distribution set at 1 standard deviation above or below the median (*abbreviation*).
41. A breath _____ nebulizer generates aerosol only during inspiration.
42. Change of state from gas to liquid.
43. A common passive humidifier (*abbreviation*).
44. A transducer that vibrates at 1.3 mHz to 2.3 mHz used to create an aerosol (*two words*).
45. The tendency of an aerosol to drop out of suspension.

Down

1. An electromechanical device that can pass liquid through a mesh or aperture plate to form droplets (*two words*).
3. _____ humidity = measured humidity ÷ water capacity × 100.
5. The change from a liquid to a gaseous state.
6. _____ humidity is 44 mg/L at 37°C.
7. A/an _____ fraction is the percent of the aerosol that is small enough to have a good chance of depositing in the lung (*two words*).
9. An electrically powered device that creates an aerosol (*abbreviation*).
11. A compact, portable, and convenient device used to produce aerosol medication (*abbreviation*).
15. The property of attracting and binding water molecules.
17. A pneumatic aerosol generator used to generate bland aerosols (*abbreviation*).
18. The mean aerodynamic diameter for particle sizes (*abbreviation*).
19. Expansion of a gas with no heat exchange with the environment.
21. A type of aerosol generator with a baffle.
22. Water cannot pass through this type of membrane.
24. _____ impaction — the tendency of a large particle to travel in a straight path and collide with an airway surface.

26. The type of humidifier that directs gas over a liquid or saturated liquid surface.
28. The mass of a drug leaving the mouthpiece of an aerosol generator (*two words*).
30. Aerosol particles settling out of suspension because of gravity.
31. A device that adds molecular water to gas.
33. Mucus that is thick and dried.
35. A breath _____ nebulizer has an inspiratory vent that closes during inspiration and forces the aerosol to exit via a 1-way valve.
38. Organization that sets design and performance standards for heat moisture exchangers, or HMEs (*abbreviation*).
42. The banned propellant (*abbreviation*).

ACHIEVING THE OBJECTIVES

1. Differentiate between the role of humidity and that of aerosol in respiratory care.

1A. What is the primary goal of humidity in respiratory care?

_____

_____

1B. What is it that necessitates humidity when supplemental oxygen is being delivered?

_____

_____

1C. List the roles that bland aerosol therapy has in respiratory care.

_____

_____

1D. What is the goal of aerosol drug therapy?

_____

_____

Think About This
Why do you get thirsty in the desert?

Helpful Web Site
■ Future Healthcare, Medical Gas Humidification — http://www.futurehealthcareus.com

2. Describe the mechanisms of humidification.

2A. How is inhaled air humidified naturally?

_____

_____

2B. What is another name for humidity?

_____

_____

2C. When a gas is warmed, what happens to its capacity to hold water?

_____

_____

2D. Name two ways in which humidity is described.

_____

_____

2E. Explain the two ways to describe humidity.

_____

_____

_____

_____

_____

2F. What would a hygrometer reading be if the relative humidity is 85% at 25°C? (*Hint:* use Table 4-1 in the textbook.)

_____

_____

_____

_____

2G. What is the relative humidity when the hygrometer reading is 15.4 mg/L at 29°C?

_____

_____

_____

_____

2H. What is the absolute humidity at body temperature when saturation is 100%?

_____

2I. List five mechanisms for artificially adding humidity to a gas.

_____

_____

_____

_____

Think About This
What is the perfect humidity level for your home?

Helpful Web Site
■ Georgia State University, Department of Physics and Astronomy, "Discussion of Relative Humidity" — http://hyperphysics.phy-astr.gsu.edu

3. Differentiate humidity from aerosol.

3A. What is humidity?

_____

_____

_____

_____

3B. What does humidity consist of?

_____

_____

3C. What is an aerosol?

_____

_____

_____

3D. How does humidity differ from aerosol?

_____

_____

_____

3E. What is humidity used for in respiratory care?

_____

_____

_____

3F. Why is humidity therapy necessary when supplemental oxygen is administered?

_____

_____

3G. What is aerosol therapy used for in respiratory care?

_____

_____

_____

_____

_____

_____

_____

Think About This

What types of aerosols are you exposed to everyday?

Helpful Web Sites

- RT for Decision Makers in Respiratory Care, "The Ins and Outs of Humidification," Stuart N. Ryan and Bryan D. Peterson — http://www.rtmagazine.com
- Medicare Health Products Co. Ltd, "What is [sic] Nebulizer?" — http://www.medicarehk.com

4. Describe the natural physiologic humidification process throughout the respiratory tract.

4A. During what part of the breath cycle does the upper airways add heat and humidity?

_____

_____

4B. During what part of the breath cycle is water reclaimed by the upper airways?

_____

_____

4C. What part of the nose increases the contact time between the inspired air and the nasal mucosa?

_____

_____

4D. Why does cold weather cause "runny" noses?

_____

_____

_____

_____

4E. Why does a stuffed nose cause a dry mouth?

_____

_____

_____

_____

Questions 4F through 4I refer to Figure 4-1.

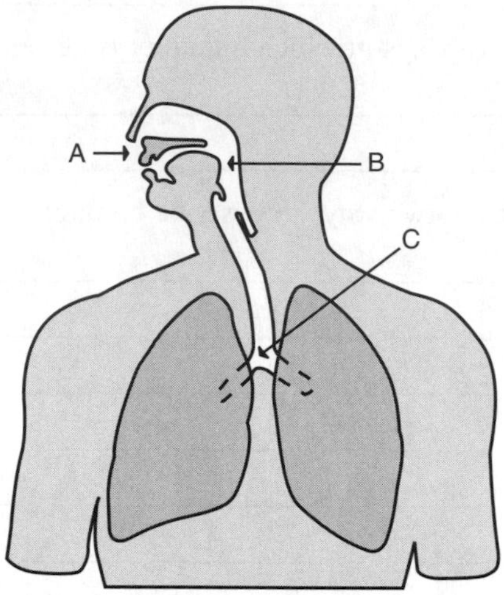

FIGURE 4-1

4F. Under ambient conditions, how much humidity is added to the inhaled air between point *A* and point *B*?

_____

_____

4G. Under ambient conditions, how much humidity is added to the inhaled air between point *B* and point *C*?

_____

_____

4H. At what point is the absolute humidity always 44 mg/L and the temperature 37°C?

_____

_____

4I. At what point is the isothermic saturation boundary (ISB)?

_____

_____

Think About This

Does the ISB change positions when a person is nose-breathing in the desert?

Helpful Web Site

- eMedicine from WebMD, "Nasal Physiology," Sanford M. Archer — http://www.emedicine.com

5. Identify the indications, contraindications, and hazards associated with humidity therapy.

5A. The presence of what seven clinical signs and symptoms, along with the administration of dry medical gas, are indications for humidity therapy?

_____

_____

_____

_____

5B. Why is heated humidity appropriate for patients who are hypothermic?

_____

_____

_____

5C. Why is heated humidity helpful during cold-induced asthma attacks?

_____

_____

5D. Regardless of whether a patient with bypassed airways is breathing spontaneously or receiving mechanical ventilation, why should humidity therapy be administered?

_____

_____

_____

_____

_____

5E. Name the seven indications for the use of cool humidified gas (bland aerosol) as mentioned in the American Association for Respiratory Care (AARC) Clinical Practice Guideline (CPG) for Bland Aerosol Administration.

_____

_____

_____

_____

_____

_____

_____

_____

5F. List the 13 hazards and complications (see AARC CPG: Humidification During Mechanical Ventilation) associated with the use of heated humidifiers.

_____

_____

_____

_____

_____

_____

_____

_____

_____

_____

_____

_____

_____

_____

_____

_____

5G. List the five contraindications for the use of HMEs.

_____

_____

_____

_____

_____

_____

5H. What are the two contraindications for the use of bland aerosol administration?

_____

_____

Think About This

What humidity level is optimum for individuals with chronic obstructive pulmonary disease (COPD)?

Helpful Web Sites

■ AARC CPG, "Bland Aerosol Administration—2003 Revision & Update" — http://www.rcjournal.com
■ AARC CPG, "Humidification During Mechanical Ventilation" (1992) — http://www.rcjournal.com

6. Describe how various types of humidifiers work.

Questions 6A and 6B refer to Figure 4-2.

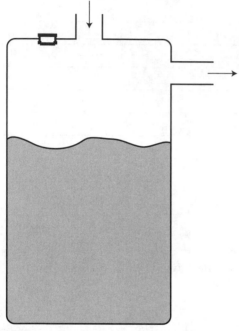

FIGURE 4-2
(Redrawn from Fink J, Cohen N: Humidity and aerosols. In Eubanks DH, Bone RC: *Principles and applications of cardiorespiratory care equipment,* St Louis, 1994, Mosby.)

6A. What type of humidifier is shown in Figure 4-2?

_____

_____

6B. How does the humidifier shown in Figure 4-2 add humidity to the gas?

_____

_____

6C. What type of humidifier brings the gas under the surface of the water?

_____

_____

Questions 6D and 6E refer to Figure 4-3.

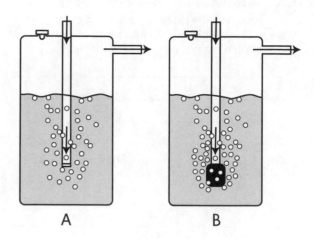

FIGURE 4-3

6D. What is the difference between the two humidifiers shown in Figure 4-3; which one is more efficient?

_____

_____

_____

6E. What would happen to one of the humidifiers shown in Figure 4-3 if the oxygen tubing connected to it becomes caught in the bed rails and is crimped off?

_____

_____

_____

_____

6F. What does adding heat do to a humidifier?

_____

_____

6G. Describe how a wick humidifier operates.

_____

_____

_____

_____

_____

_____

_____

_____

6H. How does a membrane-type humidifier operate?

_____

_____

_____

_____

_____

_____

6I. How does a large-volume jet nebulizer add humidity to a gas?

_____

_____

_____

_____

_____

_____

_____

6J. How does an ultrasonic nebulizer operate?

_____

_____

_____

_____

_____

_____

6K. How can particle size and aerosol density be altered on an ultrasonic nebulizer?

_____

_____

_____

_____

_____

_____

6L. Explain the operation of a generic HME.

_____

_____

_____

6M. Explain the operation of a condenser HME.

_____

_____

_____

_____

_____

_____

6N. How does a hygroscopic condenser HME operate?

_____

_____

_____

_____

_____

_____

6O. Explain the operation of a hygroscopic HME filter (HHMEF).

_____

_____

_____

_____

_____

_____

Think About This

What are the different types of room humidifiers?

Helpful Web Sites

■ Cardinal Health, Respiratory Abstracts, "Comparison of Vapotherm 2000i With a Bubble Humidifier for Humidifying Flow Through an Infant Nasal Cannula," Brian K. Walsh — http://www.cardinal.com

- PubMed Central, *Archives of Disease in Childhood,* "Membrane Humidification — a New Method for Humidification of Respiratory Gases in Ventilator Treatment of Neonates," "Hanssler L, Tennhoff W, and Roll C, — http://www.pubmedcentral.nih.gov
- *Chest* journal, "Comparing Two Heat and Moisture Exchangers, One Hydrophobic and One Hygroscopic, on Humidifying Efficacy and the Rate of Nosocomial Pneumonia," Thomachot et al. — http://www.chestjournal.org

7. Compare and contrast low-flow and high-flow humidifiers.

7A. What is the maximum flow rate that should be used with a low-flow humidifier?

_____

_____

7B. Name a low-flow humidifier.

_____

_____

7C. What type of oxygen devices are used with low-flow humidifiers?

_____

_____

7D. Why shouldn't a low-flow humidifier be used with a patient who has a bypassed airway?

_____

_____

_____

_____

_____

_____

7E. What are the two main structural differences between a low-flow humidifier and a high-flow humidifier?

_____

_____

_____

_____

7F. What flow rates can a high-flow humidifier handle?

_____

_____

7G. Label the following humidifiers as either low-flow or high-flow humidifiers:

1. Bubble humidifier:

   _____

   _____

2. Heated passover humidifier:

   _____

   _____

3. HME:

   _____

   _____

4. Passover humidifier on a nasal cannula:

   _____

   _____

5. Diffuser bubble humidifier:

   _____

   _____

7. Large-volume nebulizer:

   _____

   _____

8. Ultrasonic nebulizer:

   _____

   _____

Think About This

Are room humidifiers high-flow or low-flow humidifiers?

Helpful Web Sites

- AARC CPG, "Humidification During Mechanical Ventilation" — http://www.rcjournal.com
- Ryan, SN and Peterson, BD: "The Ins and Outs of Humidification" — http://www.rtmagazine.com

8. Explain the importance of monitoring and maintaining humidity therapy.

8A. Why is inspecting the water level of a bubble humidifier important?

_____

_____

_____

8B. Compare the humidity output of a bubble humidifier at 4 L/min versus one at 10 L/min.

_____

_____

_____

8C. Why is inspecting the ventilator circuit for condensation important when a heated humidification system is being used?

_____

_____

_____

_____

_____

_____

8D. List and explain four ways to reduce the collection of condensation in a ventilator circuit.

_____

_____

_____

_____

_____

_____

8E. What device may be used to accurately and reliably ensure that patients are receiving gas at the expected temperature and humidity level?

_____

_____

8F. What factors should a respiratory therapist monitor when using an HME during mechanical ventilation of a patient?

_____

_____

_____

_____

_____

8G. According to the AARC, what factors should a respiratory therapist monitor when a patient is receiving humidity therapy via a large-volume nebulizer?

_____

_____

_____

_____

_____

Think About This
What causes ground fog?

Helpful Web Sites
- AARC CPG: "Bland Aerosol Administration–2003 Revision & Update" — www.rcjournal.com
- AARC CPG: "Humidification During Mechanical Ventilation" — www.rcjournal.com
- *Clinical Foundations,* "Humidification During Mechanical Ventilation: Current Trends and Controversies," Tim Op't Holt — http://www.teleflexmedical.com

9. Describe the physical characteristics of an aerosol.

9A. Aerosols consisting of particles of a similar size are known as:

_____

_____

9B. Aerosols containing particles of many different sizes are known as:

_____

_____

9C. The average aerosol particle size expressed by the measure of central tendency for cascade impaction is known as _____ _____; for laser diffraction it is called _____.

9D. As the geometric standard deviation becomes greater, what happens to the range of particle sizes?

_____

_____

_____

_____

9E. What size particles usually remain in suspension and will be cleared with exhaled gas?

_____

_____

9F. What characteristic causes aerosol particles to increase in size as they age?

_____

_____

9G. What characteristic causes aerosol particles to decrease in size as they age?

_____

_____

Think About This

How much aerosol are you exposed to during a normal day?

Helpful Web Sites

■ National Aeronautics and Space Administration (NASA), Langley Research Center, "Atmospheric Aerosols: What Are They, and Why Are They So Important?" — http://oea.larc.nasa.gov

■ University of Colorado at Boulder, "Interactions Between Aerosols and Fog," Robert Tardif — http://www.rap.ucar.edu

10. Discuss factors that influence aerosol deposition.

10A. How does aerosol particle size influence its deposition?

_____

_____

10B. What is the primary mechanism for deposition of particles in the 1- to 5-μm range?

_____

_____

_____

_____

_____

10C. What is the primary mechanism for the deposition of aerosol particles that are less than 3 μm in size?

_____

_____

10D. List five patient factors that influence the deposition of aerosols.

_____

_____

_____

_____

Questions 10E through 10H refer to Figure 4-4

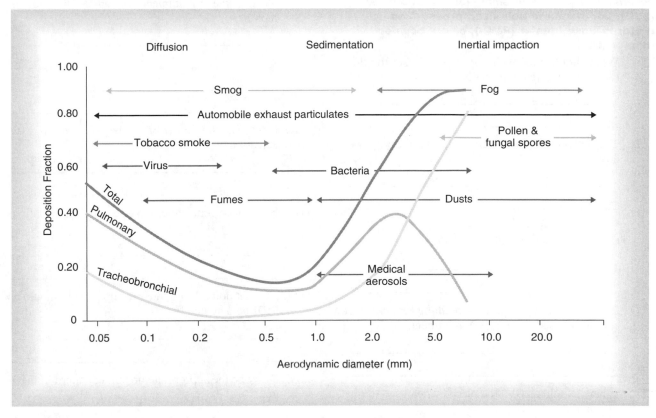

FIGURE 4-4
(From Wilkins RL, Stoller JK, Kacmarek RM. *Egan's fundamentals of respiratory care,* ed 9, St Louis, 2009, Mosby. Modified from Yu CP, Nicolaides P, Soong TT: Effect of random airway sizes on aerosol deposition. *Am Ind Hyg Assoc J* 40:999–1005, 1979.)

10E. What five common aerosols are primarily deposited in the lungs by sedimentation?

_____

_____

_____

_____

10F. Inertial impaction is the sole cause of deposition in the lungs for:

_____

_____

10G. What size particles have maximum deposition in the lungs?

_____

_____

10H. Viruses are primarily deposited in the lungs by what mechanism?

_____

_____

Think About This
What types of particles will high-efficiency particulate air (HEPA) filters remove from the air?

Helpful Web Sites
■ International Diabetes Monitor Archives, "The Physiology of Inhaled Insulin," Per Wollmer — http://www.d4pro.com
■ *Medical Design Technology* magazine, "Achieving Optimal Particle Size Distribution in Inhalation Therapy," Bob Bruno — http://www.mdtmag.com
■ Lexington Pulmonary and Critical Care, "Aerosol Therapy," Donald R. Elton — http://www.lexingtonpulmonary.com

11. Determine the optimal technique for administering aerosol: small-volume nebulizer (SVN), large-volume nebulizer, pressurized metered-dose inhaler (PMDI), or dry powder inhaler (DPI).

11A. What should the respiratory therapist set the flow rate at for a pneumatic SVN?

_____

_____

11B. The SVNs that use electrical or battery power are:

_____

_____.

11C. What is the most effective position for a patient taking a treatment with an SVN?

_____

_____

11D. Describe the appropriate breathing pattern that should be used during SVN treatment.

_____

_____

11E. Where should an SVN be placed when used during mechanical ventilation?

_____

_____

11F. What ventilator parameters need to be adjusted when an SVN is being used with mechanical ventilation?

_____

_____

_____

_____

11G. What type of SVN can aerosolize medication without increasing the patient's tidal volume?

_____

_____

11H. What patient interface should be used with continuous bronchodilator therapy through a large-volume nebulizer?

_____

_____

11I. When should a pressurized metered-dose inhaler be primed?

_____

_____

11J. What technique may be used as an alternative to placing the mouthpiece of an MDI into the mouth?

_____

_____

_____

11K. How long should the breath be held after an MDI actuation?

_____

_____

11L. How much time should elapse between actuations from an MDI?

_____

_____

11M. At what point during the breathing cycle should an MDI be actuated?

_____

_____

11N. Describe the appropriate breathing pattern for MDI use.

_____

_____

11O. What technique should be used if a breath hold is not possible when a patient is using an MDI with a valved holding chamber?

_____

_____

_____

_____

_____

11P. What is the most critical factor in the use of a DPI?

_____

_____

11Q. What types of patients would not be able to use a DPI?

_____

_____

Think About This
Which aerosol delivery device is ideal?

Helpful Web Sites
- University of Texas Policy and Procedure for Small-Volume Nebulizer (SVN) Treatment — http://www.dmz.utmb.edu
- Tri-anim Health Services, Inc, Hope™ Nebulizer Sample Protocol — http://www.tri-anim.com
- Cleveland Clinic Health System, "How to Use Your Diskus Dry Powder Inhaler (DPI)" — http://www.cchs.net

12. Describe the therapeutic indications for aerosol therapy.

12A. State the goal of medical aerosol therapy.

_____

_____

_____

_____

12B. Why is administering medications by aerosol beneficial to patients with pulmonary disorders?

_____

_____

_____

_____

For questions 12C through 12G, match the aerosolized medication with its indication.

___12C.	mucokinetic agents	a	Presence of reversible airflow obstruction
___12D.	mediator-modifying compounds	b	Management of COPD
___12E.	β-adrenergic agent	c	Reduce the accumulation of airway secretions
___12F.	anticholinergic agents	d	Maintenance of persistent asthma and severe COPD
___12G.	anti-inflammatory agent	e	Prophylactic management of mild to moderate persistent asthma

12H. What are the indications for the use of aerosol delivery devices that target the lung parenchyma?

_____

_____

12I. What are the seven indications for bland aerosol therapy?

_____

_____

_____

_____

_____

_____

_____

Think About This
Observe someone you know using a pressurized MDI. Do they use it properly?

Helpful Web Sites
- Association for Aerosol Research, "Therapeutic Aerosols: Today and Tomorrow," Gerhard Scheuch — http://www.gaef.de
- National Jewish Health, "Devices for Inhaled Medications" — http://www.nationaljewish.org

13. Explain how pneumatic, ultrasonic, and vibrating mesh aerosol generators work.
Questions 13A through 13F refer to Figure 4-5.

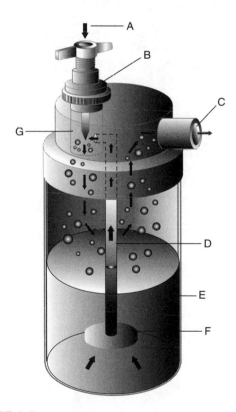

FIGURE 4-5
(From Wilkins RL, Stoller JK, Kacmarek RM. *Egan's fundamentals of respiratory care*, ed 9, St Louis, 2009, Mosby.)

13A. What type of device is shown in Figure 4-5?

_____

_____

13B. Label Figure 4-5.

    A. _____

    B. _____

    C. _____

    D. _____

    E. _____

    F. _____

    G. _____

13C. How does the device in Figure 4-5 create aerosol particles?

_____

_____

_____

_____

_____

_____

_____

13D. What flow rate should be used to operate the device in Figure 4-5?

_____

_____

13E. What is the total water output of the device in Figure 4-5 when unheated?

_____

_____

13F. What is the total water output of the device in Figure 4-5 when heated?

_____

_____

Questions 13G through 13M refer to Figure 4-6.

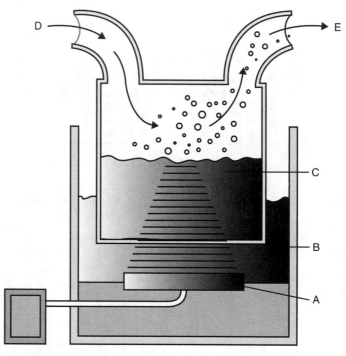

FIGURE 4-6

(From Wilkins RL, Stoller JK, Kacmarek RM. *Egan's fundamentals of respiratory care,* ed 9, St. Louis, 2009, Mosby. Modified from Barnes TA: *Core textbook of respiratory care practice,* ed 2, St Louis, 1994, Mosby.)

13G. What type of device is shown in Figure 4-6?

_____

_____

13H. Label Figure 4-6.

A. _____

B. _____

C. _____

D. _____

E. _____

13I. How does the device in Figure 4-6 create aerosol particles?

_____

_____

_____

_____

_____

_____

_____

13J. On the device in Figure 4-6, particle size is dictated by:

_____

_____

13K. The rate of aerosol production by the device in Figure 4-6 is directly related to:

_____

_____

13L. What do the flow and amplitude settings for the equipment shown in Figure 4-6 determine?

_____

_____

13M. What is the maximum total water output for the device in Figure 4-6?

_____

_____

13N. How does a vibrating mesh nebulizer create an aerosol?

_____

_____

_____

_____

13O. What is the difference between a passive vibrating mesh nebulizer and an active vibrating mesh nebulizer?

_____

_____

_____

_____

_____

_____

_____

_____

_____

_____

_____

_____

Think About This

Do pets have a need for nebulizers?

Helpful Web Sites

- American Association for Respiratory Care, *Respiratory Care* journal, "Nebulizers: Principles and Performance," Dean Hess — http://www.aarc.org
- L. Vecellio: "The Mesh Nebulizer: A Recent Technical Innovation for Aerosol Delivery." *Breathe*, March 2006 2(3) — http://www.ers-education.org
- Cystic fibrosis information, "Nebulizers and Compressors" (links page), Norma Kennedy Plourde — http://www3.nbnet.nb.ca

14. Discuss criteria for device selection.

14A. What are the five factors that should be considered when selecting the appropriate aerosol delivery device for a given patient?

_____

_____

_____

_____

_____

_____

14B. An alert and oriented elderly patient with arthritis requires the use of an aerosol delivery device at home for a bronchodilator; what are the pros and cons of each delivery device?

_____

_____

_____

_____

_____

_____

_____

_____

_____

14C. A patient with asthma arrives at the emergency department in respiratory distress. Which type of delivery system is most appropriate to treat this patient with an aerosolized bronchodilator? Why?

_____

_____

_____

_____

_____

_____

14D. What types of aerosol delivery device(s) are most appropriate for a young child? Why?

_____

_____

_____

_____

14E. A respiratory therapist has decided that a 6-year-old actively cooperative child is able to use an MDI with a valved holding chamber (VHC) to take her aerosolized medication. The child's parents, however, insist on an SVN with a compressor. What is the most appropriate action for the respiratory therapist to take? Why?

_____

_____

_____

_____

_____

_____

14F. A patient receiving mechanical ventilation requires an aerosolized medication. What are the most appropriate aerosol delivery devices for this situation? Why?

_____

_____

_____

_____

_____

_____

_____

_____

_____

14G. What device should be used to deliver ribavirin to a child with respiratory syncytial virus?

_____

_____

14H. Name three brands of SVNs that are made to deliver aerosolized pentamidine?

_____

_____

Think About This

How do aerosol deposition and dispersion change in an environment with altered gravity?

Helpful Web Sites

- *Chest* journal, "Device Selection and Outcomes of Aerosol Therapy: Evidence-Based Guidelines: American College of Chest Physicians/American College of Asthma, Allergy, and Immunology," Myrna B. Dolovich et al. — http://www.chestjournal.org
- American College of Allergy, Asthma & Immunology, "New Guidelines on Aerosol Therapy Devices" (press release) — http://www.acaai.org

15. Describe how each type of device should be set up, used, and maintained.

15A. When should an MDI be primed?

_____

_____

_____

_____

15B. What is the proper technique for priming an MDI?

_____

_____

15C. When should the MDI open-mouth technique be used?

_____

_____

15D. Describe how an MDI should be cleaned.

_____

_____

_____

_____

15E. When should an MDI be discarded?

_____

_____

_____

15F. How should a VHC be maintained?

_____

_____

15G. What is the procedure for priming a new Turbuhaler?

_____

_____

_____

_____

15H. What are the steps for the use of a Turbuhaler?

_____

_____

_____

_____

_____

_____

_____

15I. How do you know when a Turbuhaler is empty?

_____

_____

_____

_____

15J. What is the technique for the use of a vibrating mesh or ultrasonic nebulizer (USN)?

_____

_____

_____

_____

_____

_____

15K. How should a nebulizer be maintained at home after each use?

_____

_____

_____

_____

15L. How often should a home nebulizer be disinfected?

_____

_____

15M. What is the procedure for disinfecting a home nebulizer?

_____

_____

_____

15N. Give three examples of disinfectant options for the home nebulizer.

_____

_____

_____

_____

_____

15O. How should a ventilator be set up for the administration of pMDI in the ventilator circuit?

_____

_____

_____

_____

_____

_____

_____

15P. How long should the respiratory therapist wait between actuations when delivering medication via pressurized MDI in a ventilator circuit?

_____

_____

Think About This
Does asthma occur in pets and other animals?

Helpful Web Site
- *Respiratory Care* journal, "Nebulizer Use and Maintenance by Cystic Fibrosis Patients: A Survey Study," Mary K. Lester et al. — http://www.rcjournal.com

16. Identify special considerations for administering aerosol therapy.

16A. How often can aerosolized bronchodilator treatments be given to a patient having a severe asthma exacerbation?

_____

_____

16B. What are the alternative strategies for bronchodilator resuscitation in the emergency department?

_____

_____

_____

_____

_____

16C. When should continuous bronchodilator therapy (CBT) be administered?

_____

_____

16D. What equipment is needed to deliver CBT?

_____

_____

_____

16E. How often should a patient receiving CBT be assessed?

_____

_____

16F. What is considered to be a positive response to CBT?

_____

_____

_____

_____

16G. How should CBT be assessed when administered to young children?

_____

_____

_____

_____

16H. Why are special SVNs (e.g., Respirgard II) used to deliver aerosolized pentamidine?

_____

_____

_____

16I. What other aerosolized medication is associated with health risks to health care providers?

_____

_____

16J. List the health risks.

_____

_____

_____

_____

16K. What other environmental precautions should be taken when ribavirin or pentamidine is administered?

_____

_____

_____

_____

_____

_____

_____

16L. A patient in the emergency department is suspected of having active tuberculosis and needs to have an aerosol treatment. How should this treatment be administered?

_____

_____

_____

_____

_____

_____

16M. How should the filters and nebulizer used in treatments with pentamidine and ribavirin be disposed of?

_____

_____

_____

_____

Think About This

What other types of medications can be aerosolized?

Helpful Web Sites

■ International Social Security Association, Health Services Section, Consensus Paper: "Occupational Risk Prevention in Aerosol Therapy (Pentamidine, Ribavirin)," Marcel Jost et al. — http://health.prevention.issa.int

■ B & B Medical Technologies, Inc, "Sample Policy and Procedure for Continuous Bronchodilator Therapy with the Hope™ Nebulizer" — http://www.bandb-medical.com

■ Wisconsin Department of Health Services, Tuberculosis Program, "Cough-inducing and Aerosol-Generating Procedures" — http://dhfs.wisconsin.gov

NATIONAL BOARD FOR RESPIRATORY CARE (NBRC)–TYPE QUESTIONS

1. What happens at the isothermic saturation boundary (ISB)?
   A. No more cilia exist
   B. Turbulent convection occurs
   C. Inspired gas reaches body humidity
   D. The largest humidity deficit exists

2. Water moves up the "wick" of a wick humidifier because of which of the following?
   A. Venturi principle
   B. Bernoulli principle
   C. Capillary action
   D. Boyle's law

3. The type of humidifier that utilizes a low thermal conductivity condensing element is which of the following?
   A. Wick humidifier
   B. Bubble humidifier
   C. Ultrasonic nebulizer
   D. Hygroscopic heat moisture exchanger (HME)

4. What is the relative humidity when the absolute humidity is 10 mg H_2O/L and the capacity is 18 mg H_2O/L?
   A. 23%
   B. 38%
   C. 41%
   D. 55%

5. A patient is receiving oxygen therapy via a simple mask at a flow of 15 L/min with a bubble humidifier. A clinical assessment reveals a nonproductive cough. The patient is reporting a dry mouth, nose, and throat. The most appropriate action(s) to take include which of the following?
   I. Decrease the oxygen flow rate to the simple mask to 10 L/min
   II. Replace the apparatus with a small-volume nebulizer (SVN)
   III. Suggest an aerosol treatment with a mucolytic agent
   IV. Check the humidifier water level
   A. IV only
   B. II only
   C. I and IV only
   D. II and III only

6. While checking a patient who is receiving oxygen, a respiratory therapist hears a high-pitched whistle coming from the bubble humidifier. The most probable cause of the problem is which of the following?

   A. The oxygen tubing is kinked
   B. The humidifier is overheated
   C. Nasal prongs are not in place
   D. Water level in the humidifier is low

7. A heated humidifier unit has a water temperature of 40°C. The humidified gas is traveling through large-bore tubing to the patient. Which of the following statements are true?
   I. Condensation will occur.
   II. The gas will remain saturated.
   III. The relative humidity will increase.
   IV. The gas will warm and expand as it travels to the patient.
   A. I and II only
   B. II and III only
   C. III and IV only
   D. I and IV only

8. Clinical signs and symptoms of inadequate airway humidification include all of the following **EXCEPT**:
   A. Atelectasis
   B. Substernal pain
   C. Productive cough
   D. Nonproductive cough

9. Which of the following statements are true concerning bubble humidifiers?
   I. At 4 L/min the absolute humidity is approximately 30 mg/L.
   II. They are more efficient at flows greater than 5 L/min.
   III. At best a bubble humidifier can deliver 20% relative humidity at body temperature and pressure saturated (BTPS).
   IV. The pressure-relief alarm sounds when pressure in the unit exceeds 2 psi.
   A. I and II only
   B. II and III only
   C. III and IV only
   D. I and IV only

10. The primary mechanism for deposition of small particles of less than 3 micrometers is which of the following?
   A. Sedimentation
   B. Inertial impaction
   C. Brownian motion
   D. Monodispersion

Chapter **4** **Humidity and Aerosol Therapy**

11. A hypothermic patient with a bypassed airway requires humidification. Which of the following humidifiers would be most appropriate for this situation?
    I. Wick humidifier
    II. Bubble humidifier
    III. Large-volume nebulizer
    IV. Hygroscopic HME
    A. I and IV only
    B. II and III only
    C. I, III, and IV only
    D. II, III, and IV only

12. The respiratory therapist should coach a patient to breathe in which of the following patterns for particle deposition in the lower airways?
    I. Inhale slowly
    II. Inhale rapidly
    III. Inhale deeply through the nose
    IV. Use a mouthpiece instead of a mask
    V. Hold the breath in for approximately 10 seconds before exhaling
    A. II and III only
    B. II and V only
    C. I, III, and V only
    D. I, IV, and V only

13. Bland aerosol therapy is most appropriately delivered to a patient with a tracheostomy tube through which of the following methods?
    A. Humidifier, oxygen tubing, and a nasal cannula
    B. Large-volume nebulizer, large-bore tubing, and a Briggs adapter
    C. Large-volume nebulizer, large-bore tubing, and a tracheostomy collar
    D. Small-volume nebulizer (SVN), oxygen tubing, and a large-volume nebulizer

14. Which of the following devices is most commonly used to deliver continuous aerosol with oxygen to a patient with a tracheostomy?
    A. Vibrating mesh nebulizer
    B. Pneumatic jet nebulizer
    C. HME
    D. Small-particle aerosol generator

15. Which of the following breathing techniques provides for more effective delivery of an aerosolized medication to the lungs?
    A. Nose-breathing
    B. Rapid inspiration
    C. Inspiratory hold
    D. Expiratory hold

16. The device selected for the administration of pharmacologically active aerosol to the lower airway should produce particles with a mass median aerodynamic diameter (MMAD) range of:
    A. 0.5 to 1 μm
    B. 1 to 5 μm
    C. 6 to 10 μm
    D. 10 to 20 μm

17. A patient with asthma and severe bronchospasm is not responding to intermittent SVN treatments with a β-adrenergic bronchodilator. The appropriate recommendation for this patient is to switch to which of the following?
    A. Dry powder inhaler (DPI) bronchodilator
    B. Continuous bronchodilator therapy (CBT)
    C. Continuous nebulized bland aerosol
    D. Metered-dose inhaler (MDI) bronchodilator with a valved holding chamber

18. To prevent the hazards of contact with ribavirin, caregivers must wear which of the following?
    I. Gown
    II. Gloves
    III. Goggles
    IV. HEPA mask
    A. III and IV only
    B. I and II only
    C. II, III, and IV only
    D. I, II, III, and IV

19. Aerosol deposition in the lungs will be increased according to all of the following EXCEPT:
    A. Health of the patient
    B. Decreased tidal volume
    C. Decreased respiratory rate
    D. Increased inspiratory to expiratory time

20. A patient is set up on a 35% aerosol mask. Several hours later, an oxygen analyzer is placed in the circuit and its reading is 60%, but the large volume nebulizer setting remains at 35%. The most appropriate action is which of the following?
    A. Shorten the aerosol tubing
    B. Increase the nebulizer flow
    C. Decrease the nebulizer flow
    D. Drain the water from the aerosol tubing

5 Principles of Infection Control

LEARNING OBJECTIVES

Upon completion of this chapter, you will be able to:
1. Identify the major groups of microorganisms associated with nosocomial pneumonia.
2. List four factors that can influence the effectiveness of a germicide.
3. Define *high-level disinfection, intermediate-level disinfection,* and *low-level disinfection.*
4. Describe the process of pasteurization and its application to the disinfection of respiratory care equipment.
5. Explain how quaternary ammonium compounds, alcohols, acetic acid, phenols, glutaraldehyde, hydrogen peroxide, and iodophors and other halogenated compounds are used as disinfectants.
6. Name the four physical methods commonly used to sterilize medical devices.
7. Discuss the principle of ethylene oxide sterilization.
8. Identify infection-risk devices used in respiratory care.
9. Describe three components of an effective infection surveillance program.
10. Compare standard precautions with transmission-based precautions.
11. List the most common agents associated with febrile respiratory illnesses that are potential causes of mass casualty events.

"No science is immune to the infection of politics and the corruption of power."
Jacob Bronowski

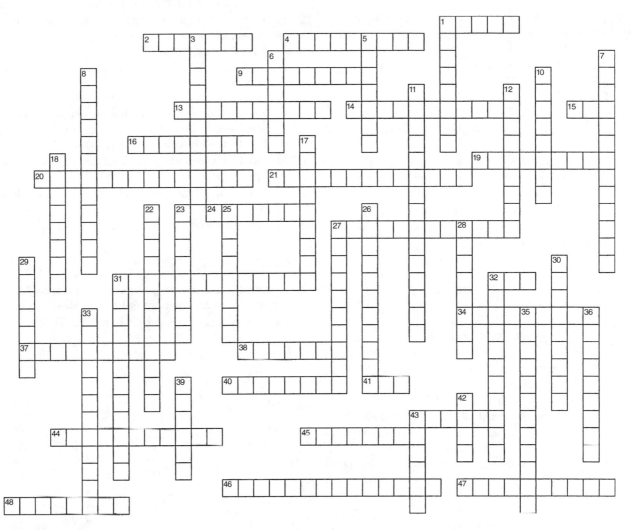

CROSSWORD PUZZLE 5-1
Created using Crossword Weaver, www.CrosswordWeaver.com.

Use the clues to complete the crossword puzzle.

Across

1. Spherical bacteria.
2. The type of precaution used to prevent the transmission of microorganisms such as *Haemophilus influenzae* type b and *Neisseria meningitidis*.
4. An agent that destroys fungi.
9. _____ precautions or techniques.
13. An infection that originates in a hospital is a _____ _____ infection.
14. An agent that kills bacteria.
15. Pneumonias caused by ventilators (*abbreviation*).
16. The type of disinfection that kills most vegetative bacteria, some fungi, and some viruses (*hyphenated word*).

19. A type of precaution designed to prevent transmission of blood-borne diseases.
20. Long chains of rod-like bacteria.
21. Complete destruction of all microorganisms.
24. Rodlike bacteria.
27. Infection _____: health facility procedures to minimize the risk of spreading infection.
31. Mutual touching of two individuals or organisms (*two words*).
32. The virus that causes acquired immunodeficiency syndrome, or AIDS (*abbreviation*).
34. An organism that requires simple inorganic nutrients to sustain itself.

37. Protozoa are an example of this type of microorganism.
38. A substance that can transmit an infectious agent.
40. A microorganism that does not require oxygen to live and grow.
41. The agency that makes infection control recommendations (*abbreviation*).
43. Cholera is in this genus.
44. Not obligatory.
45. A microbe that stains violet in color is said to be *gram-*_____.
46. The process of applying moist heat for a specific time to kill or retard the development of pathogenic bacteria.
47. Spherical bacteria that occur in pairs.
48. A microbe that has the pink color of the counterstain is said to be *gram-*_____.

Down

1. The use of hot water, soap, detergents, and enzymatic products to remove foreign material from objects.
3. Capable of producing disease.
5. A type of precaution recommended for patients infected with pathogenic organisms that can be spread by touching directly or indirectly.
6. The type of flora that live within a body and that compete with disease-producing microorganisms.
7. A genus of nonmotile, spherical, violet-staining bacteria that occur in irregular clusters.
8. The process of destroying at least the vegetative phase of a pathogenic microorganism by physical or chemical means.
10. The type of contact that occurs when the transmission of microorganisms takes place when a caregiver touches an inanimate object in a patient's environment.
11. Removal of contaminants.
12. An agent that destroys pathogenic microorganisms.
17. A chemical agent that destroys all living organisms, including viruses, in a material.
18. A type of precaution that is used for all patients.
22. _____-level disinfection removes vegetative bacteria and some viruses and fungi, but does not kill spores.
23. An agent that destroys or inactivates viruses.
25. Carried in the air via aerosol droplets, droplet nuclei, or dust particles.
26. Unicellular organisms that range in size from 0.5 to 50 micrometers.
27. A spiral bacterium.
28. A stain that enables the identification of the genus *Mycobacterium* (*two words*).
29. Organisms that require oxygen to live.

30. To sterilize by using steam under pressure.
31. Rodlike bacteria that occur in pairs.
32. Bacteria that require complex organic nutrients.
33. A genus of nonmotile, violet-staining, spherical bacteria that occur in chains.
35. _____-based precautions are used when patients have a documented or suspected infection with a highly transmissible pathogen.
36. The type of disinfection that occurs when chemical sterilants are used at reduced exposure times, usually less than 45 minutes (*hyphenated word*).
39. Nonliving material that may transmit pathogenic organisms.
42. The stain that uses violet color to identify microorganisms.
43. An insect that carries an infection.

ACHIEVING THE OBJECTIVES

1. Identify the major groups of microorganisms associated with nosocomial pneumonia.

1A. Identify the bacteria in Figure 5-1.

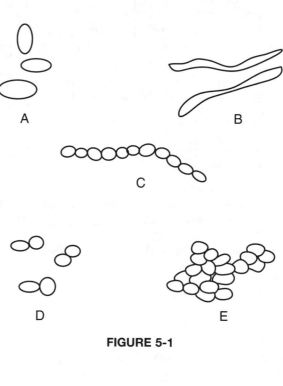

FIGURE 5-1

A. _____

B. _____

C. _____

D. _____

E. _____

1B. What is the size range for bacteria?

_____

_____

1C. How are bacteria generally classified?

_____

_____

1D. List five bacteria that will appear blue or violet following a Gram stain.

_____

_____

_____

_____

1E. List eight gram-negative pathogens.

_____

_____

_____

_____

_____

1F. What stains are used to identify *Mycobacterium*?

_____

_____

1G. Within what temperature range do pathogenic organisms typically grow?

_____

_____

1H. Why are bacteria that produce endospores a constant source of concern for infection control personnel?

_____

_____

_____

1I. The two most notable sources of bacterial endospores are:

_____

_____

1J. Which species of bacteria are gram-positive aerobes?

_____

_____

_____

1K. Which species of bacteria are gram-negative aerobes?

_____

_____

_____

_____

_____

1L. What is the size range for viruses?

_____

1M. Name three ways that viruses are classified.

_____

_____

1N. List four viruses that can cause pneumonia.

_____

_____

1O. Which virus causes severe acute respiratory syndrome?

_____

1P. Which organism causes typhus, Rocky Mountain spotted fever, and Q fever?

_____

_____

1Q. The intracellular parasite that is associated with pneumonia, sinusitis, pharyngitis, and bronchiolitis is:

_____

1R. The protozoa that causes pneumonia in individuals with human immunodeficiency virus (HIV) is:

_____

_____

71

1S. Two fungi that cause opportunistic infections are:

_____

_____

1T. Name five bacteria commonly associated with ventilator-associated pneumonia.

_____

_____

1U. Name the four routes of transmissions for infectious particles.

_____

_____

1V. Define the term *fomite*.

_____

_____

1W. Complete the following table:

Disease-causing organism	Route of transmission
Legionella pneumophila	
Mycobacterium tuberculosis	
Streptococcus pneumoniae	
Pseudomonas aeruginosa	
Staphylococcus aureus	

1X. Why are patients with endotracheal tubes, surgical wounds, intravenous catheters, Foley catheters, and burns at risk for developing nosocomial infections?

_____

_____

_____

_____

Think About This

How do "super bacteria" develop?

Helpful Web Sites

■ ERA-NET, PathoGenoMics, "What Causes the Disease?" — http://www.ict-science-to-society.org

■ *Morbidity and Mortality Weekly Report,* Centers for Disease Control and Prevention, "Guidelines for the Prevention of Nosocomial Pneumonia" (1997 update) — http://www.cdc.gov

2. List four factors that can influence the effectiveness of a germicide.

2A. Define the term *germicide.*

_____

_____

2B. How do these agents destroy the pathogenic microorganisms?

_____

2C. What is the difference between a germicide and a disinfectant?

_____

_____

_____

_____

_____

2D. The elimination of all forms of microbial life is called:

_____

_____.

2E. How do the number and location of microorganisms affect the ability of a germicide to work?

_____

_____

_____

_____

_____

2F. Name the microbe that is most resistant to disinfection and sterilization.

_____

_____

2G. As a disinfectant's concentration increases, what happens to its potency?

_____

_____

2H. Which gram-negative aerobic organism shows greater resistance to some disinfectants?

_____

_____

2I. Increasing the temperature of a germicide will ___ _____ its activity.

2J. Which two types of disinfectants increase antimicrobial activity when the pH is increased?

_____

_____

2K. Which three types of disinfectants decrease antimicrobial activity when the pH is increased?

_____

_____

2L. Relative humidity will affect the disinfectant activity of which gaseous disinfectants?

_____

_____

2M. What is the first step in the decontamination process?

_____

_____

Think About This
What other industries use germicides?

Helpful Web Site
■ University of North Carolina–Chapel Hill, "Disinfection and Sterilization in Healthcare Facilities," William A. Rutala and David J. Weber —http://www. unc.edu

3. Define *high-level disinfection, intermediate-level disinfection,* and *low-level disinfection.*

3A. How does disinfection differ from sterilization?

_____

_____

3B. What is a disinfectant that can eliminate spores called?

_____

_____

3C. Define *high-level disinfection.*

_____

_____

_____

_____

3D. How does intermediate-level disinfection differ from high-level disinfection?

_____

_____

3E. What are low-level disinfectants?

_____

_____

Think About This
Why should germicides be used in the cleaning of equipment used for tattooing, ear-piercing and body-piercing, acupuncture, and hair removal by electrolysis?

Helpful Web Site
■ Centers for Disease Control and Prevention, "Sterilization or Disinfection of Patient-Care Equipment" — http://www.cdc.gov

4. Describe the process of pasteurization and its application to the disinfection of respiratory care equipment.

4A. What happens to cell proteins during pasteurization?

_____

_____

4B. Describe flash process pasteurization.

_____

_____

4C. What is flash process pasteurization usually used for?

_____

_____

4D. Describe batch process pasteurization.

_____

_____

4E. Why is batch process pasteurization used with respiratory care equipment?

_____

_____

_____

_____

_____

73

Think About This
Other than milk, what foods and liquids are pasteurized?

Helpful Web Site
- Johns Hopkins Hospital, Interdisciplinary Clinical Practice Manual — http://www.hopkinsmedicine.org

5. Explain how quaternary ammonium compounds (quats), alcohols, acetic acid, phenols, glutaraldehyde, hydrogen peroxide, and iodophors and other halogenated compounds are used as disinfectants.

5A. What germicidal properties do quaternary ammonium compounds have?

_____

_____

5B. What is the mode of action for disinfection by quats?

_____

_____

_____

_____

5C. What are quats used for in the hospital?

_____

_____

5D. What germicidal properties do ethyl and isopropyl alcohol have?

_____

_____

5E. What is the mode of action for disinfection by alcohols?

_____

_____

5F. According to the Centers for Disease Control and Prevention (CDC), what surfaces, devices and equipment should be disinfected with alcohol?

_____

_____

5G. What are alcohols used to disinfect in the hospital?

_____

_____

_____

_____

_____

5H. What germicidal properties does acetic acid have?

_____

_____

5I. What is the mode of action for disinfection by acetic acid?

_____

_____

5J. What is the optimum concentration of acetic acid for disinfection use?

_____

_____

5K. Why is acetic acid useful in decontaminating home care respiratory equipment?

_____

_____

_____

_____

5L. What germicidal properties do phenols have?

_____

_____

5M. What is the mode of action for disinfection by phenols?

_____

_____

5N. What are phenols used to disinfect in the hospital?

_____

_____

5O. What germicidal properties does glutaraldehyde have?

_____

_____

5P. What is the mode of action for disinfection by glutaraldehyde?

_____

_____

5Q. Compare acid and alkaline glutaraldehyde.

Alkaline glutaraldehyde	Acid glutaraldehyde

5R. What germicidal properties does hydrogen peroxide have?

_____

_____

5S. What is the mode of action for disinfection by hydrogen peroxide?

_____

_____

_____

_____

5T. How can hydrogen peroxide be a sterilizing agent?

_____

_____

5U. What germicidal properties do iodophors have?

_____

_____

5V. What is the mode of action for disinfection by iodophors?

_____

_____

5W. What are iodophors used for in the hospital?

_____

_____

5X. What disinfecting agent is recommended by the CDC to clean blood spills?

_____

_____

Think About This
How do you clean your kitchen and bathrooms?

Helpful Web Site
■ *Morbidity and Mortality Weekly Report,* Centers for Disease Control and Prevention, "Appendix A: Regulatory Framework for Disinfectants and Sterilants" — http://www.cdc.gov

6. Name the four physical methods commonly used to sterilize medical devices.

6A. List the four physical methods commonly used to sterilize medical devices.

_____

_____

_____

6B. Which physical method is used to sterilize contaminated disposable equipment?

_____

6C. Which physical method is used to sterilize laboratory glassware and surgical instruments?

_____

6D. Which physical method of sterilization has questionable effectiveness against spores?

_____

6E. Which physical method of sterilizaton is highly effective, inexpensive, creates no air pollution, and is most versatile?

_____

6F. How does an autoclave increase the temperature of steam above 100°C?

_____

_____

6G. How long does contaminated equipment need to be autoclaved to be sterilized at 121°C and at 132°C?

_____

_____

6H. What is done to ensure the quality control of the autoclaving process?

_____

_____

_____

_____

_____

_____

Think About This

Why should disposable equipment not be reused?

Helpful Web Site

- LEMO S.A., "Medical Sterilization Methods" (white paper), Mehul Patel — http://www.lemo.com

7. Discuss the principle of ethylene oxide sterilization.

7A. Describe the properties of ethylene oxide (ETO).

_____

_____

7B. What is the mode of action for ETO as a sterilant?

_____

_____

_____

7C. Upon what does the effectiveness of ETO depend?

_____

_____

_____

_____

_____

_____

7D. What two factors can decrease sterilization time?

_____

_____

7E. The materials that can be used to package equipment for ETO sterilization are:

_____

_____

7F. List the stages of automated ETO sterilization.

_____

_____

_____

7G. What conditions are necessary for the mechanical aeration of equipment that is sterilized with ETO?

_____

_____

7H. Why is aeration of ETO-sterilized equipment at room temperature dangerous?

_____

_____

7I. How is the effectiveness of ETO sterilization monitored?

_____

_____

7J. What is the Occupational Safety & Health Administration (OSHA) standard for ETO exposure?

_____

_____

Think About This

What type of protective equipment should be worn when working with ETO?

Helpful Web Site

- Ethylene Oxide Sterilization Association — http://eosa.org

8. Identify infection-risk devices used in respiratory care.

8A. What are the three categories described by Spaulding for stratfying the risk of infection from reusable patient care equipment?

_____

_____

8B. Give examples of equipment in each of the risk-infection categories, and explain why they are included there.

Category	Types of equipment	Reason for category

8C. Why is sterility not necessary with equipment that comes in contact with only the skin?

_____

_____

8D. What method(s) of processing is/are recommended for respiratory care equipment?

_____

_____

8E. If the aforementioned processing (in question 8D) is not feasible, what should be done?

_____

_____

8F. What setup should be used to monitor an intubated patient with a respirometer?

_____

_____

8G. Describe the recommended steps for processing bronchoscopes.

_____

_____

_____

_____

_____

_____

8H. What are the recommendations for changing or replacing large-volume jet nebulizers and medication nebulizers and their reservoirs and tubing?

_____

_____

8I. How should water in a ventilator circuit or nebulizer tubing be disposed of?

_____

_____

Think About This
How is soiled linen decontaminated in a hospital?

Helpful Web Sites
■ Johns Hopkins, Respiratory Therapy Equipment Guidelines (complete policy available) — http://www.epitool.org/prevention/respiratory.html
■ American Association for Respiratory Care (AARC), *Respiratory Care* journal, "Clinical Practice Guideline: Care of the Ventilator Circuit and its Relation to Ventilator-Associated Pneumonia" — http://www.rcjournal.com

9. Describe three components of an effective infection surveillance program.
9A. What is the purpose of an infection surveillance program?

_____

_____

9B. Complete the following table:

	Surveillance components	Description (give example)
1		
2		
3		

9C. Why is identifying the cause of nosocomial infections important?

_____

_____

Think About This

How is respiratory care equipment in the home monitored for infection control?

Helpful Web Site

■ *Infection Control Today* magazine, "Approaches to Infection Control: Active Surveillance Culture as a Promising New Tool," Gerri Hall and Diane Flayhart —http://www.infectioncontroltoday.com/articles/621feat2.html

10. Compare standard precautions with transmission-based precautions.

10A. When should standard precautions be used in the hospital?

_____

_____

10B. From what particular substances are standard precautions providing protection?

_____

_____

10C. What is the goal of standard precautions?

_____

_____

_____

10D. What needs to be done by the respiratory care practitioner to ensure standard precautions are followed?

_____

_____

10E. When should transmission-based precautions be used in the hospital?

_____

_____

_____

_____

10F. What is the goal of transmission-based precautions?

_____

_____

_____

_____

10G. When does hand-washing (hand hygiene) need to be performed?

_____

_____

_____

_____

10H. When do gloves need to be worn?

_____

_____

_____

10I. When do gowns need to be worn?

_____

_____

_____

10J. When do face shields or masks with protective eyewear need to be worn?

_____

_____

_____

_____

10K. What are the five components of respiratory hygiene/cough etiquette?

_____

_____

_____

_____

_____

10L. What are the main components of safe injection practices?

_____

_____

_____

_____

10M. Complete the followng table:

Precaution type	Pathogen known/suspected or procedure	Precautions
Airborne precautions		
Droplet precautions		
Contact precautions		

Think About This

How often do you wash your hands when caring for a sick family member or friend?

Helpful Web Site

■ Centers for Disease Control and Prevention, "Guideline for Isolation Precautions: Preventing Transmission of Infectious Agents in Healthcare Settings 2007," Jane D. Siegel et al. — http://www.cdc.gov

11. List the agents most commonly associated with febrile respiratory illnesses that are potential causes of mass casualty events.

11A. What does an effective disaster infection control plan include?

_____

_____

_____

_____

11B. Name two intentional causes of febrile respiratory illness (FRI) that can lead to a mass casualty event.

_____

_____

11C. Name five contagious causes of FRI that can lead to a mass casualty event.

_____

_____

_____

_____

11D. Which biological agents are transmitted person-to-person through the inhalation of droplets or aerosol?

_____

_____

11E. Airborne infection isolation placement is recommended for use with patients infected with which three biological agents?

_____

_____

Think About This

I was vaccinated against smallpox before 1980; am I still protected?

Helpful Web Sites

■ Centers for Disease Control and Prevention, "Bioterrorism Case Definitions" — http://www.bt.cdc.gov

■ Centers for Disease Control and Prevention, "Emergency Preparedness & Response: Agents, Diseases, and Other Threats" — http://www.bt.cdc.gov

■ U.S. Department of Health and Human Services, Agency for Healthcare Research and Quality, "Bioterrorism and Other Public Health Emergencies: Altered Standards of Care in Mass Casualty Events" — http://www.ahrq.gov

79

NATIONAL BOARD FOR RESPIRATORY CARE (NBRC)–TYPE QUESTIONS

1. A sputum specimen is received in the lab. A smear is made, and the specimen is subjected to Gram staining. A microscopic examination reveals spherical purple-staining clusters. Which of the following characteristics can reasonably be assumed about this organism?
   I. Gram-negative
   II. In the bacilli family
   III. In the streptococci family
   IV. Associated with causing pneumonia
   A. I, II, and III only
   B. I, III, and IV only
   C. II and III only
   D. IV only

2. Which of the following statements are true about the amount of time required to kill microorganisms?
   I. The time decreases as the strength of the germicide increases.
   II. The time is directly proportional to the number of pathogens.
   III. The time increases as the microbial population increases.
   IV. Time varies with the resistance of the organism.
   A. II, III, and IV only
   B. III and IV only
   C. I and III only
   D. II and III only

3. The medical states that increase patient susceptibility to nosocomial infection include which of the following?
   A. Hypoglycemia
   B. Altered B cells
   C. Hyperbilirubinemia
   D. Hypogammaglobulinemia

4. Bacterial spores can be inactivated by exposure to which of the following?
   A. 10 hours of iodophors
   B. 8 hours of glutaraldehyde
   C. 30 minutes of isopropyl alcohol
   D. 6 hours of quaternary ammonium compounds

5. The household item that is useful for disinfection of respiratory home care equipment is which of the following?
   A. Peroxide
   B. Vinegar
   C. Bleach
   D. Lye

6. At high altitudes, sterilization by boiling must be prolonged primarily because of which of the following?
   A. Increased oxygen content
   B. Reduced oxygen content
   C. Increased normal boiling point
   D. Reduced normal boiling point

7. Which of the following viruses will cause bronchiolitis?
   A. Influenza
   B. Rhinovirus
   C. Herpes zoster
   D. Respiratory syncytial

8. Hepatitis B is spread by which type of transmission?
   A. Droplet nuclei
   B. Direct contact
   C. Indirect contact
   D. Food-borne vehicle

9. A highly effective, versatile, and inexpensive method of sterilization consists of the use of which of the following?
   A. Phenols
   B. Alcohol
   C. Autoclaving
   D. Ethylene oxide

10. A patient arrives in the emergency department with a history of increasing dyspnea on exertion, weight loss, and a positive cough history. The physician suspects tuberculosis. The most appropriate type of precaution to use for this patient is which of the following?
    A. Contact precautions
    B. Standard precautions
    C. Droplet precautions
    D. Airborne precautions

6 Airway Management Devices

Upon completion of this chapter, you will be able to:
1. Describe a complete airway exam.
2. Understand normal airway anatomy.
3. Describe ways to displace the tongue to improve gas exchange in unconscious patients.
4. List patient characteristics that may contribute to a difficult mask ventilation or intubation.
5. List several complications from improper placement of oral and nasopharyngeal airways.
6. Explain how to place the laryngeal mask airway and the Combitube in unconscious patients.
7. Describe the appropriate sequence of steps to insert an endotracheal tube to provide a secure airway.
8. Identify three ways to confirm that an *endotracheal tube* (ETT) lies in the trachea.
9. List three airway devices that can aid in placing an ETT in the event of a difficult laryngoscopic procedure.
10. Identify the airway risks facing intubated patients and identify strategies and equipment for the prevention of each.
11. List the equipment necessary to perform invasive ventilation (transtracheal or surgical airway), and describe a procedure for airway entry.
12. List the complications related to invasive airway access and the treatment of each.
13. Review the equipment and steps necessary for obtaining sputum samples from patients with tracheostomy tubes.
14. Describe three ways to wean patients from tracheostomy tubes.
15. List three methods to allow patients with tracheostomy tubes to speak.
16. Identify various types of manual resuscitators, and discuss hazards commonly associated with the use of these devices.

"There is a single light of science, and to brighten it anywhere is to brighten it everywhere."
Isaac Asimov

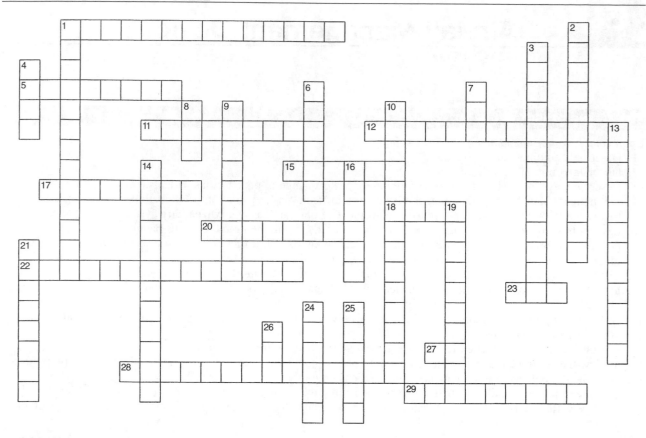

CROSSWORD PUZZLE 6-1
Created using Crossword Weaver, www.CrosswordWeaver.com.

Use the clues to complete the crossword puzzle.

Across

1. An intubation technique that uses an angiocath as a guide.
5. A locking device used to prevent the disconnection of catheters (*hyphenated word*).
11. After a failed intubation, this type of tube may be used to provide a patent upper airway; it has two cuffs.
12. An airway inserted into the mouth.
15. An oropharyngeal airway without a protected central channel.
17. A type of airway that allows ventilation during intubation.
18. A type of manual resuscitator valve.
20. A type of manual resuscitator valve that resembles a fowl.
22. A type of one-way valve.
23. A common way of providing access directly into the trachea for long-term airway management (*abbreviation*).
27. Tube used for invasive mechanical ventilation (*abbreviation*).
28. A nasal trumpet airway.
29. A curved blade used with a laryngoscope.

Down

1. Type of devices used to revive patients.
2. The type of tube that is placed directly in the trachea.
3. A valve that has a spring so it closes automatically (*hyphenated word*).
4. The type of endotracheal tube that is used for independent lung ventilation (*abbreviation*).
6. An upper airway device used to provide air passage.
7. The cuff of this airway is seated laterally in the pyriform fossa (*abbreviation*).
8. Manually ventilating a patient noninvasively (*abbreviation*).
9. Another name for *duckbill*.
10. The type of intubation that goes through the larynx.
13. An endoscope used to examine the larynx.
14. Intubation with the nose as the entry point for placement of a tube in the airway.

16. A straight blade used with a laryngoscope.

19. The type of bronchoscope that is used to intubate "difficult" airways.

21. The position that opens the airway for intubation.

24. A scale used to delineate the external diameter of catheters.

25. A trap used to collect sterile samples of sputum.

26. What is done during a cardiac/respiratory arrest (*abbreviation*).

ACHIEVING THE OBJECTIVES

1. Describe a complete airway examination.

1A. Why is an airway examination important?

_____

_____

1B. List four important points that may be obtained from an airway history, either from the patient or from review of the past medical records.

_____

_____

_____

_____

1C. Name the common components of an airway examination.

_____

_____

_____

_____

1D. The thyromental distance that is of concern when assessing the airway is

_____

_____

_____

_____.

1E. What type of external neck anatomy is of concern with respect to a difficult airway?

_____

_____

1F. List indicators in the dentition that suggest intubation might be difficult.

_____

_____

_____

_____

1G. The Mallampati class for the airway shown in Figure 6-1 is _____.

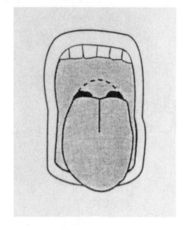

FIGURE 6-1

(In MacIntyre NR, Branson RD: *Mechanical ventilation*, Philadelphia, 2001, WB Saunders. From Mallampati SR, Gatt SP, Gugino LD, et al: A clinical sign to predict difficult tracheal intubation: a prospective study. *Can Anaesth Soc J* 32:429–434, 1985).

1H. List six predictors of a difficult intubation.

_____

_____

_____

_____

_____

Think About This

Should a person with a "difficult" airway wear a Medi-Alert bracelet with that information?

Helpful Web Site

■ Internet Scientific Publications, *The Internet Journal of Anesthesiology*, "The Dilemma of Airway Assessment and Evaluation," Magboul M. Ali Magboul — http://www.ispub.com

2. Understanding normal airway anatomy.

2A. Label the parts of Figure 6-2.

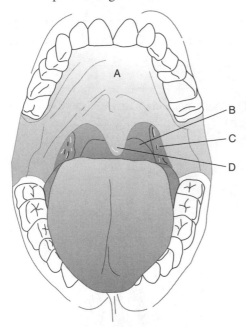

FIGURE 6-2

A. _____

B. _____

C. _____

D. _____

2B. Label the parts of Figure 6-3.

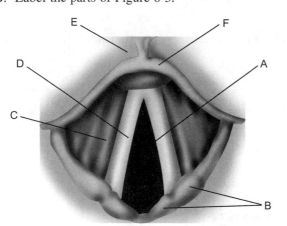

FIGURE 6-3

A. _____

B. _____

C. _____

D. _____

E. _____

F. _____

2C. The narrowest portion of an adult's airway is

_____.

2D. The narrowest portion of a child's airway until age 6 is the

_____.

2E. Match the following upper airway anatomy with its nerve innervations.

Anatomic structure	Nerve
___(1) Anterior portion of the tongue	(a) Recurrent laryngeal nerves (CN X)
___(2) Posterior third of the tongue	(b) External branch of superior laryngeal nerve (CN X)
___(3) Vocal cords	(c) Internal branch of superior laryngeal nerve (CN X)
___(4) Underside of the epiglottis	(d) Trigeminal nerve (CN V)
___(5) Trachea below the vocal cords	(e) Glossopharyngeal nerve (CN IX)
___(6) Muscles of larynx	(f) Superior laryngeal nerve
___(7) Cricothyroid muscles	

Think About This

How do the vocal cords produce sound?

Helpful Web Site

- *Gray's Anatomy* online, "The Larynx" — http://www.theodora.com

3. Describe ways to displace the tongue to improve gas exchange in unconscious patients.

3A. What can happen to the airway when the pharyngeal and tongue muscles lose tone in the supine positon?

_____

_____

3B. Describe the patient position that should be used to help open an obstructed or closed airway.

_____

_____

_____

_____

3C. Name and describe the two types of oropharyngeal airways available to displace the tongue.

_____

_____

_____

_____

_____

_____

3D. How should an oropharyngeal airway be placed in an unconscious person?

_____

_____

_____

_____

_____

_____

_____

3E. What device should be used to noninvasively ventilate and oxygenate a patient with apnea after the airway is opened?

_____

_____

3F. How should this device (from question 3E) be applied when used on the patient?

_____

_____

_____

_____

3G. List four techniques that can be used to facilitate successful ventilation of a patient with apnea.

_____

_____

_____

_____

Think About This

What causes snoring?

Helpful Web Sites

- University of Iowa, Department of Anesthesia, "Answers to Questions for *'Pearls' of Airway Management* Lecture at the Annual EMS Association Conference Nov. 14, 2003" — http://www.anesth.uiowa.edu
- American Eagle Medical, "Pi's Pillow and Sniff or Magill Position" [question-and-answer format] — http://www.americaneaglemedical.org

4. List characteristics of the patient that may contribute to a difficult mask ventilation or intubation.

4A. The body mass index (BMI) that decreases the success of face mask ventilation (FMV) is a BMI of

_____

_____.

4B. Which Mallampati airway classes are associated with an increased risk of difficulty in providing FMV?

_____

_____

4C. The age at which increased difficult in FMV may begin is

_____

_____.

4D. The type of chin structure that is associated with increased difficulty in FMV is

_____

_____.

4E. Name three additional factors that are associated with increased difficulty in FMV.

_____

_____

4F. The only easily modifiable risk factor for poor FMV is the presence of

_____

_____.

Think About This

Why should face masks accompany all intubated patients during transport?

Helpful Web Sites

- National Heart, Lung, and Blood Institute, Obesity Education Initiative, "Calculate Your Body Mass Index" — http://www.nhlbisupport.com

■ University of Virginia Health System, Department of Anesthesiology, "Airway Equipment" [video] — http://www.healthsystem.virginia.edu

5. List several complications from improper placement of oral and nasopharyngeal airways.

5A. What is the consequence of the use of a Guedel or Berman airway that is one size too small?

_____

_____

5B. What will happen if oropharyngeal airway placement is attempted on a patient with intact airway protective reflexes?

_____

_____

5C. If a patient forcibly bites an oropharyngeal airway, what may happen?

_____

_____

5D. What complication is caused by a nasopharyngeal airway that is too long for a patient?

_____

_____

5E. A major complication of inserting a nasopharyngeal tube is _____.

5F. What is the long-term risk of nasopharyngeal tube placement?

_____

_____

Think About This

Should a nasotracheal airway be used in a patient with cranial trauma?

Helpful Web Site

■ Corexcel, "Adult Ventilation Management: Artificial Airways" [continuing education course] — http://www.corexcel.com

6. Explain how to place the laryngeal mask airway and the Combitube in unconscious patients.

6A. How does a laryngeal mask airway (LMA) provide an airway for manual ventilation?

_____

_____

_____

6B. List five reasons why the LMA is a useful emergency airway device.

_____

_____

_____

_____

_____

6C. How should an LMA be checked for leaks?

_____

_____

6D. Describe how an LMA is inserted.

_____

_____

_____

_____

_____

_____

6E. The three methods that check for correct placement of an LMA are:

_____

_____

_____

_____

6F. What size of LMA should be used for an 85-kg male patient?

_____

_____

6G. When is it appropriate to use a Combitube?

_____

_____

6H. What type of artificial airway would be most beneficial to use with a bloodied airway?

_____

_____

_____

_____

6I. How is a Combitube inserted?

_____

_____

_____

_____

_____

6J. Label the parts of the Combitube in Figure 6-4.

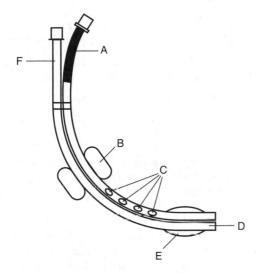

FIGURE 6-4

A. _____

B. _____

C. _____

D. _____

E. _____

F. _____

Think About This

Why are there so many different types of artificial airways?

Helpful Web Sites

■ Newest Information About the Combitube — http://www.combitube.org
■ The Airway Carnival, Information on the LMA — http://www.airwaycarnival.com/LMA.htm
■ The Airway Carnival, Information on the Intubating LMA — http://www.airwaycarnival.com/ILMA.htm
■ The Airway Carnival, Information on the Combitube — http://www.airwaycarnival.com/COM.htm

7. List the appropriate sequence of steps to insert an *endotracheal tube* (ETT) to provide a secure airway.

7A. What needs to be done for an apneic patient before intubation?

_____

_____

7B. Label the parts of the ETT in Figure 6-5.

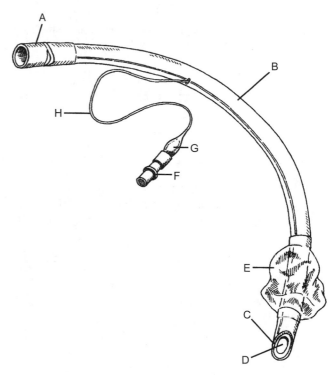

FIGURE 6-5
(From Sills JR: *Advanced respiratory therapist exam guide: the complete resource for the written registry and clinical simulation exams*, ed 3, St Louis, 2006, Mosby.)

A. _____

B. _____

C. _____

D. _____

E. _____

F. _____

G. _____

H. _____

7C. Name and describe the two types of laryngoscope blades.

_____

_____

7D. How should a laryngoscope be held?

_____

_____

_____

7E. What is the correct placement for each of the two types of laryngoscope blades?

_____

_____

_____

_____

_____

_____

7F. Once in the appropriate place, how should the laryngoscope be moved to bring the epiglottis into view?

_____

_____

7G. List the equipment needed for endotracheal intubation.

_____

_____

_____

_____

_____

_____

_____

_____

7H. What size of laryngoscope blade should be used for an average adult? _____

_____

7I. Place the sequence of events for intubation in the order that they should occur.

___ Pass the ETT through the vocal cords.
___ Check the placement of the ETT.
___ Check laryngoscope, and check ETT cuff.
___ Place lubricated stylet into the ETT.
___ Lubricate the ETT with water-soluble lubricant.
___ Inflate the cuff.
___ Visualize the laryngeal structures with the laryngoscope.

7J. Why should cuff pressure be kept below 25 cm H_2O? _____

_____

Think About This

How many intubations should a respiratory therapist perform in the operating room in order to become certified by her hospital?

Helpful Web Sites

- Joint Project of the University of Nebraska Medical Center, Penn State University, and TATRC, Virtual Disaster Medicine Training Center (VDMTC), "Module 1: Basic Review of Endotracheal Intubation for Providers at a Mass Casualty; Technique for Orotracheal Intubation" — http://vdmtc.org
- University of Virginia Health System, Anesthesiology Department, "Introduction to Airway Tutorial" [here you can access a video on how to intubate] — http://www.healthsystem.virginia.edu

8. Identify at least three ways to confirm that an ETT lies in the trachea.

8A. Why is confirmation of ETT placement important?

_____

_____

8B. What is the most sensitive method to confirm ETT placement?

_____

_____

8C. How does a color-change capnometer work?

_____

_____

8D. After intubation a color-change capnometer is attached to the ETT, but it does not indicate a change in color. Give two reasons why this would happen.

_____

_____

_____

_____

8E. How does the esophageal detection device work?

_____

_____

_____

_____

8F. With what types of patients have false-positive and false-negative results been reported when esophageal detection devices are used?

_____

_____

8G. Auscultation after intubation should be done in how many areas?

_____

_____

8H. Why can chest auscultation be misleading?

_____

_____

_____

_____

8I. An anterior-posterior chest radiograph enables the identification of

_____

_____.

8J. A lateral chest radiograph enables the identification of

_____

_____.

8K. Direct visualization with a _____
_____ is another way to confirm correct ETT placement.

Think About This

Why should ETT placement be confirmed by more than one method?

Helpful Web Sites

- Wolfe Tory Medical, Inc, "Esophageal Intubation Detector (EID)" — http://www.wolfetory.com
- PER$_{SYS}$ Medical, "PosiTube (PT-100) Esophageal Intubation Detector" — http://www.ps-med.com

9. List three airway devices that can aid in placing an ETT in the event of difficult laryngoscopy.

9A. How is a Lightwand or lighted stylet used to facilitate intubation of a difficult airway?

_____

_____

_____

_____

_____

_____

_____

9B. List the situations when the use of a Lightwand or lighted stylet is appropriate.

_____

_____

_____

_____

9C. The type of device that relies on lenses, mirrors, or fiberoptic technology to obtain a clear view of the glottic opening and cords is known as _____

_____.

9D. What is the "gold standard" for a known difficult airway or an unstable neck?

_____

_____

9E. Describe how the retrograde intubation technique is performed.

_____

_____

_____

_____

_____

_____

_____

_____

9F. Complete the following table:

Alternative airway device	Complications
Lighted stylet	
Laryngoscope, indirectly applied	
Flexible fiberoptic bronchoscope	
Retrograde wire	

Think About This

Why is airway management the most important initial element in trauma management?

Helpful Web Site

■ The University of Florida, Department of Anesthesiology, The Virtual Airway Device Intubation Techniques and Tutorials, "Difficult Airway Management & Airway Devices" — http://vam.anest.ufl.edu

10. Identify the airway risks facing intubated patients and identify strategies and equipment for the prevention of each risk.

10A. An increase in mucus production or thickness can do what to an ETT?

10B. What is incorporated into the tip of ETTs that will decrease the likelihood of an ETT becoming occluded?

10C. What will happen to the airway of a patient with an ETT that bent in half?

10D. Where do plastic ETTs tend to collapse?

10E. What type of equipment may be used to prevent a bend/kink in the ETT?

10F. Why are patients with ETTs at risk for dried secretions?

10G. What equipment should be used with intubated patients to prevent the drying of secretions?

10H. What other normal physiologic function is compromised because of the presence of an ETT?

10I. How can secretions be mobilized in a patient who has an endotracheal or tracheostomy tube?

10J. How can inadvertent movement or extubation of ETTs be prevented?

_____

_____

_____

_____

10K. What will happen to the airway if the ETT cuff fails to hold pressure?

_____

_____

10L. The most appropriate action to take when there is a cuff failure is to _____

_____ by using a/an _____

_____.

10M. What happens to the integrity of the airway when there is a leak in the pilot balloon?

_____

_____

10N. What equipment and method may be used to overcome a leaky pilot balloon?

_____

_____

_____

_____

Think About This

How is an artificial airway secured on a giraffe?

Helpful Web Site

■ *Canadian Journal of Anesthesia*, "Intratracheal Kinking of Endotracheal Tube," [letter], Y-W Lee et al — http://www.cja-jca.org

11. List the equipment necessary to perform invasive ventilation (i.e., a transtracheal or surgical airway), and describe a procedure for airway entry.

11A. In case of an unsuccessful intubation attempt, where a patent airway has not been established and manual ventilation is not possible, what method should be used to establish an emergency airway?

_____

_____

11B. Where, on Figure 6-6, should this emergency airway be located?

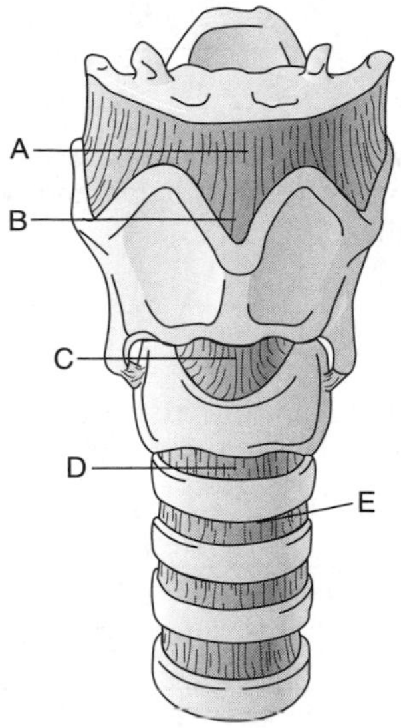

_____

_____

FIGURE 6-6
(From Kacmarek RM, Dimas S: *The essentials of respiratory care*, ed 4, St Louis, 2005, Mosby.)

11C. List the equipment necessary to establish this emergency airway.

_____

_____

_____

_____

11D. Describe the procedure for establishing this emergency airway.

_____

_____

_____

_____

_____

_____

_____

_____

_____

_____

_____

_____

11E. Identify the location for a percutaneous dilatory tracheostomy (PDT) on Figure 6-6.

_____

11F. List the equipment necessary for the Ciaglia PDT method.

_____

_____

11G. What equipment may be used to help prevent inadvertent injury of the membranous posterior tracheal wall?

_____

_____

11H. What is the main difference between the Ciaglia PDT method and the tracheostomy method described by Griggs?

_____

_____

_____

_____

_____

_____

11I. A single, tapered dilator that is used instead of sequential dilators is known as the _____

_____.

Think About This
Can non-human animals live with tracheotomies?

Helpful Web Sites
- *Update in Anaesthesia* journal, "Percutaneous Tracheostomy," A. Rudra — http://www.nda.ox.ac.uk
- eMedicine from WebMD, "Percutaneous Tracheostomy," Scott E. Brietzke et al — http://www.emedicine.com

12. List the complications related to invasive airway access and the treatment of each.

12A. How can subglottic or laryngeal stenosis be prevented after a cricothyroidotomy?

_____

_____

12B. Trauma to the tissues during the insertion of a tracheostomy tube may be prevented by using what?

_____

_____

12C. Continual cuff-pressure monitoring with cuffed tracheostomy tubes and ETTs helps prevent _____

_____.

12D. What complication is seen most often with lengthy intubations and use of a large-diameter ETT? How can this complication be prevented?

_____

_____

_____

_____

_____

12E. How is tracheomalacia treated?

_____

_____

_____

_____

Think About This
Can chest radiography enable the detection of a potential problem due to high cuff pressures?

Helpful Web Sites
- The Johns Hopkins Hospital, "Ears, Nose & Throat: Tracheostomy Complications" — http://www.hopkinshospital.org
- *Chest* journal, "Complications of Tracheostomy Performed in the ICU: Subthyroid Tracheostomy vs Surgical Cricothyroidotomy," Bruno François et al — http://www.chestjournal.org
- *Respiratory Care* journal, "Early Complications of Tracheostomy," Charles G. Durbin Jr. — http://www.rcjournal.com

13. Review the equipment and steps necessary for obtaining sputum samples from patients with tracheostomy tubes and ETTs.

13A. What physiologic functions are bypassed with invasive artificial airways?

_____

_____

_____

_____

13B. What vacuum pressures must the vacuum system be able to generate?

_____

_____

13C. What personal protective equipment should be available for suctioning patients by using invasive artificial airways?

_____

_____

13D. The respiratory therapist should be continually observing what three factors during the suctioning process?

_____

_____

13E. To prevent hypoxemia during the suctioning, what should be done before beginning the process?

_____

_____

13F. How far down into the trachea should the catheter be placed?

_____

_____

13G. When should suctioning be applied?

_____

_____

13H. Suction should be applied for how long in the trachea?

_____

_____

13I. Place the sequence of events in order for suctioning the airway of a patient by using an invasive artificial airway.

____ Preoxygenate with 100% oxygen for 30 to 60 s.
____ Don personal protective wear.
____ Repeat the procedure as needed.
____ Check equipment.
____ Gently withdraw the catheter with suction.
____ Suction the patient's mouth and nose.
____ Explain procedure to the patient.
____ Allow the patient to rest.
____ Attach the catheter to the vacuum system by using the aseptic technique.
____ Advance catheter without suctioning until obstruction is detected.
____ Note baseline heart rate, electrocardiographic rhythm, and pulse oximeter saturation.
____ Wash hands.

13J. A size 7.5 (inner diameter) tracheostomy tube requires what size of suction catheter?

_____

_____

Think About This

What should you do if the electrocardiogram shows premature ventricular contractions during suctioning?

Helpful Web Site

■ American Association for Respiratory Care, *Respiratory Care* journal, "Clinical Practice Guideline: Endotracheal Suctioning of Mechanically Ventilated Adults and Children with Artificial Airways" — http://www.rcjournal.com

14. Describe three ways to wean patients from tracheostomy tubes (TTs).

14A. Describe the fastest way for a tracheostomy patient to be weaned from the TT.

_____

_____

14B. In what situation should a stoma be maintained?

_____

_____

14C. What types of TTs can be used to maintain tracheal access while the patient is being "weaned" from the larger TT?

_____

_____

14D. What other device is available to maintain a tracheostomy stoma?

_____

_____

14E. Which device used to maintain a tracheostomy stoma has more advantages?

_____

_____

Think About This

How do patients with permanent tracheostomies humidify inspired air?

Helpful Web Sites

■ eMedicine from WebMD, "Tracheostomy," Jonathan P. Lindman et al — http://www.emedicine.com
■ Stanford Hospital and Clinics, *Patient Care Manual*, "Tracheostomy Weaning and Decannulation Protocol" — http://scalpel.stanford.edu

15. List three methods that allow patients with TTs to speak

Questions 15A through 15C refer to Figure 6-7.

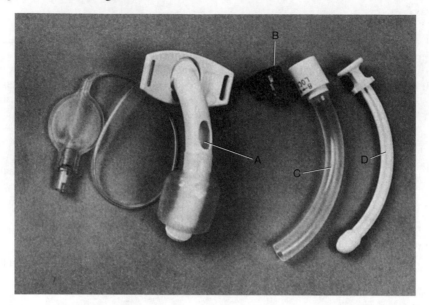

FIGURE 6-7

(From Wilkins RL, Stoller JK, Kacmarek RM: *Egan's fundamentals of respiratory care*, ed 9, St Louis, 2009, Mosby.)

15A. What type of TT is shown in Figure 6-7?

_____

_____

15B. Label the following parts of Figure 6-7:

A. _____

B. _____

C. _____

D. _____

15C. Explain how the TT in Figure 6-7 is used to allow speech.

_____

_____

_____

_____

_____

_____

_____

15D. Name two other devices available to allow patients with TTs who are capable of initiating and maintaining spontaneous ventilation to speak.

_____

_____

15E. List two ways to create an open upper airway with a TT.

_____

_____

15F. What device is designed to allow speech in patients who are unable to sustain unaided ventilation?

_____

_____

15G. How does the device mentioned in 15F function?

_____

_____

_____

_____

15H. What are the benefits of restoring the ability to speak to a patient with a TT?

_____

_____

_____

_____

Think About This

Can patients with ETTs speak during ventilation?

Helpful Web Sites

- Passy-Muir, "Benefits of the Passy-Muir Tracheostomy & Ventilator Swallowing and Speaking Valves" — http://www.passy-muir.com
- Bess Medizintechnik GmbH, "Montgomery Tracheostomy Speaking Valve" — http://www.trachs.com
- Smiths Medical, "Portex Trach-Talk™ Blue Line Tracheostomy Tubes" — http://www.smiths-medical.com

16. Describe various types of manual resuscitators, and discuss hazards commonly associated with the use of these devices.

16A. What is the function of a manual resuscitator?

_____

_____

_____

16B. How are manual resuscitators classified?

_____

Questions 16C through 16F refer to Figure 6-8.

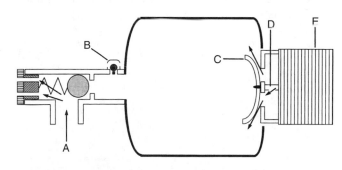

FIGURE 6-8
(Redrawn from *Mosby's respiratory care equipment*, ed 8, St. Louis, 2009, Mosby.)

16C. Label the parts of Figure 6-8.

A. _____

B. _____

C. _____

D. _____

E. _____

16D. What type of manual resuscitator is shown in Figure 6-8? _____

16E. Which phase of ventilation is shown in Figure 6-8?

_____

16F. Describe how the manual resuscitator in Figure 6-8 works.

_____

_____

_____

_____

_____

_____

_____

_____

_____

_____

_____

Questions 16G through 16J refer to Figure 6-9.

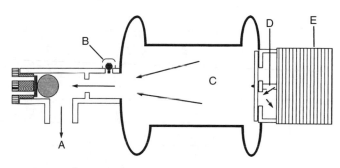

FIGURE 6-9
(Redrawn from *Mosby's respiratory care equipment*, ed 8, St. Louis, 2009, Mosby.)

16G. Label the parts of Figure 6-9.

A. _____

B. _____

C. _____

D. _____

E. _____

16H. What type of manual resuscitator is shown in Figure 6-9?

_____

16I. Which phase of ventilation is shown in Figure 6-9?

_____

16J. Describe how the manual resuscitator in Figure 6-9 works.

_____

_____

_____

_____

_____

_____

_____

16K. The American Hospital Association specifies that a manual resuscitator should deliver a tidal volume of _____ to a patient.

16L. List six causes of hypoventilation during manual ventilation.

_____

_____

_____

_____

_____

_____

_____

16M. When would high airway pressures most likely be encountered during manual ventilation?

_____

_____

16N. Excessively high pressures during manual ventilation increases the patient's risk of developing

_____

_____.

Think About This

Should manual resuscitators be kept with every automated external defibrillator?

Helpful Web Sites

- Internet Scientific Publications, *The Internet Journal of Anesthesiology*, "Manual Resuscitators (Ambu Bags) Can Ventilate the Lungs Adequately Despite Big Subatmospheric Pressure in the Breathing Circuit," Ahmad Elsharydah — http://www.ispub.com
- ECRI Institute, Medical Device Safety Reports, "Mislocated Pop-Off Valve Can Produce Airway Overpressure in Manual Resuscitator Breathing Circuits" — http://www.mdsr.ecri.org

NATIONAL BOARD FOR RESPIRATORY CARE (NBRC)–TYPE QUESTIONS

1. The most reliable and rapid method for confirming endotracheal tube placement during a cardiac arrest involves the use of which of the following?
   A. Lateral chest radiography
   B. Bilateral chest auscultation
   C. An esophageal detection device
   D. A color-change capnometric device

2. The most appropriate device to facilitate the intubation of a patient with an unstable neck is which of the following?
   A. Tracheostomy tube
   B. Carlens' tube
   C. Fiberoptic bronchoscope
   D. Laryngeal mask airway (LMA)

3. The device that allows visualization of the larynx without requiring alignment of the various axes of the airways is which of the following?
   A. Bullard laryngoscope
   B. Retrograde wire
   C. Laryngoscope
   D. LMA

4. A patient with a tracheostomy tube requires continuous mechanical ventilation and is frustrated with the fact that he is unable to speak. The respiratory therapist should recommend the use of which of the following speaking devices?
   A. Fenestrated tracheostomy tube
   B. Olympic Medical
   C. Pitt speaking tracheostomy tube
   D. Passy-Muir valve

5. A patient sustained trauma to the right chest. The patient has developed right-sided pulmonary contusion and requires intubation. The most appropriate type of artificial airway to use is which of the following?
   A. LMA
   B. Combitube
   C. Double-lumen tube
   D. RAE tube

6. An intubated patient being manually ventilated continues to have a low partial pressure of arterial oxygen (PaO_2) despite the oxygen flow being 15 L/min. The respiratory therapist should check which of the following for proper function?
   I. Pop-off valve
   II. Safety air inlet
   III. Safety oxygen outlet

IV. Reservoir bag connection
   A. I, II, and IV
   B. II, III, and IV
   C. I, II, and III
   D. I, III, and IV

7. During mask ventilation the patient's chest is not rising. The most appropriate immediate action for the respiratory therapist to take is which of the following?
   A. Reposition the mask
   B. Open the pop-off valve
   C. Change resuscitator bags
   D. Increase the flow to the reservoir

8. During oral endotracheal intubation the most appropriate head and neck position for a patient is which of the following?
   A. In a flat position
   B. In the "sniff" position
   C. In a chin-down position
   D. With a maximally flexed back

9. The airway examination component that suggests that a patient may have a difficult airway is which of the following?
   A. Flat palate
   B. Mallampati class III
   C. Interincisor distance of 4 cm
   D. Four-finger thyromental distance

10. During cardiopulmonary resuscitation, a patient is intubated. The most accurate means to confirm correct placement of the endotracheal tube involves which of the following?
   A. Capnography
   B. Auscultate for bilateral breath sounds
   C. An esophageal detection device
   D. Visualization of fog in the tube with each breath

7   Lung Expansion Devices

Upon completion of this chapter, you will be able to:
1. Compare volume-displacement and flow-dependent incentive spirometers.
2. Describe two types of machines used to administer intermittent positive pressure breathing therapy.
3. Discuss how expiratory positive airway pressure, continuous positive airway pressure, and positive expiratory pressure therapies are used to mobilize secretions and treat atelectasis.
4. Identify the major components of pneumatically and electrically powered percussors.
5. Describe the theory of operation of four devices that enhance clearance of airway secretions by producing high-frequency oscillations to the lungs and chest wall.
6. Discuss how mechanical insufflation-exsufflation devices can enhance airway secretions in patients with respiratory muscle weakness or paralysis.

"Nothing in life is to be feared. It is only to be understood."
Marie Curie

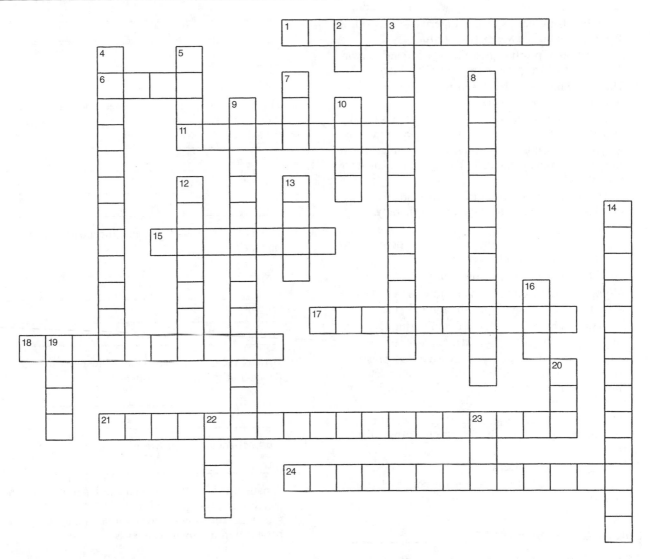

CROSSWORD PUZZLE 7-1
Created using Crossword Weaver, www.CrosswordWeaver.com.

Use the clues to complete the crossword puzzle.

Across

1. The type of nebulizer that introduces the jet stream into the main flow of gas.

6. Creates positive pressure only during expiration (*abbreviation*).

11. A device housed within a Percussionaire Intrapulmonary Percussive Ventilator that increases and decreases air pressures.

15. A valve that uses a steel ball to create a series of high-frequency oscillations on exhalation.

17. A/an_____ seal resistor consists of a column of water.

18. The type of nebulizer in which the aerosol cloud is formed outside of the main gas flow.

21. A type of lung expansion device that displays and measures the patient's inhaled gas.

24. A type of lung expansion device that requires the patient to achieve a certain inspiratory flow rate to raise the indicator, which is a ball.

Down

2. A lung expansion technique designed to mimic natural sighing by encouraging patients to take slow, deep breaths (*abbreviation*).

3. A type of resistor that relies on a spring to hold a disk or diaphragm down over the expiratory port.

4. A device that consists of a counterweighted hollow drum with attached vanes (*two words*).

5. Application of positive pressure to a patient's airway throughout the respiratory cycle (*abbreviation*).

7. The breathing maneuver used to perform incentive spirometry (*abbreviation*).

8. A type of threshold resistor that uses a specially milled steel ball placed over a calibrated orifice.

9. A type of resistor that contains a bar magnet that attracts a ferromagnetic disk seated on the expiratory port of a circuit.

10. A device commonly used to provide positive pressure breaths to aid in lung expansion therapy.

12. A/an _____ regulator is an adjustable reducing valve that regulates the gas pressure delivered to a patient by a Puritan Bennett PR-2.

13. Providing a negative baseline (*abbreviation*).

14. A type of exhalation valve that allows exhaled gases to be measured through one directional port.

16. A less-cumbersome way of delivering positive airway pressure (*abbreviation*).

19. A type of machine that is patient-triggered, pressure-limited, and time-limited; and pressure-cycled or flow-cycled; and that is used for bronchial hygiene therapy (*abbreviation*).

20. A collection of techniques used to help clear airway secretions and improve the distribution of ventilation (*abbreviation*).

22. Bird _____ 10 series.

23. A device that replaces or augments cough clearance (*abbreviation*).

ACHIEVING THE OBJECTIVES

1. Compare volume-displacement and flow-dependent incentive spirometers.

1A. What is incentive spirometry?

_____

_____

1B. List three indications for incentive spirometry.

_____

_____

_____

_____

_____

_____

1C. Define sustained maximum inspiration (SMI).

_____

_____

_____

_____

1D. How does a volume-displacement incentive spirometer operate?

_____

_____

_____

_____

1E. How does a flow-dependent incentive spirometer operate?

_____

_____

_____

_____

1F. How is volume displacement achieved with a flow-dependent incentive spirometer?

_____

_____

1G. An SMI should be how long?

_____

1H. A patient using a flow-dependent incentive spirometer holds an inspiratory flow of 900 mL/s for 1.5 seconds. The amount of volume inhaled by the patient during this maneuver is

_____

_____.

Think About This

What types of breathing patterns can occur when a person is under stress?

Helpful Web Sites

■ The Cleveland Clinic, "How to Use an Incentive Spirometer" — http://www.clevelandclinic.org

■ American Association for Respiratory Care, *Respiratory Care* journal, "Clinical Practice Guideline: Incentive Spirometry" — http://www.rcjournal.com

2. Describe two types of machines used to administer intermittent positive pressure breathing (IPPB) therapy.

2A. Define *intermittent positive pressure breathing (IPPB)*.

_____

_____

2B. List the indications for IPPB therapy.

_____

_____

_____

_____

_____

_____

2C. What should be monitored during IPPB therapy?

_____

_____

_____

_____

_____

_____

_____

2D. Which types of devices are used to deliver IPPB therapy?

_____

_____

2E. What types of IPPB devices does Puritan Bennett manufacture?

_____

_____

2F. Which Puritan Bennett IPPB devices could also be used to provide short-term ventilation for patients with apnea?

_____

_____

2G. Describe the IPPB devices mentioned in question 2F in terms of their phase variables.

_____

_____

2H. What types of IPPB devices does Bird manufacture?

_____

2I. What is the basic operational principle of the Bird IPPB devices?

_____

_____

2J. Describe the Bird IPPB devices in terms of their phase variables.

_____

_____

2K. Describe the VORTRAN-IPPB™ device in terms of its phase variables.

_____

_____

_____

_____

Think About This

Why is IPPB therapy so controversial?

Helpful Web Sites

- VORTRAN-IPPB "User's Guide" — http://www.vortran.com
- University of Medicine and Dentistry of New Jersey, Respiratory Care Program, "Assembly and Trouble-shooting of IPPB Equipment" — http://www.umdnj.edu

3. Discuss how expiratory positive airway pressure (EPAP), continuous positive airway pressure (CPAP), and positive expiratory pressure (PEP) therapies are used to mobilize secretions and treat atelectasis.

3A. Four indications for the use of positive airway pressure (PAP) devices are:

_____

_____

_____

_____

_____.

3B. How CPAP does operate?

_____

_____

3C. Describe how EPAP works.

_____

_____

_____

_____

3D. Describe how PEP operates.

_____

_____

_____

_____

3E. How does PEP therapy prevent atelectasis?

_____

_____

_____

_____

Think About This

What do the pressure-time waveforms look like for EPAP and PEP?

Helpful Web Site

■ Respironics, Inc, "User Guide for the Threshold PEP Device" — http://global.respironics.com

4. Identify the major components of pneumatically and electrically powered percussors.

4A. How do both electrically and pneumatically powered percussors clear airway secretions?

_____

_____

_____

_____

4B. How much gas pressure is necessary to power pneumatic percussors? _____

4C. What are the major components of a pneumatically powered percussor?

_____

_____

_____

_____

4D. What type of electrical current is necessary to power an electric percussor?

_____

_____

4E. What major components are common to electrically powered percussors?

_____

_____

4F. Which type or types of percussors are able to be used in home care?

_____

_____

Think About This

Can you think of a household item that can be used to improvise a manual percussor?

Helpful Web Sites

■ Med Systems, "Fluid Flo" Percussor, Model 2500 — http://www.medsystems.com

■ General Physiotherapy, Inc, Information on the G5 "Flimm-Fighter" Percussor — http://www.g5.com

5. Describe the theory of operation of four devices that enhance clearance of airway secretions by producing high-frequency oscillations to the lungs and chest wall.

5A. What factors are thought to enhance clearance of airway secretions by high-frequency oscillation devices?

_____

_____

_____

_____

_____

5B. Name the two devices that transmit high-frequency oscillation through the airway opening.

_____

_____

5C. Name the two devices that deliver high-frequency oscillation to the chest wall.

_____

_____

5D. Describe how the Percussionaire Intrapulmonary Percussive Ventilator (IPV-1) unit operates.

_____

_____

_____

_____

_____

_____

_____

_____

5E. What is the main advantage of the Acapella valve over the Flutter valve?

_____

_____

_____

5F. How many breaths should be exhaled through the Flutter valve or the Acapella valve?

_____

5G. Explain how The Vest operates.

_____

_____

_____

_____

_____

5H. Explain the operation of the Hayek Oscillator.

_____

_____

_____

_____

_____

_____

_____

_____

Think About This

How have chest physiotherapy devices improved the lives of individuals with cystic fibrosis?

Helpful Web Sites

- Percussionaire Corporation, "Intrapulmonary Percussive Ventilation Clinical Resources Manual" — http://www14.inetba.com
- RT for Decision Makers in Respiratory Care, "Review of Airway Clearance Technologies 2006," Jonathan Finder — http://www.rtmagazine.com
- Medivent International, Information on the Hayek Oscillator and More [question and answer format] — http://www.mediventintl.com
- Hill-Rom Services, Inc, "The Vest" — http://www.thevest.com

6. Discuss how mechanical insufflation-exsufflation devices (MI-E) can enhance airway secretions in patients with respiratory muscle weakness or paralysis.

6A. What is the purpose of the MI-E?

_____

_____

_____

6B. How does the MI-E device (Respironics CoughAssist) operate?

_____

_____

_____

_____

_____

_____

6C. For what disease process has the Respironics CoughAssist been shown to be most effective?

_____

_____

Think About This

What could happen if a patient with emphysema used an MI-E device?

Chapter **7** Lung Expansion Devices

Helpful Web Sites

- Respironics, Inc, CoughAssist — http://coughassist.respironics.com
- Respironics, Inc, "CoughAssist User's Guide; Models CA-3000 and CA-3200" — http://global.respironics.com
- *Chest* journal, "Mechanical Insufflation-exsufflation. Comparison of Peak Expiratory Flows with Manually Assisted and Unassisted Coughing Techniques," J.R. Bach — http://www.chestjournal.org

NATIONAL BOARD FOR RESPIRATORY CARE (NBRC)–TYPE QUESTIONS

1. Contraindications for incentive spirometry include which of the following?
   A. Postthoracic surgery
   B. Vital capacity < 10 mL/kg
   C. Restrictive pulmonary disease
   D. Inspiratory capacity > predicted value

2. A patient reports that during incentive spirometry she becomes light-headed and dizzy and must stop the maneuver when this happens. The most probable cause is that the patient is:
   A. Hypoventilating
   B. Hyperventilating
   C. Becoming fatigued
   D. Having a bronchospasm

3. Myasthenia gravis is causing a patient to have respiratory muscle weakness. This patient has a vital capacity of 5 mL/kg and is unable to cough effectively. What therapy would you recommend to help prevent pulmonary complications?
   A. Incentive spirometry
   B. Positive expiratory pressure
   C. Mechanical insufflation-exsufflation
   D. Intermittent positive pressure breathing (IPPB)

4. Which of the following intermittent positive pressure breathing (IPPB) machines is unable to provide short-term ventilatory support?
   A. Bird Mark 7
   B. Bird Mark 14
   C. Puritan Bennett AP-4
   D. Puritan Bennett PR-2

5. The therapy that mobilizes retained secretions, through the use of devices similar to continuous positive airway pressure (CPAP) resistors but that are less cumbersome, is:
   A. Expiratory positive airway pressure (EPAP)
   B. Intermittent positive pressure breathing (IPPB)?
   C. Intrapulmonary percussive ventilation (IPV)
   D. Positive expiratory pressure (PEP)

6. During a PEP therapy session, what directions should be given to the patient?
   A. "Stop after 20 to 30 breaths."
   B. "Place your lips into the mouthpiece."
   C. "Take a deep breath, then actively exhale."
   D. "Breathe normally through the mouthpiece."

7. What type of therapy is recommended to reduce air-trapping?
   A. IPV and chest physiotherapy
   B. IPPB and chest physiotherapy
   C. Positive airway pressure with PEP
   D. Positive airway pressure with CPAP of 15 cm H_2O

8. The type of adjunctive therapy that aids in the mobilization of airway secretions through high-frequency percussive breaths applied inside the patient's airways is known as:
   A. Intrapulmonary percussive ventilation (IPV)
   B. Continuous positive airway pressure (CPAP)
   C. Expiratory positive airway pressure (EPAP)
   D. Positive expiratory pressure (PEP)

9. IPV mobilizes airway secretions by:
   A. Generating subatmospheric pressure on inspiration, then expiratory resistance.
   B. Applying a positive pressure to a patient's airways throughout the respiratory cycle.
   C. Delivering high-frequency percussive breaths into the patient's airways.
   D. Applying an expiratory resistance to exhaled flow from the patient.

10. To apply positive airway pressure to a manual resuscitator bag during patient transport, which of the following are most appropriate?
    I. Spring-loaded valve
    II. Underwater seal
    III. Magnetic valve
    IV. Weighted ball
       A. I and II only
       B. I and III only
       C. II and IV only
       D. III and IV only

Chapter **7** Lung Expansion Devices

8 Assessment of Pulmonary Function

Upon completion of this chapter, you will be able to:
1. Identify three types of volume-collecting spirometers.
2. Explain the operational theory of thermal flowmeters.
3. Name three types of pneumotachometers.
4. Describe three types of body plethysmographs.
5. Discuss the American Thoracic Society/European Respiratory Society standards for lung function testing.
6. Compare the nitrogen washout and the helium dilution techniques for measuring functional residual capacity and residual volume.
7. Explain the operational theories of strain gauge, variable-inductance, and variable-capacitance pressure transducers.
8. Describe various conditions that interfere with the operation of impedance pneumographs.
9. List and describe measured and derived variables that are commonly used to assess respiratory mechanics.
10. Compare the operational principles of the two types of oxygen analyzers used in the clinical setting.
11. Describe two techniques for monitoring nitrogen oxides in the clinical setting.
12. Identify the components of a normal capnogram.
13. Assess an abnormal capnogram and suggest possible pathophysiologic processes that could contribute to the contour of the carbon dioxide waveform.
14. Compare closed-circuit and open-circuit indirect calorimeters.
15. Calculate energy expenditure by using measurements obtained during indirect calorimetry.
16. Explain how indirect calorimetry can be used to determine substrate use patterns in healthy subjects and in those with cardiopulmonary dysfunctions.

"The answer, my friend, is blowin' in the wind. The answer is blowin' in the wind."
Bob Dylan

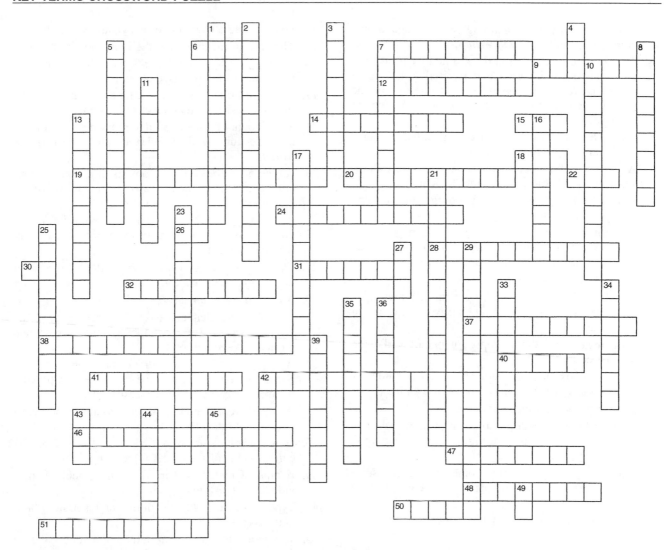

CROSSWORD PUZZLE 8-1
Created using Crossword Weaver, www.CrosswordWeaver.com.

Use the clues to complete the crossword puzzle.

Across

6. The factor derived from the number of milliliters of gas that must be displaced to cause a kymographic pen to move 1 mm.

7. A type of cart that measures the oxygen consumed and carbon dioxide produced by the patient, then calculates the energy expenditure of the patient.

9. The _____ effect is used by ultrasonic pneumotachographs to quantify the airflow velocity.

12. Electrical _____ is opposition to the flow of an alternating current.

14. Does not participate in gas exchange (*two words*).

15. A derived value that is opposition to air movement in the lungs (*abbreviation*).

18. The maximum volume of air that a person can breathe over a 1-minute period (*abbreviation*).

19. Body _____, or use of a body box.

20. The type of water-sealed spirometer that uses a plastic bell to measure volume changes in the airway opening (*two words*).

22. When lungs are normal, this equals functional residual capacity, or FRC (*abbreviation*).

107

24. Indirect _____ measures energy expenditure.

26. The volume of gas remaining in the lungs after a complete exhalation (*abbreviation*).

28. The volume of oxygen is determined by measuring the volumes of inspired and expired gases, along with the fractional inspired oxygen (F_iO_2) in the inspired and expired gases (*two words*). **See 24 across.**

30. The total amount of air that can be exhaled after a maximum inspiration (*abbreviation*).

31. A type of flowmeter that uses a temperature-sensitive, temperature-resistant element.

32. A device for graphically recording lung volume changes during spirometry.

37. Electromechanical _____ may be classified as a strain gauge device, a variable-inductance device, or a variable-capacitance device.

38. Old term for *repeatability*.

40. An effect that occurs when light interacts with gas molecules to cause rotational energy changes in the gas molecules.

41. A tracing that shows the proportion of carbon dioxide in exhaled air.

42. A type of oxygen analyzer that uses the flow of electric current between a cathode and an anode.

46. Ability to repeat a measurement.

47. A chemiluminescence monitoring system measures _____ oxide during nitric oxide administration.

48. The _____ manometer is a pressure-measuring device that compares a reference pressure to an observed pressure.

50. A stainless-steel screen with a mesh size of 400 wires/in.

51. A gauge for determining the force or speed and sometimes the direction of the wind or air.

Down

1. _____ system compliance normally averages 0.1 L/cm H_2O.

2. Patient breathes in and out of a container prefilled with oxygen. (*The opposite of 28-across.*)

3. Usually undetected residual pressure above atmospheric pressure remaining in the alveoli at end-exhalation due to dynamic air-trapping.

4. Maximum pressure in the patient circuit (*abbreviation*).

5. A type of capnograph that pulls the gas to be sampled away from the airway.

7. A type of capnograph that analyzes carbon dioxide at the airway.

8. The expression of an instrument's ability to reproduce a measurement.

10. A type of oxygen analyzer that uses a magnetic field.

11. Diminishing a chemical or enzymatic reaction.

13. The ease of movement of the lung and chest wall.

16. _____ ventilation is the volume of air that ventilates all the perfused alveoli.

17. A type of bridge that has a particular arrangement of multiple resistors in an electrical circuit.

21. The amount of force needed to move a given volume into the lung with a relaxed chest wall (*three words*).

23. A type of spirometer that consists of a canister containing a piston that is sealed to it with a rolling diaphragm-like seal (*three words*).

25. Pneumo_____, an instrument that incorporates a pneumotachometer to record variations in respiratory gas flow.

27. The amount of gas in the lungs after a maximum inspiration (*abbreviation*).

29. A type of oxygen analyzer.

33. A manometer that consists of a vacuum chamber with a flexible cover or a diaphragm that flexes when pressure is applied to it.

34. A/an_____ pneumotachograph uses a bundle of brass capillary tubes arranged in a parallel manner to create the known resistance.

35. A graphic representation of lung volumes and ventilatory flow rates.

36. How closely a measured value is related to the correct value of the quantity measured.

39. A type of meter used in the management of individuals with asthma.

42. Type of pressure obtained during an inspiratory hold maneuver.

43. The total amount of gas left in the lungs after a normal, quiet exhalation (*abbreviation*).

44. _____ transformation is based on the fact that nitrogen is not used or given off by the body.

45. The type of ventilation derived from multiplying tidal volume by respiratory rate.

49. Measures the metabolic cost of various forms of physical activity (*abbreviation*).

ACHIEVING THE OBJECTIVES

1. Identify three types of volume-collecting spirometers.

1A. How do volume-collecting spirometers operate?

_____

_____

_____

_____

1B. Identify the spirometer in Figure 8-1.

_____

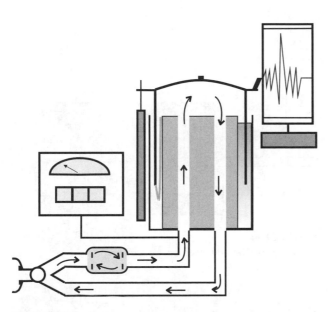

FIGURE 8-1
(From Ruppel G: *Manual of pulmonary function testing*, ed 8, St. Louis, 2009, Mosby.)

1C. Describe how the spirometer in Figure 8-1 operates.

_____

_____

_____

_____

_____

_____

_____

_____

_____

1D. Identify the spirometer in Figure 8-2.

_____

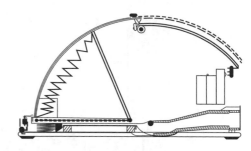

FIGURE 8-2
(Modified from Vitalograph, Shawnee Mission, Kansas)

1E. Describe how the spirometer in Figure 8-2 operates.

_____

_____

_____

_____

_____

_____

_____

_____

109

1F. What are the similarities and differences between the spirometers in Figure 8-1 and Figure 8-3?

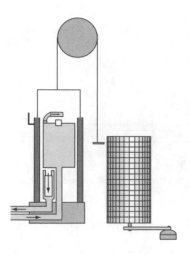

FIGURE 8-3
(Modified from Collins Medical, Braintree, Massachusetts)

_____

_____

_____

_____

_____

_____

_____

_____

_____

_____

_____

_____

_____

_____

_____

1G. Identify the spirometer in Figure 8-4.

_____

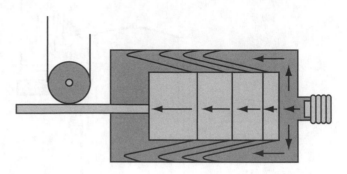

FIGURE 8-4
(From Datex-Ohmeda, Madison, Wisconsin)

1H. Describe how the spirometer in Figure 8-4 operates.

_____

_____

_____

_____

_____

_____

_____

1I. What are the three types of volume-collecting spirometers?

_____

_____

Think About This

Are volume-collecting spirometers appropriate for use with young children and infants?

Helpful Web Sites

- SpirXpert, "Lung Function Testing: Spirometers" — http://www.spirxpert.com/technical6.htm
- Morgan Scientific, Inc, Morgan SpiroAir Device — http://www.morgansci.com/pulmonary-testing-products/spiroair-pft

2. Explain the operational theory of thermal flowmeters.

Questions 2A and 2B refer to Figure 8-5.

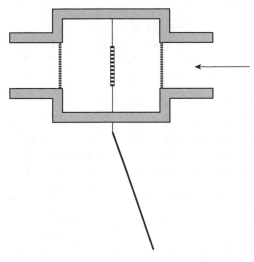

FIGURE 8-5
(From Cairo J: *Mosby's respiratory care equipment*, ed 7, St. Louis, 2008, Mosby.)

2A. Label Figure 8-5. (1) _____,

   (2) _____, and

   (3) _____.

2B. How does this type of flowmeter operate?

_____

_____

_____

_____

_____

2C. List four sources of errors that could interfere with the operation of a thermal flowmeter.

_____

_____

_____

_____

2D. How can the amount of cooling of the hot wire be affected?

_____

_____

Think About This
What other uses do hot-wire anemometers have?

Helpful Web Site
■ SpirXpert, "Lung Function Testing: Hot Wire Anemometer" — http://www.spirxpert.com/technical5.htm

3. Name three types of pneumotachometers.

Questions 3A through 3D refer to Figure 8-6.

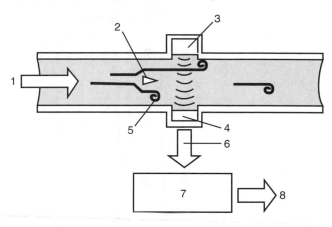

FIGURE 8-6
(Redrawn from Sullivan WJ, Peters GM, Enright PL: Pneumotachography: theory and clinical application, *Respir Care* 29:736, 194.)

3A. What type of pneumotachometer is shown in Figure 8-6?

_____

_____

3B. Identify the parts labeled in Figure 8-6.

1.	
2.	
3.	
4.	
5.	
6.	
7.	
8.	

3C. How does the pneumotachograph shown in Figure 8-6 operate?

_____

_____

_____

_____

_____

3D. Can the pneumotachograph shown in Figure 8-6 measure inspiratory and expiratory flow simultaneously?

_____

3E. What type of pneumotachograph measures flow by using a variable area and flexible obstruction for measuring flow as a function of the pressure differential generated by the obstruction?

_____

Questions 3F through 3H refer to Figure 8-7.

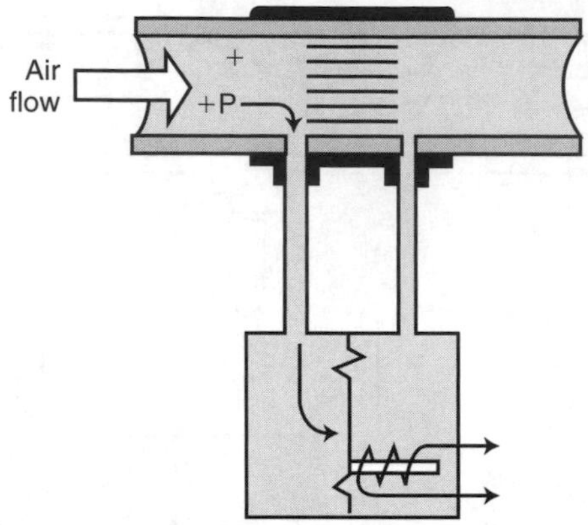

FIGURE 8-7
(Redrawn from Sullivan WJ, Peters GM, Enright PL: Pneumotachography: theory and clinical application, *Respir Care* 29:736, 194.)

3F. What type of pneumotachograph is shown in Figure 8-7?

_____

_____

3G. How does the pneumotachograph in Figure 8-7 operate?

_____

_____

_____

_____

_____

_____

3H. What is the purpose of having a heater in the pneumotachograph in Figure 8-7?

_____

_____

_____

_____

3I. The type of pneumotachograph that uses ceramic parallel channels instead of brass capillary tubes is the

_____

_____.

3J. What type of pneumotachograph uses a Monel screen as the main resistive component with a heating element?

_____

_____

3K. The pneumotachograph that uses sound waves that are projected parallel to the flow of gas and that can be used to measure bidirectional flows is the

_____

_____.

Think About This

What use would a pneumotachograph have during speech therapy?

Helpful Web Sites

- SpirXpert, "Lung Function Testing: Fleisch Type Pneumotachometer" — http://www.spirxpert.com
- SpirXpert, "Lung Function Testing: Lilly Type Pneumotachometer" — http://www.spirxpert.com
- SpirXpert, "Lung Function Testing: Hot Wire Anemometer" — http://www.spirxpert.com
- Phipps & Bird, "Fleisch Pneumotachograph" — http://www.phippsbird.com

4. Describe three types of body plethysmographs.

4A. What variables can be measured with a body plethysmograph?

_____

_____

_____

4B. The most common type of body plethysmograph is the

_____

_____.

4C. How does the body plethysmograph in Question 4B operate?

_____

_____

_____

_____

_____

_____

4D. How does a volume-displacement plethysmograph operate?

_____

_____

4E. To measure airflow changes during constant-pressure (volume-displacement) plethysmography, what equipment is incorporated into the body box?

_____

_____

4F. What additional calculations can be made by measuring these airflow changes?

_____

_____

4G. What gas law is being applied during the use of body plethysmography?

_____

_____

Think About This

How has body plethysmography been changed over the years to reduce claustrophobia?

Helpful Web Sites

- Cook, R: Disease Management with Body Plethysmography — http://www.touchrespiratorydisease.com
- RT for Decision Makers in Respiratory Care, "Whole-body Plethysmography," John D. Zoidis — http://www.rtmagazine.com
- Johns Hopkins School of Medicine Interactive Respiratory Physiology Encyclopedia, "Body Plethysmography" — http://oac.med.jhmi.edu

5. Discuss the American Thoracic Society/European Respiratory Society (ATS/ERS) standards for lung function testing.

5A. The ATS/ERS documents provide guidance for which pulmonary function tests?

_____

_____

5B. Define the term *repeatability* as it relates to lung function testing.

_____

_____

_____

5C. What is the repeatability standard for forced expiratory volume in 1 second (FEV_1)?

_____

5D. What is the repeatability standard for peak expiratory flow (PEF)?

_____

_____

5E. How often should spirometry equipment be checked for volume and leaks?

_____

_____

5F. What methods are used to perform the volume and leak tests on spirometry equipment?

_____

_____

5G. How frequently should the volume linearity of a spirometer be checked? How should this be accomplished?

_____

_____

_____

5H. What are the six diagnostic indications for spirometry according to ATS/ERS standards?

_____

_____

_____

_____

_____

5I. What are the four monitoring indications for spirometry according to ATS/ERS standards?

_____

_____

_____

_____

5J. How often should flow-measuring spirometers be checked for flow? How is this calibration check done?

_____

_____

_____

Think About This

How does testing technique affect the ability to detect change in lung function?

Helpful Web Sites

■ *European Respiratory Journal*, "General Considerations for Lung Function Testing," M. R. Miller et al — http://erj.ersjournals.com

■ *European Respiratory Journal*, "Standardisation of Spirometry," M. R. Miller et al — http://erj.ersjournals.com

6. Compare the nitrogen washout and the helium dilution techniques for measuring functional residual capacity (FRC) and residual volume.

6A. What gas is inhaled by the patient during a nitrogen washout test? _____

6B. What gas is inhaled by the patient during a helium dilution test? _____

6C. Describe how the nitrogen washout test enables you to measure FRC.

_____

_____

_____

_____

_____

_____

_____

_____

_____

_____

_____

_____

6D. Describe how the helium dilution test enables you to measure FRC.

_____

_____

_____

_____

_____

_____

_____

_____

_____

6E. What problems could a patient with chronic obstructive pulmonary disease (COPD) have when being tested with the nitrogen washout procedure or the helium dilution test?

_____

_____

_____

_____

_____

Think About This

What does the difference between a total lung capacity (TLC) measurement obtained by means of body plethysmography and a TLC measurement obtained by means of helium dilution represent?

Helpful Web Sites

■ Morgan Scientific, Inc, "What is a Pulmonary Function Test?" — http://www.morgansci.com

■ "Residual Volume Measurement," Professor K.S. Park — http://kspark.kaist.ac.kr

7. Explain the operational theories of strain gauge, variable-inductance, and variable-capacitance pressure transducers.

7A. How does a strain gauge operate?

_____

_____

_____

_____

_____

Questions 7B through 7D refer to Figure 8-8.

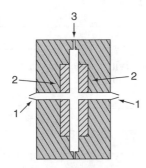

FIGURE 8-8
(Courtesy Snow M: Instrumentation. In Clausen JL, editor: *Pulmonary function testing: guidelines and controversies*, New York, 1982, Academic Press.)

7B. What type of pressure transducer is shown in Figure 8-8?

_____

7C. Label Figure 8-8.

_____
_____
_____
_____

7D. Explain how the pressure transducer in Figure 8-8 operates.

_____
_____
_____
_____
_____

Questions 7E through 7G refer to Figure 8-9.

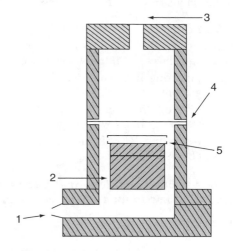

FIGURE 8-9
(Courtesy Snow M: Instrumentation. In Clausen JL, editor: *Pulmonary function testing: guidelines and controversies*, New York, 1982, Academic Press.)

7E. What type of pressure transducer is shown in Figure 8-9?

_____
_____

7F. Label Figure 8-9.

_____

7G. Explain the operation of the pressure transducer in Figure 8-9.

_____
_____
_____
_____
_____

7H. Which two types of pressure transducers are most commonly used for measuring respiratory and cardiovascular pressures?

_____
_____
_____

Think About This

In what other industries are pressure transducers used?

Helpful Web Sites

- RDP Electrosense, "How it Works — Strain Gauge Pressure Transducer" — http://www.rdpe.com
- Omega Engineering, Inc, "The Strain Gauge" — http://www.omega.com
- Engineers Edge, "Inductance Type Transducer — Instrumentation" — http://www.engineersedge.com
- HowStuffWorks, Inc, "How Inductors Work" — http://electronics.howstuffworks.com

8. Describe various conditions that interfere with the operation of impedance pneumographs.

8A. Define *electrical impedance*.

_____

_____

_____

8B. How is electrical impedance determined?

_____

_____

_____

8C. How does electrical impedance enable the measurement of lung volumes?

_____

_____

_____

_____

_____

_____

_____

8D. What is the most common use for impedance pneumography?

_____

_____

8E. What alarms are incorporated into impedance pneumographs?

_____

_____

8F. Why is sensitivity of the impedance pneumographs an important setting?

_____

_____

_____

_____

8G. What conditions can interfere with the proper operation of impedance pneumographs?

_____

_____

8H. How do these conditions interfere with impedance pneumographs?

_____

_____

_____

_____

_____

_____

_____

8I. What other noninvasive method is used to measure respiratory function?

_____

_____

Think About This

What other uses does impedance plethysmography have?

Helpful Web Site

- *Chest* journal, "Impedance Pneumography: Comparison Between Chest Impedance Changes and Respiratory Volumes in 11 Healthy Patients," Ake Grenvik et al — http://www.chestjournal.org

9. List and describe measured and derived variables that are commonly used to assess respiratory mechanics.

9A. Label the volumes and capacities represented in Figure 8-10.

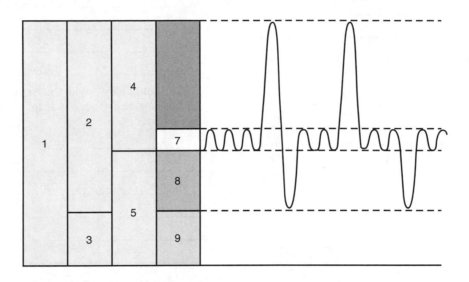

FIGURE 8-10
(From Comroe J: *The lung*, ed 3, Chicago, 1986, Mosby.)

9B. What volume measurements are included in simple spirometry?

_____

_____

9C. What are the formulas for the ventilatory capacities calculated from simple spirometry?

_____

_____

_____

9D. What dynamic lung volumes can be measured with simple spirometry?

_____

_____

_____

9E. Compare simple spirometry with full lung-volume tests.

_____

_____

_____

_____

_____

_____

_____

9F. How are mechanically ventilated patients tested to assess their pulmonary progress and their ability to breathe spontaneously? What is the significance of the finding?

_____

_____

_____

_____

_____

_____

9G. What airway pressure measurements are usually performed on spontaneously breathing patients?

_____

_____

_____

_____

_____

9H. How are these typical airway pressure measurements obtained?

_____

_____

_____

_____

_____

_____

9I. Define the two airway pressures that are most commonly measured while a patient is receiving mechanical ventilation.

_____

_____

_____

_____

_____

9J. What are the peak inspiratory pressure and the plateau pressure values in Figure 8-11?

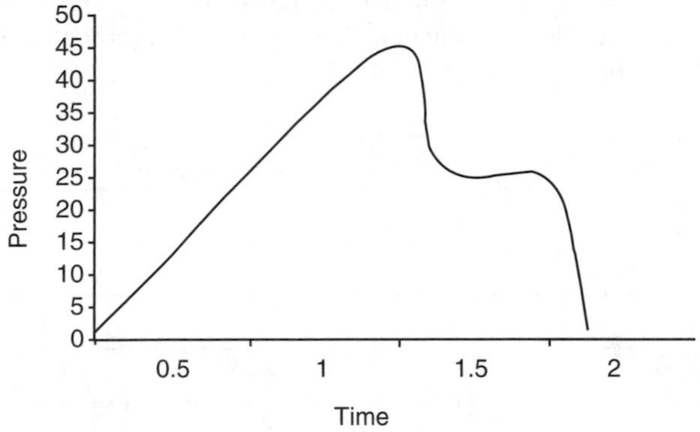

FIGURE 8-11

9K. What is the formula for calculating airway resistance?

_____

_____

9L. What information does airway resistance give about the status of the airways? What is the normal range of values for airway resistance?

_____

_____

_____

_____

9M. What is respiratory system compliance? What is the normal range of values for respiratory system compliance?

_____

_____

_____

_____

9N. What pulmonary conditions cause changes both in airway resistance and in respiratory system compliance?

_____

_____

_____

_____

_____

_____

Think About This

How are respiratory mechanics assessed in newborns?

Helpful Web Sites

- SpirXpert, "Lung Function Indices — Spirographic indices: An Overview" — http://www.spirxpert.com
- Johns Hopkins School of Medicine Interactive Respiratory Physiology Encyclopedia, "Compliance" — http://oac.med.jhmi.edu
- Morgan Scientific Inc, "What is a Pulmonary Function Test?" — http://www.morgansci.com

10. Compare the operational principles of the two types of oxygen analyzers used in the clinical setting.

10A. What type of cathode and anode are used in polarographic oxygen analyzers?

_____

_____

10B. In what type of fluid are the polarographic cathode and anode immersed?

_____

_____

10C. What happens at the anode and cathode of the polarographic analyzer?

_____

_____

_____

_____

10D. What type of anode and cathode are used in the galvanic oxygen analyzers?

_____

_____

10E. In what type of fluid are the galvanic cathode and anode immersed?

_____

_____

10F. What is the major difference between the polarographic analyzer and the galvanic analyzer?

_____

_____

_____

_____

_____

10G. List three clinical uses for galvanic and polarographic oxygen analyzers.

_____

_____

_____

10H. What situations can affect the readings of a galvanic or polarographic oxygen analyzer?

_____

_____

_____

10I. The electrodes of which type of analyzer last longer and why?

_____

_____

_____

_____

10J. Label the galvanic analyzer shown in Figure 8-12.

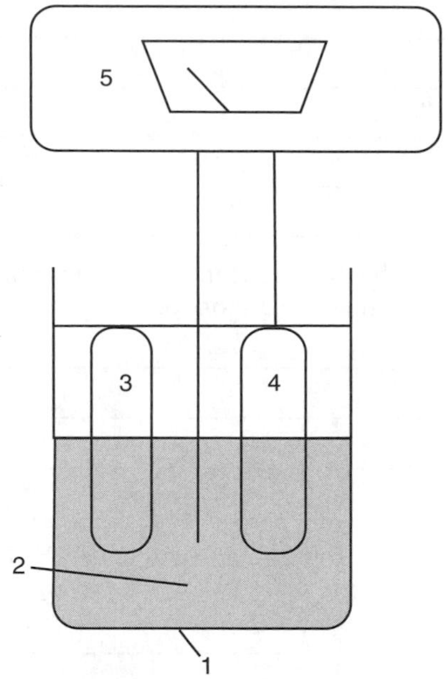

FIGURE 8-12

_____

_____

_____

Think About This
In what other industries are oxygen analyzers used?

Helpful Web Site
■ Alpha Omega Instruments, "Oxygen Analyzer Sensor Types" — http://www.aoi-corp.net

11. Describe two techniques for monitoring nitrogen oxides in the clinical setting.

11A. The administration of what therapeutic gas necessitates monitoring of nitrogen oxides?

_____

_____

11B. What happens to gases sampled by a chemiluminescence monitor?

_____

_____

_____

_____

_____

_____

119

11C. How is nitrogen (NO_2) dioxide converted to nitric oxide within the chemiluminescence monitor?

_____

_____

_____

_____

11D. How is the NO_2 concentration determined by the chemiluminescence monitor?

_____

_____

_____

11E. Name four sources of error in a chemiluminescence monitor.

_____

_____

_____

_____

11F. Electrochemical monitoring of nitrogen oxides is based on what principle?

_____

_____

11G. Describe the structure of an electrochemical nitric oxide (NO) analyzer.

_____

_____

_____

_____

_____

_____

11H. Name two sources of inaccuracy with an electrochemical NO analyzer.

_____

_____

_____

_____

11I. According to the proposed U.S. Food and Drug Administration standards for NO and NO_2 monitoring devices, what should the monitoring range, accuracy, and response time be?

_____

_____

_____

_____

_____

_____

_____

11J. Which type of NO monitoring device is easy to use and the most accurate, but also the most expensive?

_____

_____

Think About This

What role does the measurement of exhaled NO play in airways disease management?

Helpful Web Sites

■ The Scientific & Technological Research Council of Turkey, *Turkish Journal of Medical Sciences*, "Nitric Oxide I: Advances in the Measurements for Clinical Applications," Ayşe Baysal — http://journals.tubitak.gov.tr

■ *British Journal of Anaesthesia*, "Formation of Nitrogen Dioxide from Nitric Oxide and Their Measurement in Clinically Relevant Circumstances," U. Schedin et al — http://bja.oxfordjournals.org

■ Mayo Clinic Proceedings, "Inhaled Nitric Oxide Therapy," Robert J. Lunn — http://www.mayoclinicproceedings.com

12. Identify the components of a normal capnogram.

12A. Define the term *capnogram*.

_____

12B. What is the fraction of inspired carbon dioxide?

_____

12C. What is the fraction of expired carbon dioxide?

_____

Questions 12D through 12H refer to Figure 8-13.

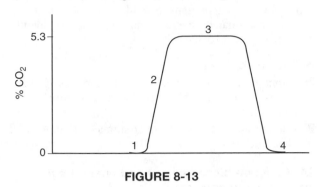

FIGURE 8-13

12D. What is happening during phase 1 of the capnogram?

_____

_____

_____

12E. Why is there an upswing in the capnogram, which is depicted in Figure 8-13 as the line labeled 2?

_____

_____

_____

_____

12F. What causes phase 3 to have a flat appearance?

_____

_____

12G. At what point on the capnogram is end-tidal partial pressure of carbon dioxide (PCO_2) read?

_____

_____

12H. Why does the capnogram fall to 0 during phase 4?

_____

_____

Think About This

Are there any other clinical uses for capnography?

Helpful Web Sites

■ American Association for Respiratory Care (AARC), *AARC Times*, "Clinical Applications of Carbon Dioxide Monitoring," Timothy B. Op't Holt— http://www.aarc.org

■ Normal capnographic waveforms — http://capno.chez-alice.fr

■ Normal capnogram — http://www.capnography.com

13. Assess an abnormal capnogram and suggest possible pathophysiologic processes that could contribute to the contour of the carbon dioxide waveform.

13A. The amount of carbon dioxide in exhaled air depends on what?

_____

_____

13B. When ventilation and perfusion in the lungs are matched, how much of a difference is there between partial pressure of arterial carbon dioxide ($PaCO_2$) and partial pressure of end-tidal CO_2 ($P_{ET}CO_2$)?

13C. When ventilation decreases relative to perfusion (V < Q), what happens to $P_{ET}CO_2$?

_____

_____

13D. When ventilation increases relative to perfusion (V > Q), what happens to $P_{ET}CO_2$?

_____

_____

13E. What are the possible pathophysiologic causes for the capnographic contour shown in Figure 8-14?

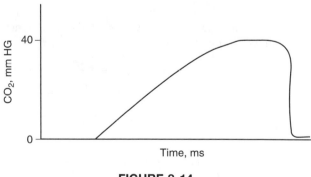

FIGURE 8-14

_____

_____

_____

_____

_____

13F. What is the most likely cause of the capnogram shown in Figure 8-15?

_____

_____

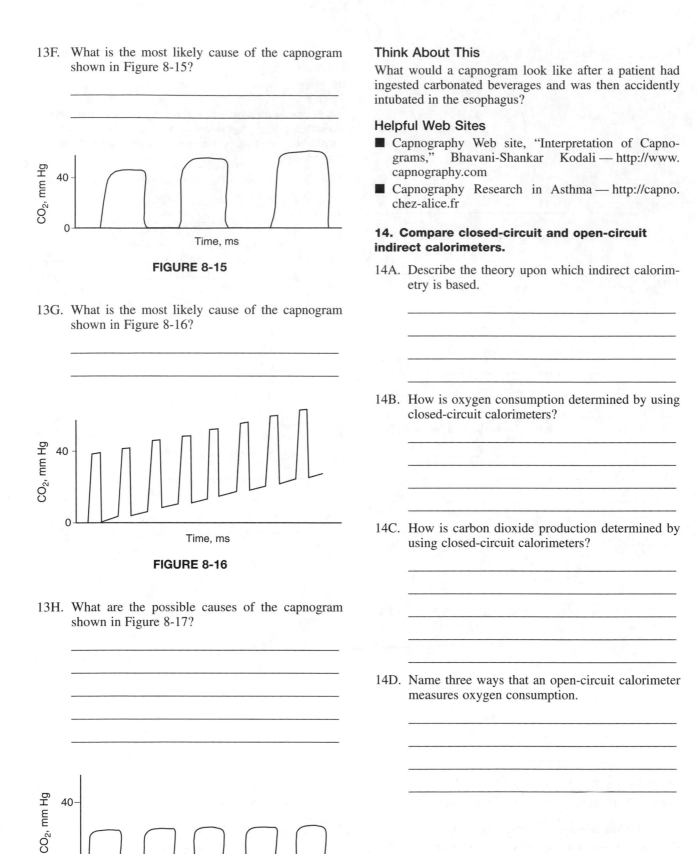

FIGURE 8-15

13G. What is the most likely cause of the capnogram shown in Figure 8-16?

_____

_____

FIGURE 8-16

13H. What are the possible causes of the capnogram shown in Figure 8-17?

_____

_____

_____

_____

_____

FIGURE 8-17

Think About This

What would a capnogram look like after a patient had ingested carbonated beverages and was then accidently intubated in the esophagus?

Helpful Web Sites

■ Capnography Web site, "Interpretation of Capno-grams," Bhavani-Shankar Kodali — http://www.capnography.com

■ Capnography Research in Asthma — http://capno.chez-alice.fr

14. Compare closed-circuit and open-circuit indirect calorimeters.

14A. Describe the theory upon which indirect calorim-etry is based.

_____

_____

_____

_____

14B. How is oxygen consumption determined by using closed-circuit calorimeters?

_____

_____

_____

_____

14C. How is carbon dioxide production determined by using closed-circuit calorimeters?

_____

_____

_____

_____

_____

14D. Name three ways that an open-circuit calorimeter measures oxygen consumption.

_____

_____

_____

_____

14E. How do each of these systems operate?

_____

_____

_____

_____

_____

_____

_____

_____

_____

_____

_____

14F. Which type of calorimeter may have problems when used with mechanically ventilated patients? Why?

_____

_____

_____

_____

_____

Think About This

How can indirect calorimetry be used to manage patients with burns?

Helpful Web Sites

- AARC, *Respiratory Care* journal, "Clinical Practice Guideline: Metabolic Measurements Using Indirect Calorimetry During Mechanical Ventilation—2004 Revision and Update" — http://www.rcjournal.com
- *Clinical Window* Web journal, "Indirect Calorimetry — Practical Applications," Chris L. Harris — http://www.clinicalwindow.net

15. Calculate energy expenditure by using measurements obtained during indirect calorimetry.

15A. In what two ways can energy expenditure be expressed?

_____

15B. What are the normal values for energy expenditure for a normal, healthy adult?

_____

_____

15C. Calculate the energy expenditure when the oxygen consumption is 250 mL/min and carbon dioxide production is 200 mL/min.

_____

_____

_____

_____

15D. A 62-year-old male patient with a history of COPD comes into the emergency department with a report of increasing shortness of breath over the last 3 days. He is hypoxemic and severely hypercapnic and is intubated and placed on mechanical ventilation. Three days later, several attempts to wean him from mechanical ventilation have failed. An indirect calorimetry study was performed and had the following results: oxygen consumption, 230 mL/min; carbon dioxide production, 220 mL/min. Calculate the patient's energy expenditure.

_____

_____

_____

_____

15E. Calculate the energy expenditure when the oxygen consumption is 270 mL/min and carbon dioxide production is 235 mL/min.

_____

_____

_____

_____

_____

_____

Think About This

What effect does infection have on energy expenditure?

Helpful Web Sites

- Internet Scientific Publications, *The Internet Journal of Internal Medicine*, "Quick Review: The Metabolic Cart," Tisha J. Fujii and Bradley J. Phillips — http://www.ispub.com

■ Sage Journals Online, *Journal of Parenteral and Enteral Nutrition Online*, "Resting Energy Expenditure During Mechanical Ventilation and its Relationship with the Type of Lesion," J. M. Raurich et al

16. Explain how indirect calorimetry can be used to determine substrate use patterns in healthy subjects and in those with cardiopulmonary dysfunctions.

16A. What are substrate use patterns?

_____

_____

_____

_____

_____

16B. What is respiratory quotient (RQ)?

_____

_____

_____

_____

16C. How does indirect calorimetry contribute to substrate use patterns?

_____

_____

16D. What is the RQ for the following under normal conditions?

Carbohydrates	
Proteins	
Fat	
Healthy adults	

16E. A mechanically ventilated patient has been unable to complete three weaning attempts. Indirect calorimetry reveals carbon dioxide production of 182 mL/min and oxygen consumption of 240 mL/min. Calculate the RQ.

_____

_____

16F. Given the circumstances in the previous question, what may be causing this patient's difficulty with weaning?

_____

_____

_____

_____

Think About This

Does malnutrition have an effect on pulmonary function?

Helpful Web Site

■ University of Tennessee at Knoxville, The Institute for Environmental Modeling, "Metabolism for Energy and the Respiratory Quotient," M. Beals et al —http://www.tiem.utk.edu

NATIONAL BOARD FOR RESPIRATORY CARE (NBRC)–TYPE QUESTIONS

1. The accuracy of an instrument depends on which of the following?
   I. The standard deviation of repeated measurements
   II. The instrument's linearity and frequency response
   III. The instrument's ability to reproduce a measurement
   IV. The instrument's sensitivity to environmental conditions
   A. I and II only
   B. I and III only
   C. II and III only
   D. II and IV only

2. The best method for accurately measuring the thoracic gas volume of a patient with emphysema is:
   A. Helium dilution
   B. Nitrogen washout
   C. Pressure plethysmography
   D. Chemiluminescence monitoring

3. After functional residual capacity (FRC) has been measured by using both body plethysmography and nitrogen washout, it is discovered that the FRC measurement from the nitrogen washout test is less than that from the body plethysmographic test. The cause of this discrepancy could be which of the following?
   A. Poor technique
   B. Severe air-trapping
   C. Restrictive lung disease
   D. Directional-valve malfunction

4. The parents of a newborn sent home with an apnea monitor call the respiratory therapist to report several apnea periods were noted by the monitor's alarm system. The respiratory therapist should check which of the following to ensure that the baby's movement was not the cause of these alarms?
   A. Sensitivity of the monitor
   B. Placement of the electrodes
   C. Amount of electrical current
   D. Frequency of the vibrations

5. Which of the following variables can be measured directly?
   A. Lung compliance
   B. Work of breathing
   C. Airway resistance
   D. Plateau pressure

6. The results of pulmonary function testing show a normal total lung capacity and decreased, but reversible, forced expiratory volume in 1 second (FEV_1) and a forced expiratory flow of 25% to 75% ($FEV_{25\%-75\%}$). The patient is a 22-year-old, non-smoking man with an intermittent history of "noisy breathing." Which of the following is most likely the cause of his problem?
   A. Asthma
   B. Emphysema
   C. Pulmonary fibrosis
   D. Severe restrictive pulmonary disease

7. What type of device can be incorporated into a ventilator to provide continuous recordings of airway pressure during the breathing cycle?
   A. Variable-capacitance transducer
   B. Inductive plethysmograph
   C. Strain gauge transducer
   D. Aneroid manometer

8. A device that can measure nitric oxide uses which of the following?
   A. Wheatstone bridge
   B. Catalytic converter
   C. Potassium hydroxide
   D. Infrared spectroscope

9. The capnograph in the ventilator circuit is giving an erroneous reading. Which of the following actions is appropriate?
   A. Change the nitrous oxide filter
   B. Increase the amplifier
   C. Change the reference cell
   D. Alter the position of the mirror

10. A 24-year-old skier with a broken femur has been in the postanesthesia care unit for 24 hours and is 12 hours postextubation with no supplemental oxygen. He is awake, alert, and oriented, and he reports shortness of breath. A capnograph shows a decreased partial pressure of end-tidal CO_2 ($P_{ET}CO2$). Which of the following may cause this patient's current status?
   A. Respiratory center depression
   B. Pulmonary embolism
   C. Muscular paralysis
   D. Alveolar shunt

Chapter **8** **Assessment of Pulmonary Function**

11. Most calorimeters are unreliable when the oxygen concentration is above 50% to 60% because of which of the following?
    A. Boyle's law
    B. Charles' law
    C. Hamburger effect
    D. Haldane effect

12. What is the expected respiratory quotient of a patient with severe sepsis?
    A. 0.7
    B. 0.8
    C. 1.0
    D. >1.0

13. In Figure 8-18, the amount of pressure required to overcome elastic and frictional forces is represented by which of the following?

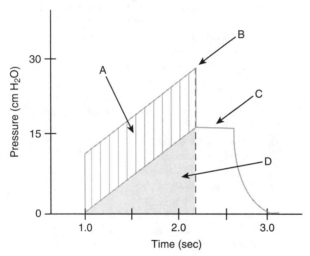

FIGURE 8-18

(From Pilbeam SP, Cairo JM: *Mechanical ventilation: physiological and clinical applications*, ed 4, St Louis, 2006, Mosby.)

    A. "A"
    B. "B"
    C. "C"
    D. "D"

14. The capnogram seen in Figure 8-19 shows which of the following?

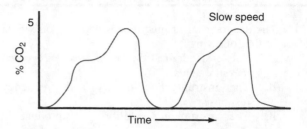

FIGURE 8-19

(From Pilbeam SP, Cairo JM: *Mechanical ventilation: physiological and clinical applications*, ed 4, St Louis, 2006, Mosby.)

    A. Excessive phase 4
    B. Deep "curare cleft"
    C. Indistinguishable phase 3
    D. Slow cardiac oscillation

15. The arterial-to–end-tidal carbon dioxide and the arterial-to–maximum expiratory partial pressure of carbon dioxide (PCO_2) gradients are both elevated and equal to each other. This finding is consistent with which of the following?
    A. Chronic obstructive pulmonary disease
    B. Left-sided heart failure
    C. Esophageal intubation
    D. Pulmonary embolism

9 Assessment of Cardiovascular Function

LEARNING OBJECTIVES

Upon completion of this chapter, you will be able to:
1. Discuss the electrophysiologic properties of the heart.
2. Explain the principles of electrocardiography.
3. Identify the major components of an electrocardiogram.
4. Demonstrate the correct placement of electrodes on a patient to obtain a 12-lead electrocardiogram.
5. Explain the various waves, complexes, and intervals that appear on a normal electrocardiogram.
6. List and describe the most common dysrhythmias encountered in clinical electrocardiography.
7. Describe the pressure, volume, and flow events that occur in the heart and major blood vessels during a typical cardiac cycle.
8. Explain the principles of operation of various noninvasive and invasive devices that are routinely used to obtain blood pressure measurements.
9. Describe various methods that are used to measure cardiac output.
10. Interpret hemodynamic measurements that are obtained from patients in a critical care setting.

"The heart has its reasons, which reason does not know."
Blaise Pascal

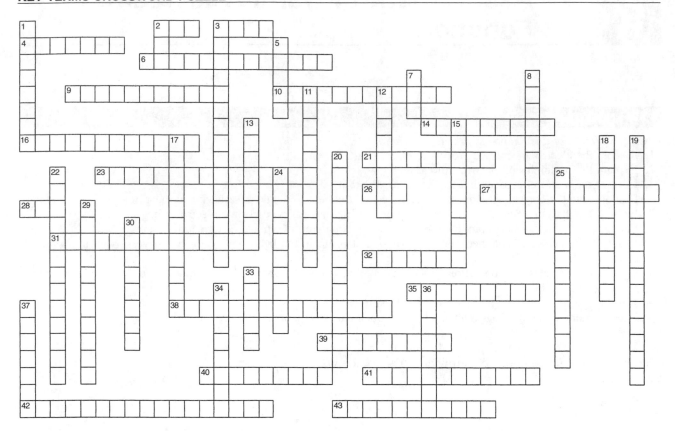

CROSSWORD PUZZLE 9-1
Created using Crossword Weaver, www.CrosswordWeaver.com.

Use the clues to complete the crossword puzzle.

Across

2. Occurs when an ectopic impulse originates in the ventricles before the normal sequence of depolarization begins at the sinoatrial node (*abbreviation*).

3. An abbreviation for a dangerous arrhythmia that should be treated immediately with cardiopulmonary resuscitation

4. Ventricular _____ is the contraction period for the cardiac ventricular muscle.

6. Associated with atrial depolarization on the electrocardiogram (*two words*).

9. Normal (*two words*) _____ _____ _____ occurs when the heart rate is 60 bpm to 100 bpm and each QRS complex is preceded by a P wave that appears to be abnormal.

10. Impedance _____ can be used to measure cardiac output by placing two pairs of electrodes on the thorax.

14. Atrial _____ depolarizations are ectopic bears that can originate in any part of the atria.

16. Ability of a cell to respond to an electrical stimulus.

21. An abbreviation for an ECG with gross irregularities in both atrial and ventricular depolarization (*two words*).

23. Heart sounds amplified and recorded graphically.

26. The resistance to left ventricular blood flow offered by the systemic circulation (*abbreviation*).

27. Ability of certain specialized cells of the heart to depolarize spontaneously.

28. The impedance to right ventricular blood flow offered by the pulmonary circulation (*abbreviation*).

31. A period of rest of the atria of the heart (*two words*).

32. A muscle cell.

35. The long period of reduced filling that typically follows the rapid-filling period during the first third of ventricular filling.

38. A self-propagating electrical impulse transmitted across the plasma membrane of nerve or muscle cells (*two words*).

39. _____ depolarization occurs within nodal tissue during phase 4.

40. _____ sounds are heard during the taking of blood pressure with a blood pressure cuff and a manometer.

41. Ability of cardiac tissue to propagate an action potential.

42. Blood pressure cuff.

43. Sinus _____ is a slow heart rate with normal electrocardiographic waves and complexes.

Down

1. Ventricular _____ is the complete absence of any ventricular electrical activity.

2. Repeated episodes of atrial tachycardia with an abrupt onset lasting from a few seconds to many hours (*abbreviation*).

3. Refers to the tissues that surround the heart and to the fact that they conduct electrical impulses (*two words*).

5. An abbreviation for a cardiac arrhythmia that is characterized by at least 3 consecutive ventricular complexes with a rate of more than 100 bpm that originates distal to the bundle of His.

7. _____ syndrome is an unusual rhythm that results from the presence of an abnormal route of conduction that bypasses the atrioventricular nodes (*abbreviation*).

8. An abnormal conduction delay (*two words*).

11. The automatic depolarization and repolarization of cardiac tissue in a repetitive and stable manner.

12. _____ refractory period begins during the middle of phase 3 and lasts until the beginning of phase 4.

13. _____ refractory period occurs when a myocyte cannot be depolarized no matter how strong the stimulus.

15. The _____ refractory period occurs when the cardiac tissue is unable to propagate an impulse.

17. Sinus _____ is a rapid heart rate with normal electrocardiographic waves and complexes.

18. _____ escape rhythm typically occurs in cases of sinus block or sinus arrest.

19. Impedance _____ is a technique that enables the detection of blood vessel occlusion that dictates volumetric changes in an area of the body.

20. _____ contraction occurs when all valves are closed.

22. An ECG with a "sawtooth" appearance (*two words*).

24. Isovolumetric _____ is the period of time between the closure of the semilunar valves and the opening of the atrioventricular valves.

25. A single heartbeat (*two words*).

29. The product of pressure and volume measurements that accompany ventricular contraction (*two words*).

30. _____ electrodes use electrolyte gel or paste.

33. _____ arrhythmia is the waxing and waning of the heart rate with the breathing cycle.

34. Ventricular _____ begins with the closure of the aortic and pulmonary valves.

36. A small negative deflection on the aortic and pulmonary artery tracing associated with a transient reversal of flow as a result of elastic recoil of the vessels.

37. Abnormal heart sounds.

ACHIEVING THE OBJECTIVES

1. Discuss the electrophysiologic properties of the heart.

1A. Define the three most important aspects of the electrophysiology of the heart.

_____

_____

_____

_____

1B. What is a polarized cell?

_____

_____

1C. Specialized cells with automaticity are located in which areas of the heart?

_____

_____

1D. Why is the inside of a cardiac cell negatively charged?

_____

_____

_____

_____

_____

129

1E. What allows ions to move across cell membranes?

_____

_____

1F. Describe the function of the sodium-potassium adenosine triphosphatase pump.

_____

_____

_____

_____

1G. What causes the change in membrane potential that results in depolarization of the cardiac cells?

_____

_____

_____

_____

1H. Use Figure 9-1 to match the following phases with their associated conditions.

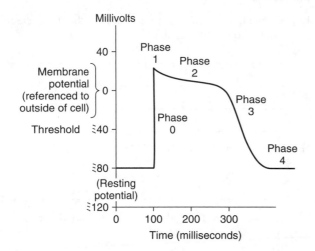

FIGURE 9-1

__1.	Phase 0	a.	Myocyte can be depolarized again by a stronger-than-normal stimulus.
__2.	Phase 1	b.	Partial repolarization occurs.
__3.	Phase 2	c.	Resting membrane potential.
__4.	Phase 3	d.	Regardless of the strength of the stimulus, the myocyte cannot be depolarized again.
__5.	Phase 4	e.	A series of slow calcium and sodium channels open.
__6.	Absolute refractory period	f.	Rapid upstroke or depolarization.
__7.	Relative refractory period	g.	Return toward the negative resting membrane potential.

1I. Within what tissues are the action potentials shown in Figure 9-1 found? What are they called?

_____

_____

_____

_____

1J. What type of cardiac tissues have slow action potentials?

_____

_____

1K. Decreasing the threshold potential of the sinoatrial (SA) node will cause _____. Increasing the threshold potential of the SA node will cause

_____.

1L. Label the heart and its electrical anatomy as depicted in Figure 9-2.

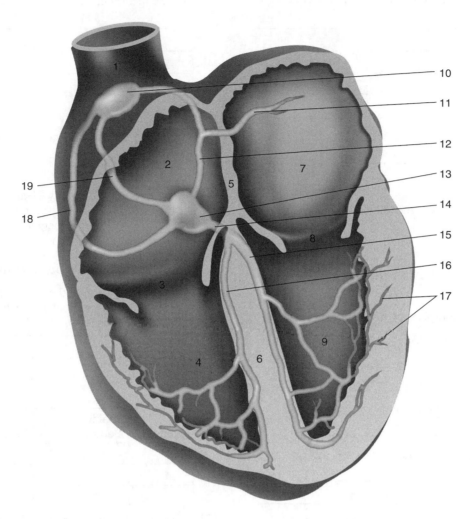

FIGURE 9-2
(From Wilkins RL, Stoller JK, Kacmarek RM: *Egan's fundamentals of respiratory care*, ed 9, St Louis, 2009, Mosby.)

1.	
2.	
3.	
4.	
5.	
6.	
7.	
8.	
9.	
10.	

11.	
12.	
13.	
14.	
15.	
16.	
17.	
18.	
19.	

Chapter **9** **Assessment of Cardiovascular Function**

1M. What is the function of the delay in conduction rate that occurs within the atrioventricular (AV) node?

_____

_____

1N. In what direction do the ventricles repolarize?

_____

_____

_____

Think About This

Can tachycardia affect cardiac output?

Helpful Web Site

■ Boston Scientific, *LifeBeat Online*, "The Heart's Electrical System" — http://www.bostonscientific.com

2. Explain the principles of electrocardiography.

2A. What does the electrocardiogram (ECG) represent?

_____

_____

2B. What is meant by a *volume conductor*?

_____

_____

_____

_____

2C. Which electrode is the sensing electrode?

_____

2D. What causes an upward deflection on the ECG's recording paper?

_____

_____

_____

_____

2E. What causes a downward deflection on the ECG's recording paper?

_____

_____

_____

_____

2F. How might heart disease affect an electrocardiographic recording?

_____

_____

_____

_____

Think About This

Why is there an electrocardiographic tracing during cardiopulmonary resuscitation?

Helpful Web Site

■ Peking (Beijing) University Health Science Center, "Basic Principles of Electrocardiographic Interpretation," Ary L. Goldberger — eMedicineHealth Electrocardiogram http://www.emedicinehealth.com

3. Identify the major components of an ECG.

3A. What is the function of the conduction jelly or electrolyte paste used on floating electrodes?

_____

_____

3B. Complete the following table for the augmented leads.

Lead	Positive electrode	Zero reference

3C. Name four causes of electrical interference that can occur during electrocardiography.

_____

_____

_____

_____

3D. How far apart are the ruled lines on an ECG's paper?

_____

_____

3E. Label the ECG machine in Figure 9-3.

_____

_____

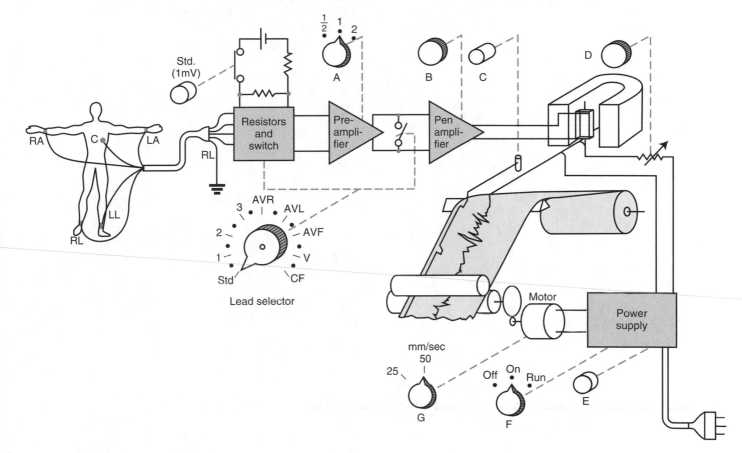

FIGURE 9-3
(Modified from Cromwell L, Weibell FJ, Pfeiffer EA: *Biomedical instrumentation and measurements*, ed 2, Englewood Cliffs, NJ, 1980, Prentice-Hall.)

Think About This

Is it possible to construct a homemade ECG machine?

Helpful Web Sites

■ Mad Scientist Software Inc, MicroEKG Manual, "What is an ECG?" — http://www.madsci.com

■ The University of Sydney (Australia), School of Electrical & Information Engineering, ECG information — http://www.eelab.usyd.edu.au

4. Demonstrate the correct placement of electrodes on a patient to obtain a 12-lead ECG.

4A. Circle and number precordial chest lead placement on Figure 9-4.

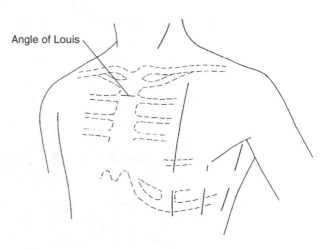

FIGURE 9-4
(From Goldberger AL: *Clinical electrocardiography: a simplified approach*, ed 7, St Louis, 2006, Mosby.)

4B. Identify the components of Einthoven's triangle in Figure 9-5.

_____

_____

_____

_____

Think About This

How would a misplaced lead effect the ECG?

Helpful Web Site

■ "Electrodes, Leads & Wires: A Practical Guide to ECG Monitoring and Recording," Mike Cowley — http://www.mikecowley.co.uk

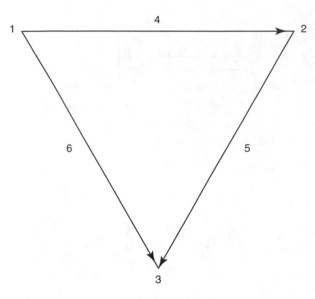

FIGURE 9-5

5. Explain the various waves, complexes and intervals that appear on a normal ECG.

Questions in this section all refer to Figure 9-6.

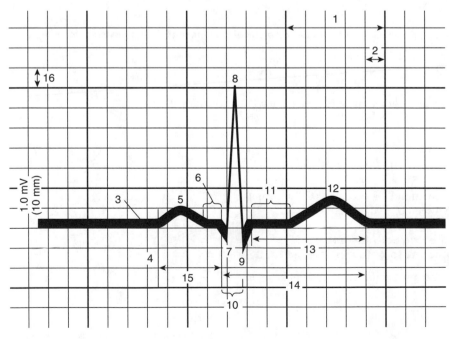

FIGURE 9-6

5A. How long is the interval represented by line 1?

_____

5B. How long is the interval represented by line 2?

_____

5C. What is the name of line 3?

_____

5D. What is the name of line 6?

_____

5E. What is the name of the portion of the ECG represented by 13?

_____

5F. How much amplitude does line 16 represent?

_____

5G. Complete the following table that refers to the waves of an ECG.

Wave/ complex/ interval	Name	Normal duration/ amplitude	Representation
5			
15			
10			
11			
12			
14			

Think About This
What is Brugada syndrome?

Helpful Web Sites
- University of Utah School of Medicine, The ECG Learning Center, Frank G. Yanowitz — http://library.med.utah.edu
- Cardiovascular Physiology Concepts, Richard E. Klabunde — http://cvphysiology.com
- ECG Library, "A Normal Adult 12-lead ECG," Dean Jenkins and Stephen Gerred — http://www.ecglibrary.com

6. List and describe the most common dysrhythmias encountered in clinical electrocardiography.

6A. What is respiratory sinus arrhythmia?

_____

6B. What are the rhythm and rate shown in Figure 9-7?

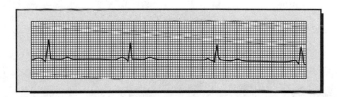

FIGURE 9-7

6C. What type of arrhythmia causes a ventricular rate of >100 bpm with the SA node as the source of cardiac excitation? _____

6D. What type of arrhythmia is shown in Figure 9-8? _____

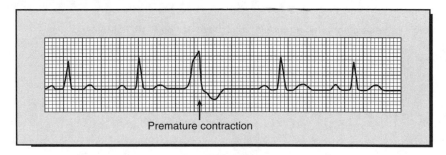

Premature contraction

FIGURE 9-8

Chapter **9** **Assessment of Cardiovascular Function**

6E. What type of arrhythmia is caused by premature atrial depolarizations with prolonged AV conduction time?

_____

6F. Impulses that originate in or near the AV node cause what type of a cardiac rhythm?

_____

6G. What type of arrhythmia is shown in Figure 9-9?

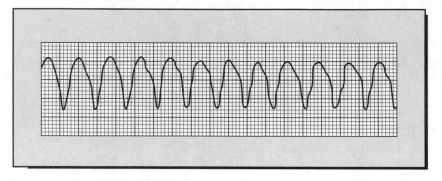

FIGURE 9-9

6H. The presence of a bypass tract in the AV nodes that causes a delta wave following the P wave is known as

_____.

6I. What arrhythmia causes gross irregularities in both atrial and ventricular depolarizations with an atrial rate between 400 bpm and 700 bpm and a ventricular rate between 120 bpm and 200 bpm?

_____

6J. What type of cardiac arrhythmia causes a "sawtooth" appearance?

_____

6K. What type of arrhythmia is shown in Figure 9-10?

_____

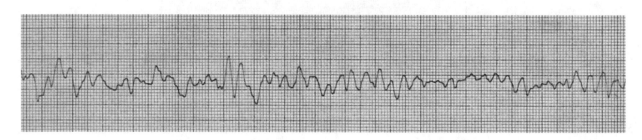

FIGURE 9-10
(From Seidel JC, ed: *Basic electrocardiography: a modular approach.* St Louis, 1986, Mosby.)

6L. What type of arrhythmia is shown in Figure 9-11?

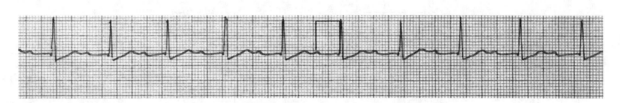

FIGURE 9-11
(From Seidel JC, ed: *Basic electrocardiography: a modular approach.* St Louis, 1986, Mosby.)

6M. Describe the difference between a Mobitz type I block and a Mobitz type II block.

6N. A complete dissociation of atrial and ventricular conduction causes what type of arrhythmia?

6O. Name five causes of right bundle branch blocks.

6P. Name two causes of left bundle branch blocks.

Think About This
What types of arrhythmias can tracheobronchial suctioning cause?

Helpful Web Site
■ The Cleveland Clinic, "Common Types of Arrhythmias" — http://my.clevelandclinic.org

7. Describe the pressure, volume, and flow events that occur in the heart and major blood vessels during a typical cardiac cycle.

7A. What are the two main parts of the cardiac cycle?

7B. What electrocardiographic waveform corresponds with isovolumetric contraction?

7C. Why does the volume in the ventricles remain constant during isovolumetric contraction of the heart?

7D. How much pressure is generated in the left and right ventricles during isovolumetric contraction?

7E. What opens the semilunar valves of the heart?

7F. What are the peak systolic pressures in the left and right ventricles?

Questions 7G through 7K refer to Figure 9-12.

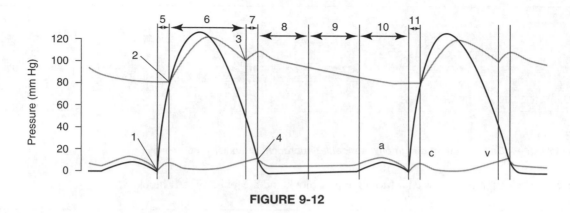

FIGURE 9-12

7G. At what points on Figure 9-12 do the following events occur?

Mitral valve closes _____ Aortic valve opens _____

Aortic valve closes _____ Mitral valve opens _____

7H. Identify the cardiac flow events that are indicated by the following points on Figure 9-12.

Point 5 _____

_____

Point 6 _____

_____

Point 7 _____

_____

Point 8 _____

_____

Point 9 _____

_____

Point 10 _____

_____

Point 11 _____

_____

7I. In Figure 9-12, the letter "a" on the atrial pressure tracing represents what atrial event?

_____

_____

7J. In Figure 9-12, the letter "c" on the atrial pressure tracing represents what atrial event?

_____

_____

7K. In Figure 9-12, the letter "v" on the atrial pressure tracing represents what atrial event?

_____

_____

Think About This

How would aortic valve leakage change the pressure, volume, and flow events of the cardiac cycle?

Helpful Web Sites

■ CTSNet Wiki Notes, "The Cardiac Cycle" — http:// wiki.ctsnet.org

■ University of Kansas, School of Nursing, Advanced Cardiac Assessment, Sharon Kumm — http://classes. kumc.edu

8. **Explain the principles of operation of various noninvasive and invasive devices that are routinely used to obtain blood pressure measurements.**

8A. How does a sphygmomanometer measure blood pressure?

_____

_____

_____

_____

_____

_____

_____

_____

_____

_____

8B. Why does the tapping sound disappear when measuring noninvasive blood pressure?

_____

_____

8C. How are pressure pulsations detected with an automated blood pressure system?

_____

_____

_____

8D. What are the errors most commonly encountered while determining arterial blood pressure with either a manual or an automated blood pressure monitoring system?

_____

_____

_____

_____

8E. What devices are used to determine intravascular and intracardiac pressures?

_____

_____

8F. What type of device is used to measure right-sided heart pressure?

_____

_____

8G. Explain the purpose of each lumen of a four-lumen thermodilution catheter.

_____

_____

_____

_____

_____

_____

_____

_____

8H. How are aortic pressure, left ventricular pressure, and left atrium pressure measured?

_____

_____

_____

8I. What is the transseptal approach to left-sided heart catheterization?

_____

_____

_____

8J. Name the three types of pressure transducers.

_____

_____

_____

8K. Which pressure transducers are the most frequently used?

_____

_____

Think About This

Why must a left-sided heart catheterization be performed in the cardiac catheterization lab, whereas right-sided heart catheterization can be performed at the bedside?

139

Helpful Web Sites

■ *Critical Care Nurse* journal, "Noninvasive Blood Pressure Monitoring," Kathleen R. Dobbin — http://ccn.aacnjournals.org

■ University of Virginia Health System, "Procedure: Placing a Pulmonary Artery Catheter" — http://www.healthsystem.virginia.edu

9. Describe various methods that are used to measure cardiac output.

9A. What information is necessary to use Fick's direct method of calculating cardiac output?

_____

_____

_____

_____

9B. What is the formula for Fick's direct method?

_____

_____

9C. How is cardiac output measured with use of the indicator dilution method?

_____

_____

_____

_____

_____

_____

_____

_____

_____

9D. How is cardiac output measured with use of the thermodilution technique?

_____

_____

_____

_____

_____

_____

9E. How is impedance plethysmography used to determine cardiac output?

_____

_____

_____

_____

_____

_____

_____

_____

9F. How is bioimpedance used to measure cardiac output?

_____

_____

_____

_____

9G. What is the difference between the Fick's direct and Fick's indirect method of calculating cardiac output?

_____

_____

_____

_____

_____

Think About This

Does respiratory variation in pulmonary blood flow cause changes in cardiac output measurements?

Helpful Web Sites

■ Medical College of Georgia, "Indirect Measurement of Cardiac Output" — http://www.lib.mcg.edu

■ Internet Scientific Publications, *The Internet Journal of Anesthesiology*, "Paradigm Shift in Hemodynamic Monitoring," Lailu Mathews — http://www.ispub.com

10. Interpret hemodynamic measurements that are obtained from patients in a critical care setting.

10A. How can tachycardia lead to decreased cardiac output?

_____

_____

10B. What factors are the focus of a hemodynamic profile?

_____

_____

10C. What measurements are used to estimate right ventricular end-diastolic pressure and left ventricular end-diastolic pressure?

_____

_____

10D. What are two reasons for a reduction in cardiac output?

_____

_____

10E. Complete the following table with the equations and normal ranges for each hemodynamic measurement:

Hemodynamic measurement	Formula	Normal range
Cardiac output ($\dot{Q}$)		
Cardiac index (CI)		
Stroke index (SI)		
Systemic vascular resistance (SVR)		
Pulmonary vascular resistance (PVR)		
Left ventricular stroke work (LSW)		
Right ventricular stroke work (RSW)		
Left ventricular stroke work index (LSWI)		
Right ventricular stroke work index (RSWI)		

10F. A 55-year-old female patient is admitted to the emergency department with ischemic heart disease requiring three coronary artery bypass grafts. After surgery the patient is being maintained on mechanical ventilation. She has an intraaortic balloon pump and a pulmonary artery catheter in place. Use the following data to calculate the patient's cardiac index, stroke index, LSWI, RSWI, SVR, and PVR.

Body surface area = 1.7 m^2 $\dot{Q} = 4.0$ L/min

Mean arterial pressure = 68 mm Hg

Mean pulmonary artery pressure = 36 mm Hg
Pulmonary capillary wedge pressure = 14 mm Hg
Central venous pressure = 18 mm Hg

Heart rate = 98 bpm

_____

_____

_____

_____

_____

_____

_____

_____

_____

_____

Think About This
Are hemodynamic profiles appropriate for all mechanically ventilated patients?

Helpful Web Site
■ "Hemodynamic Calculations," M. L. Cheatham — http://www.surgicalcriticalcare.net

NATIONAL BOARD FOR RESPIRATORY CARE (NBRC)–TYPE QUESTIONS

1. β-adrenergic blocking agents, such as propranolol, can cause which of the following?
   A. Sinoatrial block
   B. Sinus tachycardia
   C. Sinus bradycardia
   D. Premature atrial beats

2. Failure of the sinoatrial node to depolarize or failure of the atrioventricular (AV) node to conduct impulses will result in which of the following cardiac arrhythmias?
   A. Atrial fibrillation
   B. Junctional escape rhythm
   C. Premature ventricular beats
   D. Paroxysmal atrial tachycardia

3. The heart block that causes "dropped" beats and that is often the result of increased parasympathetic tone is which of the following?
   A. Sinoatrial block
   B. Mobitz type I block
   C. First-degree AV block
   D. Left bundle branch block

4. "Pressure rises in the ventricles, but no blood is ejected" is the definition of which of the following?
   A. Ventricular systole
   B. Ventricular diastole
   C. Isovolumetric relaxation
   D. Isovolumetric contraction

5. The right ventricle peak systolic pressure is how many mm Hg?
   A. 15
   B. 25
   C. 80
   D. 120

6. Closure of the semilunar valves and opening of the AV valves is associated with which heart sound?
   A. S1
   B. S2
   C. S3
   D. S4

7. The respiratory therapist is unable to "wedge" the pulmonary artery catheter 24 hours after insertion. The problem is most likely caused by which of the following?
   A. Pneumothorax
   B. Balloon rupture
   C. Catheter knotting
   D. Pulmonary artery rupture

8. Use Fick's direct method to calculate cardiac output for a patient with the following hemodynamic values:

Partial pressure of arterial oxygen (PaO_2) = 80 mm Hg	Hemoximetry oxygen saturation (SaO_2) = 90%	Hemoglobin = 14 gm/dL
Partial pressure of oxygen in mixed venous blood ($P_{\bar{V}}O_2$) = 35 mm Hg	Saturation of oxygen in mixed venous blood ($S_{\bar{V}}O_2$) = 65%	P_{bar} = 760 mm Hg
	Oxygen consumption ($\dot{V}O_2$) = 210 mL/min	

   A. 3.5 mL/min
   B. 4.38 mL/min
   C. 5.83 mL/min
   D. 6.15 mL/min

9. Calculate cardiac index when cardiac output = 5.0 mL/min and body surface area = 2.9 m^2.
   A. 1.72 L/min/m^2
   B. 1.67 L/min/m^2
   C. 2.10 L/min/m^2
   D. 12.5 L/min/m^2

10. Calculation of systemic vascular resistance is 1700 dyne sec/cm^{-5}. Which of the following is consistent with this value?
    A. Elevated left ventricular afterload
    B. Elevated right ventricular afterload
    C. Decreased left ventricular preload
    D. Decreased right ventricular preload

10 Blood Gas Monitoring

Upon completion of this chapter, you will be able to:
1. Describe how to perform and evaluate the modified Allen test.
2. Identify various sites used to obtain samples for blood gas analysis.
3. Label the components of a modern, in vitro blood gas analyzer.
4. Compare the operational principles of the pH, partial pressure of carbon dioxide (PCO_2), and partial pressure of oxygen (PO_2) electrodes.
5. Apply values for PO_2 at which 50% saturation of hemoglobin occurs (P_{50}), as well as for bicarbonate, buffer base, and base excess, in the interpretation of arterial blood gases (ABGs).
6. Explain the operational principle of carbon monoxide (CO)–oximetry.
7. Name the components of a quality assurance program for blood gas analysis.
8. Compare the effect of hyperthermia and hypothermia on ABGs.
9. Describe physiologic and technical factors that can affect pulse oximeter readings.
10. Identify various factors that can influence transcutaneous PO_2 and PCO_2 measurements.
11. State the criteria for identifying four types of acid-base disorders.

"You know you're old if they have discontinued your blood type."
Phyllis Diller

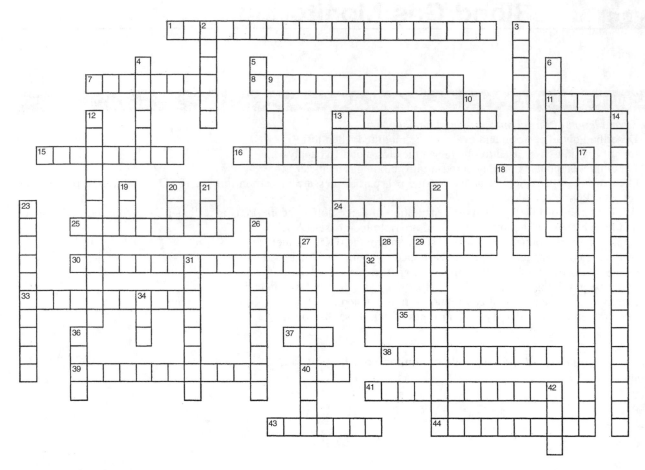

CROSSWORD PUZZLE 10-1
Created using Crossword Weaver, www.CrosswordWeaver.com.

Use the clues to complete the crossword puzzle.

Across

1. The use of light waves to detect changes in the volume of an organ or tissue.

7. Optical _____ does not allow light to come in contact with the vascular bed, causing pulse oximetry readings to be erroneously high or low.

8. The partial pressure of this gas is normally between 35 mm Hg and 45 mm Hg.

11. The standard pH electrode.

13. _____ hemoglobin saturation equals oxyhemoglobin divided by the concentration of hemoglobin capable of carrying oxygen.

15. A contact for the induction or detection of electrical activity.

16. Procedures that do not require access to the inside of the body are said to be _____.

18. Requires access to the inside of the body.

24. Occurring in laboratory apparatus (*two words*).

25. The total amount of this substance is capable of binding hydrogen ions (*two words*).

29. An equation that expresses the relationship between the electrical potential across a membrane and the concentration ratio between permeable ions on either side of the membrane.

30. This chemical formula uses the ratio of the conjugate base to the weak acid (*two words*). **See 28 down.**

33. Testing outside of the main hospital laboratory by using portable devices (*three words*).

35. A calibration that involves adjusting the electronic output to two known standards (*two words*).

37. Used in instruments to display digital data (*abbreviation*).

38. Too little alkalinity is known as _____ (*two words*).

39. Charts that are used as a method of recording quality control data (*two words*).
40. Blood drawn from a capillary to check for acid-base status and oxygenation status (*abbreviation*).
41. Refers to measuring an electric current at a single applied potential.
43. A type of plethysmography that is used to define systolic and diastolic time periods during the cardiac cycle.
44. Temperature _____ applies mathematical formulae to adjust blood gas tensions to more accurately reflect the patient's core temperature.

Down

2. When the partial pressure of this gas is low, the patient requires a supplement.
3. This is equal to what is attached to the hemoglobin plus what is dissolved in the plasma (*two words*).
4. Occurring in a living organism (*two words*).
5. A planned, systematic approach to designing, measuring, assessing, and improving performance (*abbreviation*).
6. A type of sensor designed to react to physical stimulation from light or other radiant energy.
9. A test to check for a patent ulnar artery.
10. Any evaluation of services provided and the results achieved as compared with accepted standards (*abbreviation*).
12. A small, transparent tube or container with specific optical properties.
13. _____ hemoglobin saturation equals oxyhemoglobin divided by the amount of all four types of hemoglobin present.
14. Yellow discoloration of the skin associated with hepatic dysfunction.
17. A nomogram used for calculating actual and standard bicarbonate concentrations (*two words*). **See also 25 across and 26 down**.
19. Has a greater affinity for oxygen than its adult counterpart (*abbreviation*).
20. All hemoglobin (*abbreviation*).
21. A type of hemoglobin that does not allow normal oxygen binding (*abbreviation*).
22. Refers to measuring voltage.
23. A calibration that should be performed every 6 months (*two words*).
26. Too much alkalinity is known as _____ (*two words*).
27. A type of sensor that uses dyes that "light up" when struck by light in the ultraviolet or near-ultraviolet visible range.
28. The scale for which the neutral value is 7.0 (*abbreviation*).

31. A calibration that involves adjusting the electronic output to a single, known standard (*two words*).
32. The electrode that measures the partial pressure of oxygen in the blood.
34. The component of a computer that controls the encoding and execution of instructions.
36. One of the cells of an electrode that measures the answer to **28 down**.
42. Amendments, developed in 1988, that require routine calibrations of instruments (*abbreviation*).

ACHIEVING THE OBJECTIVES

1. Describe how to perform and evaluate the modified Allen test.

1A. When should the modified Allen's test be used?

_____

_____

1B. Why does a patient need to clench her fist during the Allen's test?

_____

_____

1C. Identify the two blood vessels depicted in Figure 10-1.

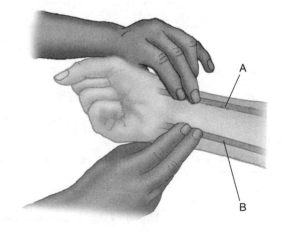

FIGURE 10-1
(From Wilkins RL, Stoller JK, Kacmarek RM: *Egan's fundamentals of respiratory care*, ed 9, St Louis, 2009, Mosby.)

_____

_____

1D. What is the purpose of applying pressure to both blood vessels shown in Figure 10-1?

_____

_____

1E. How should the hand appear when the patient releases his fist while the vessels are occluded?

_____

_____

1F. Which blood vessel is released first?

_____

1G. How do you assess a negative result for the Allen's test?

_____

_____

_____

1H. How do you assess a positive result for the Allen's test?

_____

_____

_____

_____

1I. What should you do if the result of the Allen's test is negative? Positive?

_____

_____

_____

_____

_____

_____

_____

Think About This

Can an Allen's test be performed on an unconscious patient?

Helpful Web Sites

■ YouTube, Arterial Blood Gas Demonstration — http://www.youtube.com

■ University of Connecticut Health Center, Acid Base Online Tutorial, "Modified Allen's Test" — http://fitsweb.uchc.edu

2. Identify various sites used to obtain samples for blood gas analysis.

2A. Identify and name the four most common percutaneous sampling sites in Figure 10-2.

_____

_____

_____

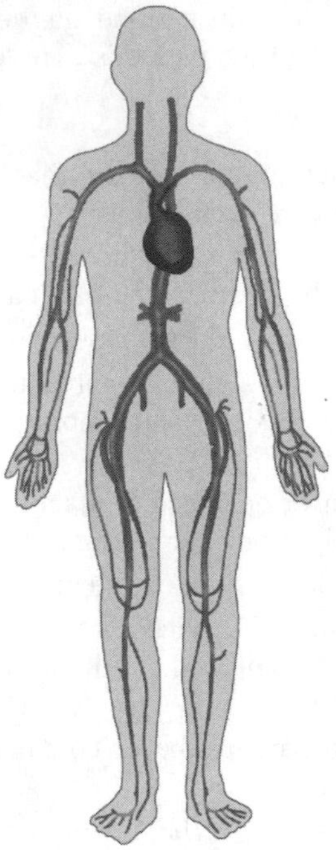

FIGURE 10-2
(From Wilkins RL, Stoller JK, Kacmarek RM: *Egan's fundamentals of respiratory care*, ed 9, St Louis, 2009, Mosby.)

2B. Through what type of catheter are mixed venous blood samples drawn?

_____

_____

2C. Capillary blood samples can be drawn from what site?

_____

_____

Think About This

Why does the bevel of the needle need to be facing up when you are drawing an arterial blood gas sample?

Helpful Web Site

■ Dalhousie University, "Arterial Blood Gas Sampling" [video] — http://www.youtube.com

3. Label the components of a modern, in vitro blood gas analyzer.

3A. Label the pH electrode shown in Figure 10-3.

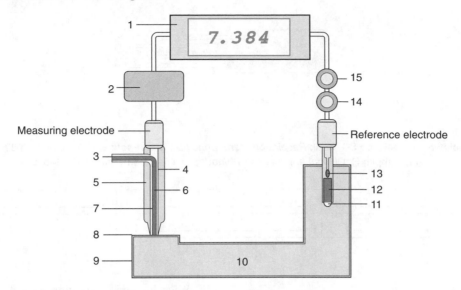

Measuring electrode

Reference electrode

FIGURE 10-3

(From Hess DR, MacIntyre NM, Mishoe SC, et al: *Respiratory care: principles and practice*, Philadelphia, 2002, WB Saunders.)

1. _____	2. _____	3. _____
4. _____	5. _____	6. _____
7. _____	8. _____	9. _____
10. _____	11. _____	12. _____
13. _____	14. _____	15. _____

3B. Label the Stowe-Severinghaus electrode shown in Figure 10-4.

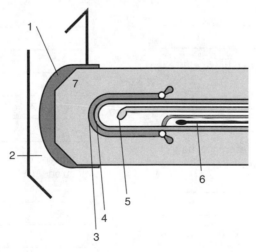

FIGURE 10-4

(Redrawn from Shapiro BA, Peruzzi WT, Templin R: *Clinical application of blood gases*, ed 5, St Louis, 1994, Mosby.)

1. _____	2. _____	3. _____
4. _____	5. _____	6. _____
7. _____		

3C. Label the Clark electrode shown in Figure 10-5.

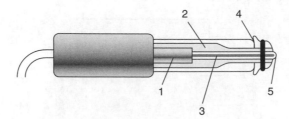

FIGURE 10-5

(From Hess DR, MacIntyre NM, Mishoe SC, et al: *Respiratory care: principles and practice*, Philadelphia, 2002, WB Saunders. From Shapiro BA, Peruzzi WT, Templin R: *Clinical application of blood gases*, ed 5, St Louis, 1994, Mosby.)

1. _____	2. _____	3. _____
4. _____	5. _____	

Think About This

What other uses do pH, partial pressure of carbon dioxide (PCO_2), and partial pressure of oxygen (PO_2) electrodes have?

Helpful Web Site

■ Anaesthetist.com, "Simply Acid-Base" — http://www.anaesthetist.com

4. Compare the operational principles of the pH, PCO_2, and PO_2 electrodes.

4A. Which electrode has a silver anode and a platinum cathode?

_____

_____

4B. Which electrode is composed of two half-cells, each composed of silver–silver chloride?

_____

_____

4C. Which electrode has a calomel reference half-cell and a silver–silver chloride electrode?

_____

_____

4D. The pH electrode uses what two immersion solutions?

_____

_____

_____

_____

4E. What immersion solution does the PCO_2 electrode use?

_____

_____

4F. What immersion solution does the PO_2 electrode use?

_____

_____

4G. What type of measurement technique is used in the pH electrode?

_____

_____

_____

_____

_____

4H. What type of measurement technique does the PCO_2 electrode use?

_____

_____

_____

_____

_____

4I. The PO_2 electrode uses what type of measurement technique?

_____

_____

_____

_____

4J. What equation represents what occurs within the pH electrode?

_____

_____

4K. The chemical reaction that occurs in the immersion solution of the PCO_2 electrode is:

_____

_____.

4L. How is pH related to the PCO_2?

_____

_____

Think About This

What other types of chemical electrodes exist?

Helpful Web Site

■ ABG Analysis — http://virtual.yosemite.cc.ca.us

5. Apply values for PO_2 at which 50% saturation of hemoglobin occurs (P_{50}), as well as for bicarbonate, buffer base, and base excess, in the interpretation of arterial blood gases (ABGs).

5A. Take the following factors into account.

pH 7.22	Partial pressure of arterial carbon dioxide ($PaCO_2$) 55 mm Hg	Bicarbonate ($HCO_3.$) 25 mEq/L	Partial pressure of arterial oxygen (PaO_2) 60 mm Hg	Hemoximetry oxygen saturation (SaO_2) 88%
Fractional inspired oxygen (F_IO_2) Nasal Cannula (NC) 3 L/min	Age 45			

Offer your interpretation of these data:

_____

_____

5B. Take the following factors into account.

pH 7.32	$PaCO_2$ 32 mm Hg	$HCO_3.$ 18 mEq/L	PaO_2 101 mm Hg	SaO_2 97%
F_IO_2 room air	Age 58			

Offer your interpretation of these data:

_____

_____

5C. Take the following factors into account.

pH 7.43	$PaCO_2$ 48 mm Hg	$HCO_3.$ 36 mEq/L	PaO_2 91 mm Hg	SaO_2 97%
F_IO_2 NC 3 L/min	Age 66			

Offer your interpretation of these data:

_____

_____

5D. Take the following factors into account.

pH 7.48	$PaCO_2$ 22 mm Hg	$HCO_3.$ 16 mEq/L	PaO_2 96 mm Hg	SaO_2 98%
F_IO_2 room air	Age 18			

Offer your interpretation of these data:

_____

_____

Use Figure 10-6 to complete questions 5E through 5G

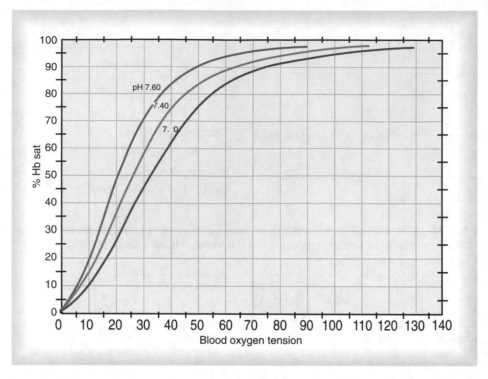

FIGURE 10-6
(From Wilkins RL, Stoller JK, Kacmarek RM: *Egan's fundamentals of respiratory care*, ed 9, St Louis, 2009, Mosby.)

5E. What is the P_{50} for a pH of 7.60?

_____

5F. What is the P_{50} for a pH of 7.40?

_____

5G. What is the P_{50} for a pH of 7.20?

_____

5H. A low P_{50} represents what type of change in the oxyhemoglobin dissociation curve?

_____

_____

5I. A high P_{50} represents what type of change in the oxyhemoglobin dissociation curve?

_____

_____

Think About This

Are the ABGs of other animals similar to those of humans?

Helpful Web Sites

■ Acid-Base Tutorial, Alan W. Grogono — http://www.acid-base.com

■ VentWorld, Oxyhemoglobin Dissociation Curve Interactive Tool — http://www.ventworld.com

6. Explain the operational principle of carbon monoxide (CO)–oximetry.

6A. What values does an in vitro CO-oximeter measure?

_____

_____

6B. What is spectrophotometry?

_____

_____

_____

6C. What law is used to determine the actual concentration of hemoglobin in an arterial blood sample?

_____

_____

_____

_____

_____

_____

6D. What is the first step in the operation of a CO-oximeter?

_____

_____

6E. What is the second step in the operation of a CO-oximeter?

_____

_____

6F. How is light transmission measured by means of the CO-oximeter?

_____

_____

_____

_____

_____

_____

6G. What factors interfere with CO-oximetry measurements?

_____

_____

_____

_____

_____

_____

Think About This

What advantage does fetal hemoglobin provide by causing a left shift in the oxygen dissociation curve?

Helpful Web Site

■ *Clinical Chemistry* journal, "Interference of Fetal Hemoglobin with the Spectrophotometric Measurement of Carboxyhemoglobin," Hendrik J. Vreman et al — http://www.clinchem.org

7. Name the components of a quality assurance program for blood gas analysis.

7A. Which agencies publish the standards that clinical blood gas laboratories must follow?

_____

_____

_____

_____

7B. What is the definition of *quality control*?

_____

_____

_____

_____

7C. What is the definition of *quality assurance*?

_____

_____

_____

_____

7D. What are the components of a quality assurance program for blood gas analysis?

_____

_____

_____

_____

_____

_____

7E. How is blood gas analyzer proficiency testing accomplished?

_____

_____

_____

_____

_____

_____

_____

7F. What are the generally acceptable limits for pH, PCO_2, and PO_2 in proficiency testing?

_____

_____

_____

_____

Think About This

What steps need to be taken to obtain a Clinical Laboratory Improvement Amendments certification for a blood gas lab?

Helpful Web Sites

■ American Association for Respiratory Care (AARC), *Respiratory Care* journal, "AARC Clinical Practice Guideline: Blood Gas Analysis and Hemoximetry:

2001 Revision & Update" — http://www.rcjournal.com

- AARC, "Critical Details of Arterial Blood Gas Laboratory Certification," John Olmstead and Brenda Wilkerson — http://www.aarc.org

8. Compare the effect of hyperthermia and hypothermia on ABGs.

8A. What effect does temperature have on the PaO_2?

_____

_____

8B. For every degree Celsius, how much will the $PaCO_2$ change?

_____

8C. For every degree Celsius, how much will the pH change?

_____

8D. What happens to the oxyhemoglobin dissociation curve when the patient is hypothermic?

_____

_____

_____

8E. What happens to the oxyhemoglobin dissociation curve when the patient is hyperthermic?

_____

_____

_____

_____

Think About This

Why is there such a controversy over temperature correction for ABG parameters?

Helpful Web Site

- "The Interactive Oxyhemoglobin Dissociation Curve," Nielufar Varjavand — http://www.ventworld.com

9. Describe physiologic and technical factors that can affect pulse oximeter readings.

9A. Why do low perfusion states cause intermittent or absent saturations when measured by pulse oximetry?

_____

_____

9B. Name three physiologic causes and one technical cause of low perfusion states.

_____

_____

_____

_____

9C. How can the problem of low perfusion states be prevented when pulse oximetry is used?

_____

_____

9D. How do high levels of carboxyhemoglobin alter pulse oximetry oxygen saturation (SpO_2) measurements?

_____

_____

_____

9E. What type of hemoglobin absorbs both red and infrared light?

_____

9F. How will this type of hemoglobin (from Question 9E) affect the pulse oximeter reading?

_____

_____

_____

_____

_____

9G. What can cause the production of the hemoglobin discussed in Questions 9E and 9F?

_____

_____

9H. During cardiac catheterizations, what might cause a false drop in the patient's SpO_2?

_____

_____

_____

_____

9I. How do dark nail polishes affect SpO$_2$ readings?

_____

_____

_____

_____

9J. What types of light sources might adversely affect heart rate and SpO$_2$ readings?

_____

_____

9K. How do pulse oximeters compensate for ambient light interference?

_____

_____

_____

_____

Think About This

What role does pulse oximetry play in the diagnosis of sleep apnea?

Helpful Web Sites

- Oximetry.org, "Principles of Pulse Oximetry Technology" — http://www.oximetry.org
- *Respiratory Care* journal, "AARC Clinical Practice Guideline: Pulse Oximetry" — http://www.rcjournal.com

10. Identify various factors that can influence transcutaneous PO$_2$ and PCO$_2$ measurements.

10A. How could a heater failure of the transcutaneous PO$_2$ electrode affect its ability to measure?

_____

_____

_____

10B. How are transcutaneous PO$_2$ (PtcO$_2$) measurements influenced by peripheral perfusion?

_____

_____

_____

10C. Which pathologic states can lead to erroneous PtcO$_2$ measurements in a patient?

_____

_____

_____

10D. What effect does a decreasing cardiac index have on the accuracy of PtcO$_2$ measurements?

_____

_____

_____

10E. Why does heating a carbon dioxide electrode cause a slightly higher reading of the PtcO$_2$ than the PaCO$_2$?

_____

_____

10F. Why should the site for the electrode placement be prepped by cleansing and (if necessary) shaving?

_____

_____

10G. What potential adverse effect can the heat at the electrode site cause?

_____

_____

_____

10H. Why should electrodes be cleaned periodically?

_____

10I. Why should the electrolyte and the sensor's membranes be checked regularly?

_____

_____

Think About This

Are there other uses for transcutaneous electrodes?

Helpful Web Site

- *Respiratory Care* journal, "AARC Clinical Practice Guideline: Transcutaneous Blood Gas Monitoring for Neonatal and Pediatric Patients—2004 Revision & Update" — http://www.rcjournal.com

11. State the criteria for identifying four types of acid-base disorders.

11A. What are the criteria for metabolic acidosis?

Type of metabolic acidosis	pH	PCO$_2$	HCO$_3$-
Acute			
Partly compensated			
Compensated			

11B. What are the criteria for respiratory acidosis?

Type of respiratory acidosis	pH	PCO$_2$	HCO$_3$-
Acute			
Partly compensated			
Compensated			

11C. What are the criteria for metabolic alkalosis?

Type of metabolic alkalosis	pH	PCO$_2$	HCO$_3$-
Acute			
Partly compensated			
Compensated			

11D. What are the criteria for respiratory alkalosis?

Type of respiratory alkalosis	pH	PCO$_2$	HCO$_3$-
Acute			
Partly compensated			
Compensated			

Interpret the following results in terms of acid-base balance:

	pH	PCO$_2$	HCO$_3$-	Interpretation
11E.	7.28	60	24	
11F.	7.38	96	32	
11G.	7.52	28	20	
11H.	7.44	28	19	
11I.	7.46	34	26	
11J.	7.28	80	37	
11K.	7.59	49	48	
11L.	7.34	40	21	
11M.	7.44	48	33	
11N.	7.36	30	15	
11O.	7.51	39	31	
11P.	7.34	34	18	

Think About This

What are the normal and abnormal acid-base values for dogs, cats, and other non-human animals?

Helpful Web Site

■ VentWorld, "Acid-Base Challenge" — http://www.ventworld.com

NATIONAL BOARD FOR RESPIRATORY CARE (NBRC)–TYPE QUESTIONS

1. What is the correct sequence of events when one is obtaining arterial blood from the radial artery of a patient?
   I. Perform a modified Allen's test.
   II. Remove any air bubbles from the sample.
   III. Apply direct pressure to the puncture site.
   IV. Clean the puncture site with a suitable antiseptic solution.
   V. Use a 23-gauge needle and a plastic syringe containing an anticoagulant.
      A. I, IV, III, V, II
      B. IV, I, V, II, III
      C. I, IV, V, III, II

2. What is the correct order of steps to perform a modified Allen's test?
   I. Pressure is applied to both the radial and ulnar arteries.
   II. The fist is opened, but the fingers are not fully extended.
   III. Pressure on the ulnar artery is removed.
   IV. The hand is clenched into a tight fist.
   V. The palm and fingers are blanched.
      A. IV, I, II, V, III
      B. IV, V, I, III, II
      C. I, IV, III, II, V
      D. IV, II, I, III, V

3. The reference half-cell of a pH analyzer is composed of which of the following?
   A. Silver anode
   B. Platinum cathode
   C. Silver–silver chloride
   D. Mercury–mercurous chloride

4. In a partial pressure of carbon dioxide (PCO_2) electrode, carbon dioxide:
   I. Reacts with potassium chloride.
   II. Reacts with water to form carbonic acid.
   III. Diffuses through a silicon elastic membrane.
   IV. Diffuses through a semipermeable plastic membrane.
      A. II and III only
      B. I and III only
      C. I and IV only
      D. II and IV only

5. Erroneous PCO_2 measurements may be caused by which of the following?
   I. A cracked electrode
   II. Wearing out of the silver anode
   III. Increased temperature of the patient
   IV. Dehydration of bicarbonate solution
      A. I and II only
      B. I and IV only
      C. II and III only
      D. III and IV only

6. Which of the following variables is measured directly?
   A. Partial pressure of oxygen at which hemoglobin is 50% saturated (P_{50})
   B. Partial pressure of arterial oxygen (PaO_2)
   C. HCO_3.
   D. Hemoximetry oxygen saturation (SaO_2)

7. Which of the following would create the highest P_{50}?
   A. pH = 7.40
   B. pH = 7.50
   C. PCO_2 = 40 mm Hg
   D. PCO_2 = 60 mm Hg

8. What type of calibration should be performed after an electrode is changed?
   A. Quality control
   B. Three-point
   C. Two-point
   D. One-point

9. Quality control includes which of the following?
   I. Analyzing unknown samples and submitting to the sponsoring organization
   II. Comparing control sample measurements against defined limits
   III. Addressing problems through corrective actions
   IV. Identifying problems
      A. I and II only
      B. III and IV only
      C. II, III, and IV only
      D. I, II, III, and IV

10. What are the two bases of operation for pulse oximetry?
    I.   Optical plethysmography
    II. Impedance plethysmography
    III. Spectrophotometry
    IV. Potentiometry
        A. I and III only
        B. II and IV only
        C. I and IV only
        D. II and III only

11. A patient is being treated with dapsone, an antibiotic, for *Pneumocystis carinii*. Which of the following ways of measuring oxygen saturation would be most appropriate?
    A. In vivo blood gas monitoring
    B. In vitro blood gas monitoring
    C. Pulse oximetry
    D. Carbon monoxide (CO)–oximetry

12. A patient undergoing continuous pulse oximetry is receiving supplemental oxygen. The pulse oximetry oxygen saturation (SpO_2) has been 93% ± 2 for the past 12 hours. The pulse oximeter suddenly sounds an alarm and reads 78%. A rapid assessment reveals cyanosis and shortness of breath. What should your immediate action be?
    A. Take an arterial blood gas measurement without delay.
    B. Recalibrate the pulse oximeter.
    C. Change the pulse oximeter probe.
    D. Decrease the supplemental oxygen.

13. Which of the following cause erroneous transcutaneous partial pressure of oxygen ($PtcO_2$) readings?
    I.   Hypovolemia
    II. Hypothermia
    III. Septic shock
    IV. Asthma
        A. I and III only
        B. I and IV only
        C. I, II, and III only
        D. II, III, and IV only

14. The following arterial blood gas results — pH = 7.37; PCO_2 = 55 mm Hg; PO_2 = 53 mm Hg; SaO_2 = 88%; HCO_3 = 31 — can be interpreted as:
    A. Compensated metabolic alkalosis with mild hypoxemia
    B. Compensated respiratory acidosis with moderate hypoxemia
    C. Partially compensated respiratory acidosis with mild hypoxemia
    D. Partially compensated respiratory acidosis with severe hypoxemia

15. Analyze the following acid-base balance: pH = 7.35; PCO_2 = 22 mm Hg; HCO_3 = 12 mEq/L. What would be your interpretation of these data?
    A. Combined alkalemia
    B. Combined acidemia
    C. Compensated respiratory alkalemia
    D. Respiratory alkalemia and metabolic acidemia

11 Introduction to Ventilators

Upon completion of this chapter, you will be able to:

1. List the two primary power sources used in mechanical ventilators.
2. Compare and contrast negative-pressure ventilation and positive-pressure ventilation.
3. Explain how a closed-loop ventilator system can perform self-adjustment.
4. Define *volume* and *pressure ventilation*.
5. Provide three alternative terms for *pressure ventilation* and *volume ventilation*.
6. Name three volume-displacement designs and three flow-control valves.
7. Compare the location of expiratory valves on current intensive care unit ventilators with that on older-model ventilators.
8. Draw the flow and pressure curves produced by linear drive and rotary drive piston ventilators.
9. Explain the two fundamental principles of fluidics.
10. Evaluate available positive end-expiratory pressure (PEEP) valves to determine whether a flow resistor or a threshold resistor is being used.
11. Evaluate patient information to determine which expiratory maneuver is indicated: negative end-expiratory pressure, continuous positive airway pressure (CPAP), PEEP, expiratory pause, or expiratory retard.
12. Troubleshoot a freestanding CPAP system.
13. Describe the four phases of a breath.
14. Explain how pressure-, flow-, and volume-triggering mechanisms work to begin the inspiratory phase of a breath.
15. Identify the graph of the flow-time, volume-time, and pressure-time curves for time-triggered, volume- or pressure-limited, and time-cycled breaths.
16. Identify a pressure-time curve showing patient-triggering.
17. Apply Chatburn's classification for ventilator modes.
18. Explain the concept of having an adjustable flow drop-off feature for ending inspiration in pressure-support ventilation.
19. Name at least one current use of CPAP.
20. Define the modes of ventilation by their triggering, limiting (controlling), and cycling mechanisms.
21. Compare the dual-control mode of ventilation to adaptive ventilation.
22. Contrast the three methods of minimum minute ventilation as achieved by current-generation ventilators.
23. Define each of the following modes of ventilation: airway pressure-release ventilation, proportional assist ventilation, neurally adjusted ventilatory assist, and adaptive support ventilation..
24. List the five common methods of delivering high-frequency ventilation.
25. Analyze ventilator graphics to determine modes of ventilation and problems commonly occurring during ventilation.

"Breathe. Let go. And remind yourself that this very moment is the only one you know you have for sure."
Oprah Winfrey

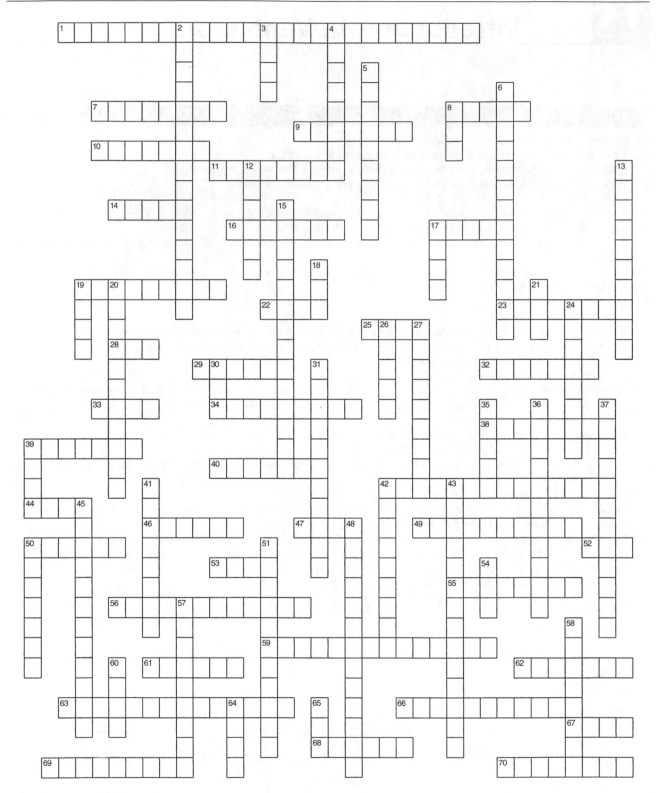

CROSSWORD PUZZLE 11-1
Created using Crossword Weaver, www.CrosswordWeaver.com.

Use the clues to complete the crossword puzzle.

Across

1. Feature of artificial airway compensation (*three words*).
7. _____ pressure ventilator; patient is in a vacuum.
8. The ventilator variables responsible for all four parts of a breath.
9. Power transmission without moving parts or electrical circuits.
10. The type of pressure obtained from an inspiratory hold maneuver.
11. Trigger _____.
14. _____ transmission systems or internal drive mechanisms.
16. The external circuit is the _____ circuit.
17. The phase variable that ends inspiration.
19. A fluidic component (*hyphenated*).
22. A mode that provides two levels of continuous positive airway pressure (*abbreviation*).
23. A/an_____-powered ventilator, which is pneumatically powered and microprocessor-controlled.
25. Inspiratory pressure during bilevel positive airway pressure ventilation (*abbreviation*).
28. A mode with pressure-targeted spontaneous breaths (*abbreviation*).
29. Compliance with no flow.
32. Direct-drive _____.
33. Mode of ventilation based on neural respiratory input (*abbreviation*).
34. A type of resistor used to create positive end-expiratory pressure (PEEP).
38. The circuit that conducts gas within the ventilator.
39. Pressure, volume, and flow are _____ variables.
40. Electrically _____.
42. Pressure or flow begins inspiration.
44. A mode that has a set pressure with targeted volume over several breaths (*abbreviation*).
46. The compliance factor used to calculate delivered tidal volume.
47. Feedback.
49. _____ bubble, a low-pressure vortex.
50. The effect that involves wall attachment.
52. Maximum pressure reached during inspiration (abbreviation).
53. Above atmosphere baseline (*abbreviation*).
55. A type of breath where all or part of inspiration or expiration is performed by the ventilator.
56. _____ solenoid valves, which are valves that use on/off switches to control flow.
59. A mode that may be triggered by the patient or the ventilator.
61. _____ drive piston, a direct-drive piston.
62. The _____ mode, which requires no patient involvement.
63. One of the principles of fluid logic (*two words*).
66. At the proximal airway.
67. Subambient pressure (*abbreviation*).
68. Flow-control _____.
69. Inadvertent pressure at the end of expiration.
70. The pressure maintained at the airway during exhalation and the pressure from which inspiration begins.

Down

2. A maneuver to measure plateau pressure (*two words*).
3. Baseline during bilevel positive airway pressure ventilation (*abbreviation*).
4. A type of patient trigger.
5. _____ breath, which is a ventilator breath.
6. The interface between operator and ventilator (*two words*).
8. A mode that assists spontaneous ventilation by adjusting the amount of work of breathing assumed by the ventilator (*abbreviation*).
12. The type of drive pistons that produce a sine-wavelike flow curve.
13. This type of waveform is produced by an oscillator.
15. _____, or computer-controlled.
17. A ventilator mode where there is spontaneous breathing with an elevated baseline (*abbreviation*).
18. The mode that allows spontaneous breathing between mandatory breaths (*abbreviation*).
19. A trigger variable that depends on the speed of the gas.
20. Pressure reading drops to plateau during this pause.
21. A mode that guarantees the delivery of a set minimum minute ventilation (*abbreviation*).
24. A large negative-pressure ventilator (*two words*).
26. A mode that has a set pressure with an inverse inspiration-to-expiration ratio (*abbreviation*).
27. Movement from one lung segment to another.
30. Inspiratory time plus expiratory time (*abbreviation*).
31. An intelligent system (*hyphenated*).
35. Confine the variable.
36. Trigger _____.
37. This type of device creates positive expiratory pressure.

39. Spontaneous breathing at above atmospheric pressure (*abbreviation*).

41. Self-adjusting mode on the Dräger EvitaXL.

42. The _____ circuit carries the gas from the gas source, through the ventilator, to the patient, then back to the exhalation valve.

43. A maneuver to measure auto-PEEP (*two words*).

45. User interface (*two words*).

48. _____-powered, or gas-powered.

50. The ventilator does all the work in this mode.

51. Type of breath controlled by the patient.

54. Advanced level of computational logic on the Hamilton GALILEO Gold and G5 (*abbreviation*).

57. The _____ system, an unintelligent ventilator system.

58. The circuit that conducts gas from the ventilator to the patient and from the patient to the expiratory valve.

60. A mode with spontaneous breathing in between synchronized ventilator breaths (*abbreviation*).

64. Ventilator-triggered.

65. A mode that has a set pressure (*abbreviation*).

ACHIEVING THE OBJECTIVES

1. List the two primary power sources used in mechanical ventilators.

1A. What is the range of gas power necessary to run a pneumatically powered ventilator?

_____

_____

1B. How does a pneumatic ventilator lower the source pressure to operating pressure?

_____

_____

1C. Name the two types of pneumatically controlled ventilators.

_____

_____

1D. What type of ventilators use alternating current to power their internal components?

_____

_____

1E. What is the most common type of intensive care unit (ICU) ventilator used today?

_____

_____

1F. The power sources for these ICU ventilators include

_____

_____.

Think About This

Which type of ventilator should be used during magnetic resonance imaging (MRI)?

Helpful Web Site

■ VentWorld, "What is a Ventilator? Part I. The Basic Components and Definition," Frank P. Primiano Jr. and Robert L. Chatburn — http://www.ventworld.com

2. Compare and contrast negative-pressure and positive-pressure ventilation.

2A. For gas to flow, what must exist?

_____

_____

2B. During normal spontaneous breathing, what initiates inspiration?

_____

_____

2C. What is the major muscle of ventilation?

_____

_____

2D. What causes gas to move into the lungs during normal spontaneous breathing?

_____

_____

_____

_____

2E. What causes expiration during normal spontaneous breathing?

_____

_____

_____

_____

2F. How do negative-pressure ventilators cause gas to enter the lungs?

_____

_____

_____

_____

_____

_____

_____

2G. What causes air to flow out of the patient during negative-pressure ventilation?

_____

_____

_____

_____

2H. Name two types of negative-pressure ventilators.

_____

_____

2I. What causes inspiration during positive-pressure ventilation?

_____

_____

_____

_____

_____

2J. Which form of ventilation is most physiologic?

_____

_____

2K. Which type of ventilation is most commonly used today?

_____

_____

Think About This

How can a vacuum cleaner become a ventilator?

Helpful Web Sites

- University of Virginia, "Emergency! An Iron Lung in a Hurry" — http://historical.hsl.virginia.edu
- Man Who Used Negative Pressure Ventilation for 50 Years in an Iron Lung—http://www.johnprestwich. btinternet.co.uk
- Corrado A, Gorini M: Negative-pressure Ventilation: is There Still a Role? — http://www.erj.ersjournals. com

3. Explain how a closed-loop ventilator system can perform self-adjustment.

3A. List three other terms for a *closed-loop system*.

_____

_____

3B. What specific type of hardware is used to control the function of a closed-loop system?

_____

_____

3C. Another word for an *open-loop system* is

_____

_____.

3D. What is it about the closed-loop ventilator system that allows it to perform self-adjustments?

_____

_____

3E. A patient who is breathing spontaneously through a mechanical ventilator becomes apneic. The ventilator alarm rings. What type of ventilator system is this?

_____

_____

3F. A patient who is breathing spontaneously through a mechanical ventilator becomes apneic. The ventilator alarm rings and begins to ventilate the patient. What type of ventilator system is this?

_____

_____

Think About This

What closed-loop systems do you use in everyday life?

Helpful Web Sites

- RT for Decision Makers in Respiratory Care, "Closing the Loop in Pediatric Mechanical Ventilation," Justin Tse — http://www.rtmagazine.com

■ *Respiratory Care* journal, "Computer Control of Mechanical Ventilation," Robert L. Chatburn — http://www.rcjournal.com

4. Define volume and pressure ventilation.

4A. What is a control circuit?

_____

_____

4B. What is a control variable?

_____

_____

4C. Name three main control variables.

_____

_____

4D. In the clinical setting, what are the two most-common variables that are controlled?

_____

_____

4E. When volume is the control variable, what happens to the pressure if there is a change in the patient's lung characteristics?

_____

_____

4F. When pressure is the control variable, what happens to the volume and flow if there is a change in the patient's lung characteristics?

_____

_____

4G. What type of ventilation controls the volume variable?

_____

_____

4H. What type of ventilation controls the pressure variable?

_____

_____

Think About This
Which type of ventilation will protect the lungs best?

Helpful Web Site
■ BESIM-Simulation of Respiratory Mechanics Version 3.01 — http://www.jicu.de

5. Provide three alternative names for pressure ventilation and volume ventilation.

5A. What are the three alternative terms for *volume ventilation*?

_____

_____

_____

_____

5B. What are the three alternative terms for *pressure ventilation*?

_____

_____

_____

_____

Think About This
Can you think of any other industry in which there is such confusion over many names having the same meaning?

6. Name three volume-displacement designs and three flow-control valves.

6A. What type of volume-displacement device normally produces a constant flow-time curve and has a single circuit?

_____

_____

6B. What type of volume-displacement device normally produces a sine-wavelike flow curve during volume delivery?

_____

_____

6C. The third type of volume-displacement design is a

_____

_____.

6D. What type of device responds rapidly and has precise control over the exact pattern of gas and pressure?

_____

_____

6E. The type of device that is based on the principle of physics that concerns electricity and magnetism is the

_____

_____.

6F. What type of device has a microprocessor-controlled motor that moves a cam against a wheel, which propels a plunger against spring tension to open and close a valve?

_____

_____

6G. The flow device that uses several valves simultaneously in the open or closed position is called

_____

_____ .

Think About This
Will MRI interfere with the operation of ventilator drive mechanisms?

Helpful Web Sites
- Animation of a Rotary Piston, R. Castelnuovo — http://www.nationmaster.com
- Animation and Information About Solenoid Valves — http://www.solenoid-valve-info.com

7. Compare the location of expiratory valves on current ICU ventilators with those on older-model ventilators.

7A. Explain the function of an expiratory valve.

_____

_____

_____

_____

7B. Why is an expiratory valve necessary?

_____

_____

_____

_____

7C. Where is the expiratory valve located in older ventilators?

_____

_____

_____

_____

7D. Where is the expiratory valve located on current ICU mechanical ventilators?

_____

_____

_____

_____

7E. Describe a current ventilator expiratory valve.

_____

_____

_____

_____

7F. Identify the expiratory valve in Figure 11-1.

_____

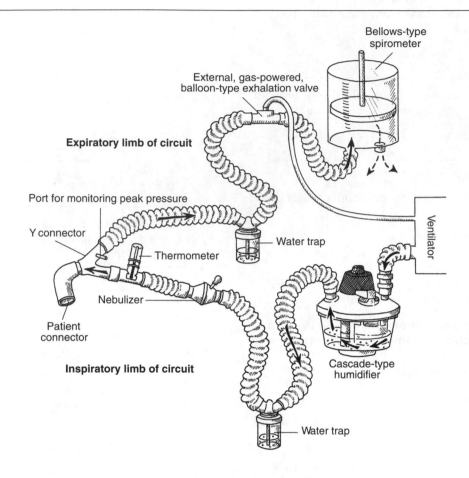

Bellows-type
spirometer

External, gas-powered,
balloon-type exhalation valve

Expiratory limb of circuit

Port for monitoring peak pressure

Y connector

Water trap

Thermometer

Ventilator

Nebulizer

Patient
connector

Inspiratory limb of circuit

Cascade-type
humidifier

Water trap

FIGURE 11-1
(From Sills JR: *Entry level respiratory therapist exam guide*, ed 4, St Louis, 2005, Mosby.)

7G. With what type of ventilator would the external circuit in Figure 11-1 be used?

_____

7H. Where is the expiratory valve located in Figure 11-2?

_____

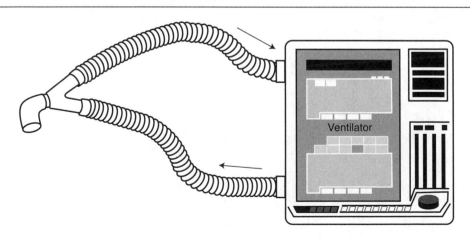

Ventilator

FIGURE 11-2
(From Sills JR: *Entry level respiratory therapist exam guide,* ed 4, St. Louis, 2005, Mosby.)

7I. With what type of ventilator would the external circuit in Figure 11-2 be used?

_____

_____

Think About This

Is it an advantage or disadvantage to have an internal expiration valve?

Helpful Web Site

- "Ventilator Failure in the ICU: Déjà Vu All Over Again," Richard C. Prielipp et al — http://www.apsf.org

8. Draw the flow and pressure curves produced by linear drive and rotary drive piston ventilators.

8A. How does a linear drive piston move forward?

_____

8B. If a flow rate is set at 40 L/min on a linear drive ventilator, what will be the flow rate at the beginning of inspiration?

_____

8C. Label and draw the flow-time curve for a linear drive ventilator with flow setting of 40 L/min.

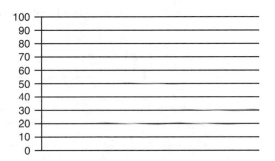

FIGURE 11-3

8D. When a linear drive piston ventilator is delivering a breath, how does the pressure increase from the beginning of inspiration to the end of inspiration?

_____

_____

8E. Label and draw the pressure-time curve for a linear drive ventilator from the beginning of inspiration to the end of inspiration with a maximum pressure of 30 cm H_2O.

FIGURE 11-4

8F. Describe the forward motion of a rotary drive piston.

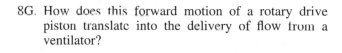

_____

8G. How does this forward motion of a rotary drive piston translate into the delivery of flow from a ventilator?

_____

_____

_____

8H. During the delivery of a breath from a rotary drive piston ventilator, when will the set flow rate (highest flow) be reached?

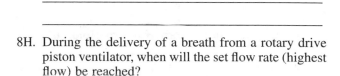

_____

8I. Label and draw the flow-time curve for a rotary drive piston ventilator with a flow rate setting of 50 L/min.

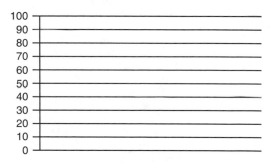

FIGURE 11-5

Chapter **11** **Introduction to Ventilators**

8J. When a rotary drive piston ventilator is delivering a breath, how does the pressure increase from the beginning of inspiration to the end of inspiration?

_____

_____

8K. Label and draw the pressure-time curve for a rotary drive ventilator from the beginning of inspiration to the end of inspiration with a maximum pressure of 30 cm H_2O.

FIGURE 11-6

Think About This
Where else are rotary and linear pistons used?

Helpful Web Site
■ "Basics of Waveform Interpretation," E. M. Collado — http://www.rtcorner.net

9. Explain the two fundamental principles of fluidics.

9A. The characteristic of fluidic ventilators that makes them suitable to be used for a patient during MRI is that fluidic-operated ventilators

_____

_____.

9B. Another name for the *Coanda effect* is

_____

_____.

9C. Describe what is shown in Figure 11-7.

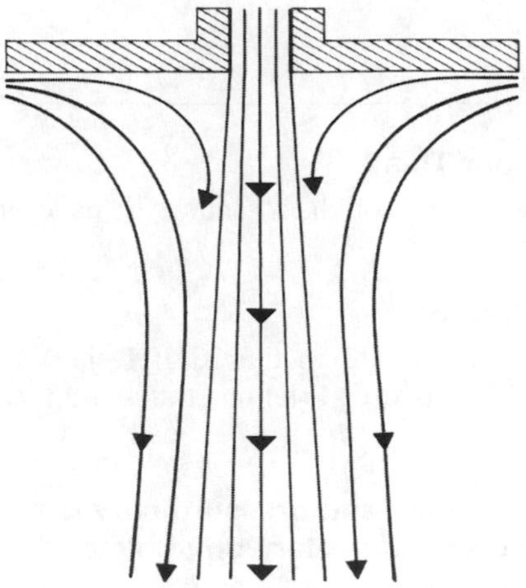

FIGURE 11-7
(From Dupuis YC: *Ventilators: theory and clinical application*, ed 2, St Louis, 1992, Mosby.)

_____

_____

_____

_____

9D. What happens to the jet stream when there is a wall on one side of it?

_____

_____

_____

_____

_____

_____

9E. Describe the phenomenon of beam deflection.

_____

_____

_____

_____

Think About This
What other applications does the Coanda effect have?

Helpful Web Sites
■ The Coanda Effect, Jean-Louis Naudin — http://jnaudin.free.fr
■ Science Toy Maker, Explanation of the Coanda Effect — http://www.sciencetoymaker.org

10. Evaluate available positive end-expiratory pressure (PEEP) valves to determine whether a flow resistor or a threshold resistor is being used.

10A. Expiratory retard can be created by what type of expiratory valve?

_____

_____

10B. Which type of expiratory valve can accommodate high expiratory flow without creating high pressure?

_____

_____

10C. What type of expiratory valve does a positive expiratory pressure (PEP) mask use?

_____

_____

10D. Why are flow resistors not commonly used for expiratory valves in ventilators?

_____

_____

_____

10E. Why are threshold resistors more commonly used as ventilator expiratory valves?

_____

_____

_____

10F. Identify the type of expiratory valve in Figure 11-8.

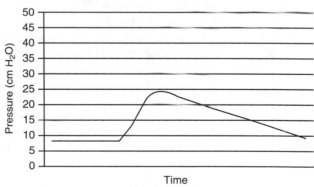

FIGURE 11-8
(Modified from Pilbeam SP, ed: *Mechanical ventilation: physiological and clinical applications*, ed 2, St Louis, 1992, Mosby.)

_____

_____

10G. What type of ventilator has the expiratory valve seen in Figure 11-8?

_____

_____

10H. Identify the type of expiratory valve in Figure 11-9.

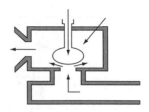

FIGURE 11-9
(Modified from Pilbeam SP, ed: *Mechanical ventilation: physiological and clinical applications*, ed 2, St Louis, 1992, Mosby.)

_____

_____

10I. What type of valve is an electromagnetic valve?

_____

_____

10J. Identify the type of expiratory valve that produces the pressure-time curve in Figure 11-10.

_____

_____

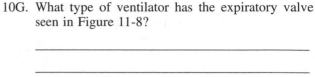

FIGURE 11-10

Chapter **11** **Introduction to Ventilators**

10K. Identify the type of expiratory valve that produces the pressure-time curve in Figure 11-11.

_____

_____

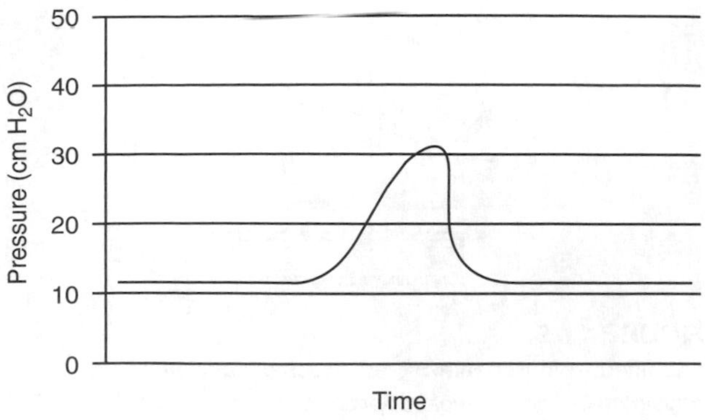

FIGURE 11-11

Think About This

What effects does expiratory resistance have on the inspiratory work of breathing?

Helpful Web Site

■ "Flow Resistance of Expiratory Positive Pressure Valve System" MJ Banner, et al. — http://www.chestjournal.org

11. Evaluate patient information to determine which expiratory maneuver is indicated: negative end-expiratory pressure (NEEP), continuous positive airway pressure (CPAP), PEEP, expiratory pause, or expiratory retard.

11A. What procedure is performed to estimate the pressure in the patient's lung and ventilator circuit due to trapped air?

_____

_____

11B. Name three causes of this trapped air.

_____

_____

_____

11C. What is this air-trapping usually called?

_____

_____

11D. The technique that was intended to counterbalance the increase in mean intrathoracic pressures caused by positive-pressure ventilation is called

_____

_____.

11E. A patient is receiving full ventilatory support. The patient's arterial blood gas shows a low oxygenation level. What expiratory maneuver is necessary?

_____

_____

11F. A spontaneously breathing patient with an oxygenation problem would benefit from what procedure?

_____

_____

11G. During what mode of ventilation is NEEP currently used?

_____

_____

11H. A patient with atelectasis or secretion retention would benefit from what type of device?

_____

_____

11I. What maneuver does an expiratory retard mimic?

_____

_____

Think About This

Why do patients with chronic obstructive pulmonary disease purse their lips to breathe?

Helpful Web Site

■ *Critical Care* journal, "Measurement of Intrinsic Positive End-expiratory Pressure," Papiris et al — http://ccforum.com

12. Troubleshoot a freestanding CPAP system.

12A. What is the purpose of the safety pressure-release valve on a CPAP system?

_____

_____

12B. How is the safety pressure release valve set?

_____

_____

12C. During the use of a freestanding CPAP unit, the safety pop-in valve is being opened on every breath. What is the most likely problem in this situation?

_____

_____

12D. A patient is using a freestanding CPAP system with a low-pressure alarm that is actively alarming. What is the most likely problem?

_____

_____

Think About This
Why is CPAP used for sleep apnea?

Helpful Web Site
■ Amcrican Sleep Apnea Association, "CPAP Trouble-shooting Guide" — http://www.sleepapnea.org

13. Describe the four phases of a breath.

13A. What is the definition of the term *breath*?

_____

_____

13B. What is the formula for total cycle time?

_____

_____

13C. The first breath phase is

_____.

13D. The second breath phase is

_____

_____.

13E. The third breath phase is

_____

_____.

13F. The fourth breath phase is

_____

_____.

13G. Define *phase variable*.

_____

_____

13H. What phase variable begins inspiration?

_____

13I. Define *cycle variable*.

_____

13J. What are the two most-common control variables?

_____

_____

13K. Define the term *limit variable*.

_____

_____

13L. During expiration, what two variables can be controlled?

_____

_____

Think About This
What controls the four variables of a spontaneous breath?

Helpful Web Site
■ Anaesthetist.com, "New Approaches to Ventilation" — http://www.anaesthetist.com

14. Explain how pressure-, flow-, and volume-triggering mechanisms work to begin the inspiratory phase of a breath.

14A. How does a patient pressure-trigger inspiration?

_____

_____

14B. What is baseline pressure?

_____

_____

14C. In what three places is pressure measured in the ventilator circuit?

_____

_____

_____

_____

_____

14D. What device measures pressure?

_____

_____

14E. The pressure baseline is set at 5 cm H_2O, and the sensitivity is set at 1.5 cm H_2O. At what pressure will the ventilator be pressure-triggered?

_____

_____

14F. Define *base flow* or *bias flow*.

_____

_____

14G. What three factors determine the flow-trigger setting?

_____

_____

_____

_____

14H. Describe how the flow trigger works.

_____

_____

_____

_____

14I. The base flow is set at 5 L/min, and the flow trigger is set at 2 L/min. The base flow must drop to what value before the ventilator will flow-trigger?

_____

_____

14J. Explain how the volume trigger operates.

_____

_____

Think About This

How does the patient's trigger effort affect work of breathing?

15. Identify the graph of the flow-, volume-, and pressure-time curves for time-triggered, volume- or pressure-limited, and time-cycled breaths.

Questions 15A through 15G refer to Figure 11-12.

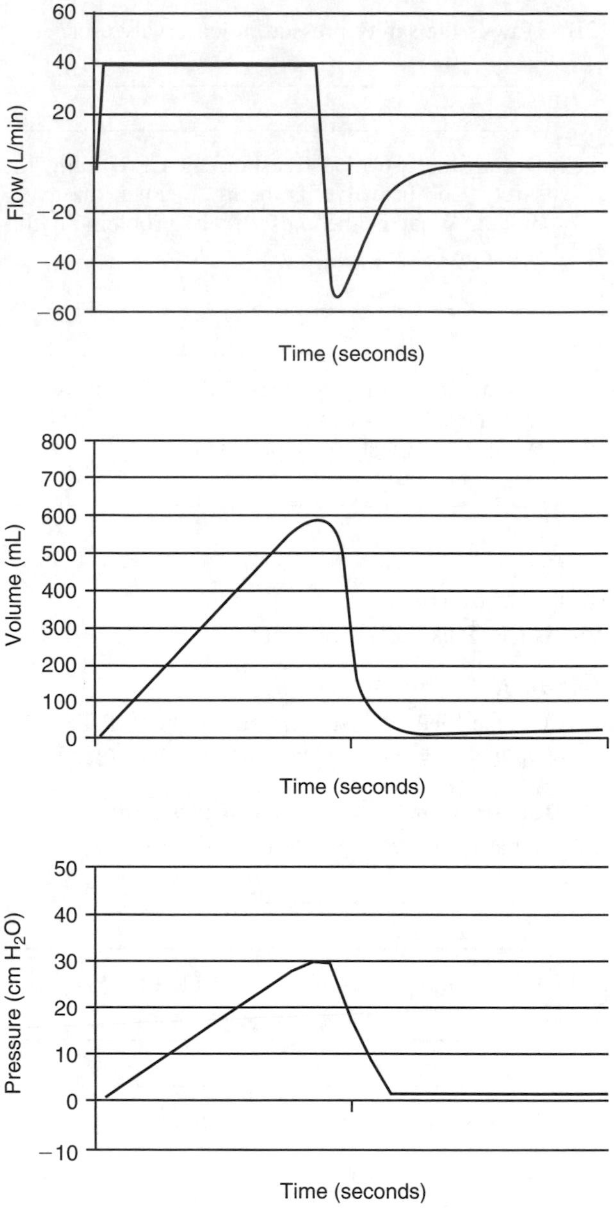

FIGURE 11-12

15A. The trigger in Figure 11-12 is

_____.

15B. What variable is limited in Figure 11-12?

_____

15C. What is the cycle variable in Figure 11-12?

_____

15D. What type of flow waveform is shown in Figure 11-12?

_____

15E. The peak inspiratory pressure in Figure 11-12 is

_____.

15F. What is the peak flow setting in Figure 11-12?

_____

15G. What volume is delivered in Figure 11-12?

_____

Questions 15H through 15N refer to Figure 11-13.

15H. The trigger in Figure 11-13 is

_____.

15I. What variable is limited in Figure 11-13?

_____

15J. What is the cycle variable in Figure 11-13?

_____

15K. What type of flow waveform is shown in Figure 11-13?

_____

15L. The peak inspiratory pressure in Figure 11-13 is

_____.

15M. What is the peak flow setting in Figure 11-13?

_____

15N. What volume is delivered in Figure 11-13?

_____

Think About This

Which do you think is the most important scalar to monitor and why?

Helpful Web Sites

- Auckland District Health Board, "Newborn Services Clinical Guideline: Ventilation Graphics and Respiratory Function Monitoring" — http://www.adhb.govt.nz
- RT for Decision Makers in Respiratory Care, "Ventilator Graphics Made Easy," William C. Pruitt — http://www.rtmagazine.com

16. Identify a pressure-time curve showing patient-triggering.

16A. Use Figure 11-14 to draw and label a pressure-time curve for a volume-cycled breath with a baseline of +5 cm H_2O, a trigger of –1 cm H_2O, and a peak inspiratory pressure of 25 cm H_2O.

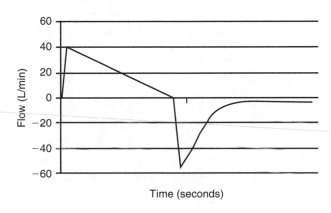

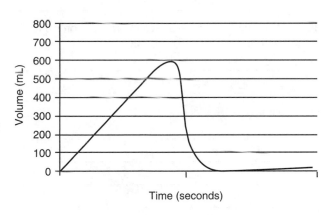

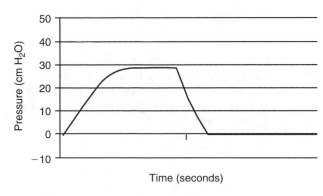

FIGURE 11-13

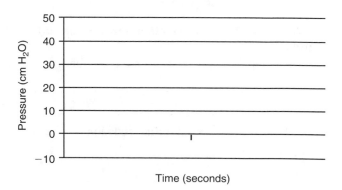

FIGURE 11-14

16B. Use Figure 11-15 to draw and label a pressure time curve for a pressure limited breath with a baseline of +10 cm H_2O, a trigger of 1.5 cm H_2O, and a pressure limit setting of 30 cm H_2O.

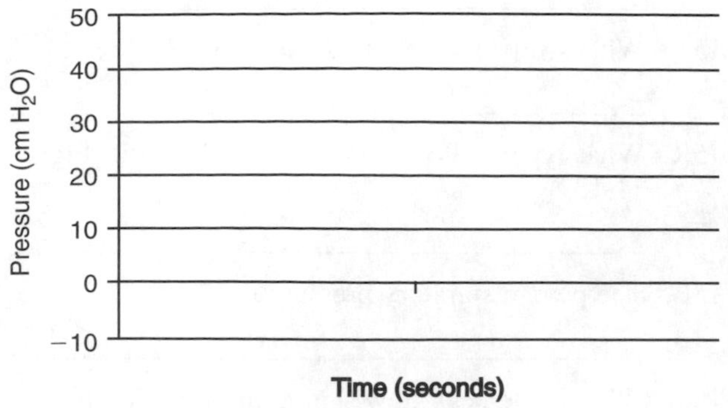

FIGURE 11-15

16C. Circle the pressure-triggered breaths in Figure 11-16.

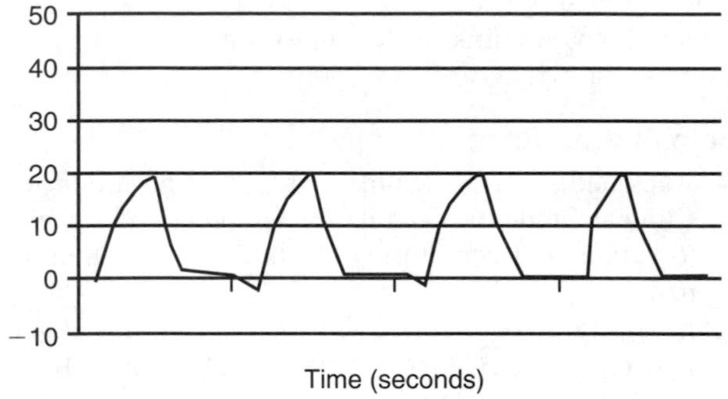

FIGURE 11-16

Think About This
What effect does intrinsic PEEP have on pressure-triggering?

Helpful Web Site
- "Ventilator Graphics," by Shakeel Amunullah — http://www.emedicine.com

17. Apply Chatburn's classification for ventilator modes.
17A. A mode description according to Chatburn is

_____

_____ .

17B. What is the key point of the equation of motion?

_____

_____

17C. What are the three main breath-control variables?

_____

_____

17D. In pressure control, _____ is constant and _____ can vary. In volume control, _____ is constant, and _____ can vary.

17E. Explain a dual-control breath variable mode.

_____

_____

_____

_____

17F. What are the three types of breath sequences?

_____

_____

_____

_____

17G. An analysis of ventilator breaths reveals that spontaneous breaths are allowed between mandatory breaths. What breath sequence is this?

_____

_____

17H. Describe the three main categories of control types used in mechanical ventilation.

_____

_____

_____

_____

_____

_____

_____

_____

_____

_____

17I. The level 1 Chatburn classification for a mode that is time-triggered or patient-triggered and switches from volume control to pressure control during ventilator breaths is

_____

_____ .

17J. The level 1 Chatburn classification for a mode that allows the patient to breathe spontaneously between mandatory ventilator breaths that are pressure-targeted is

_____

_____.

17K. The level 1 Chatburn classification for a mode that provides pressure-targeted spontaneous breaths is

_____

_____.

17L. The control type for pressure-control continuous spontaneous ventilation where the pressure-support level is automatically adjusted to maintain appropriate breathing frequency, tidal volume, and end-tidal carbon dioxide (CO_2) depending on the type of patient is

_____

_____.

Think About This

Can you think of items in your everyday life that do the same thing but have different names?

Helpful Web Site

■ Chatburn's Classification of Ventilators — http://www.aic.cuhk.edu.hk

18. Explain the concept of having an adjustable flow drop-off feature for ending inspiration in pressure-support ventilation.

18A. The level 1 Chatburn classification for pressure-support ventilation is

_____

_____.

18B. What are the phase variables for pressure-support ventilation?

_____

_____

18C. Describe the flow-time curve for pressure-support ventilation.

_____

_____

18D. What is the reason for the specific appearance of the flow-time curve?

_____

_____

18E. Which ventilators allow the operator to change the cycle level (% flow)?

_____

_____

18F. Use Figure 11-17 to draw the flow-time graph for a pressure-support breath with a peak flow of 35 L/min and a flow cycle of 30%.

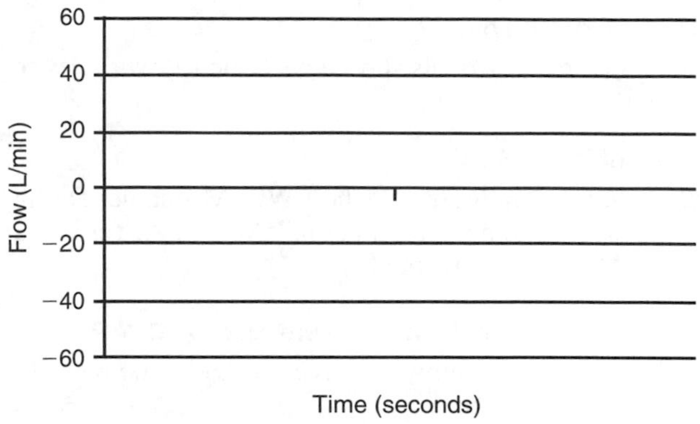

FIGURE 11-17

18G. What happens to the flow cycle if there is a leak in the system during the delivery of a pressure-support breath?

_____

_____

_____

_____

_____

18H. During pressure-support ventilation the patient coughs. What happens with the ventilator in this situation?

_____

_____

_____

18I. What three factors determine how much volume will be delivered during a pressure-support breath?

_____

_____

_____

18J. Why would a patient with a nasal intubation benefit from the use of pressure-support ventilation while breathing spontaneously?

_____

_____

_____

_____

Think About This
Which types of patients should have their flow cycles set higher?

Helpful Web Site
■ *Critical Care* journal, "Chest Wall Mechanics During Pressure Support Ventilation," Andrea Aliverti et al — http://ccforum.com

19. Name at least one current use of CPAP.
19A. Define *continuous positive airway pressure*.

_____

_____

19B. What does CPAP do to functional residual capacity?

_____

19C. What does CPAP do to mean airway pressure?

_____

19D. How does CPAP reverse atelectasis?

_____

19E. What are the two main uses for CPAP?

_____

_____

Think About This
Will you float better in a pool if you breathe as if you were receiving CPAP?

Helpful Web Site
■ WebMD — http://www.webmd.com

20. Define the modes of ventilation by their triggering, limiting (controlling), and cycling mechanisms.
Questions 20A through 20D refer to Figure 11-18.

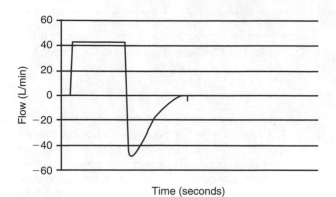

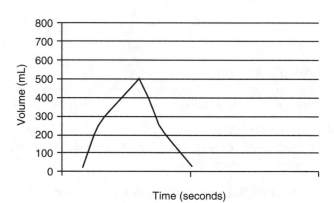

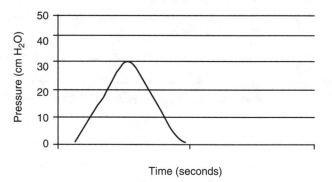

FIGURE 11-18

20A. What variable is the trigger in Figure 11-18?

_____

20B. What variable is the limit in Figure 11-18?

_____

20C. What variable is the cycle in Figure 11-18?

_____

20D. What mode of ventilation is shown in Figure 11-18?

_____

Questions 20E through 20H refer to Figure 11-19.

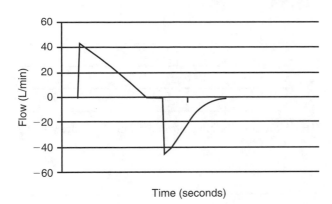

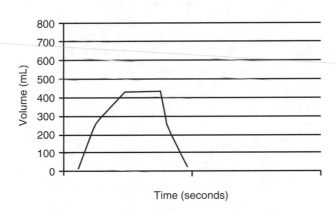

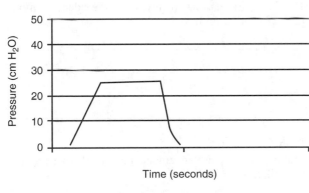

FIGURE 11-19

20E. What variable is the trigger in Figure 11-19?

_____

20F. What variable is the limit in Figure 11-19?

_____

20G. What variable is the cycle in Figure 11-19?

_____

20H. What mode of ventilation is shown in Figure 11-19?

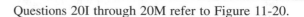

Questions 20I through 20M refer to Figure 11-20.

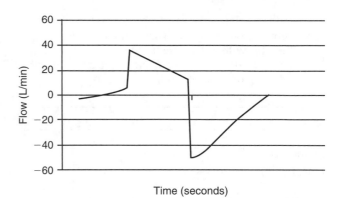

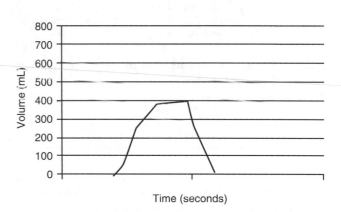

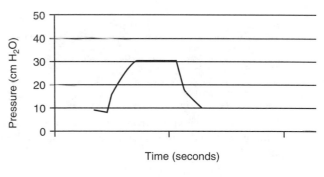

FIGURE 11-20

20I. What variable is the trigger in Figure 11-20?

_____

20J. What variable is the limit in Figure 11-20?

_____

20K. What variable is the cycle in Figure 11-20?

_____

20L. What is the baseline pressure?

_____

20M. What mode of ventilation is shown in Figure 11-20?

_____

20N. Flow-triggered, pressure-limited, flow-cycled breaths with intermittent flow or time-triggered, pressure-limited, time-cycled breaths describes what mode of ventilation?

_____

_____

Think About This

Trigger, limit, cycle = start, contain, end.

Helpful Web Site

- Critical Care Medicine Tutorials, "A System for Analysing Ventilator Waveforms," Patrick Neligan — http://www.ccmtutorials.com

21. Compare the dual-control mode of ventilation to adaptive ventilation.

21A. Define *dual-control mode*.

_____

_____

_____

21B. Give examples of dual control modes

_____

_____

_____

_____

21C. Why would switching from pressure control to volume control during a breath be beneficial to the patient?

_____

_____

_____

_____

_____

_____

21D. How does the dual-control mode of ventilation ensure volume delivery?

_____

_____

_____

_____

_____

_____

21E. How does the adaptive control mode ensure volume delivery?

_____

_____

_____

_____

_____

_____

_____

21F. Which ventilators have adaptive modes?

_____

_____

_____

21G. What limitations, if any, does the adaptive mode of ventilation have?

_____

_____

_____

_____

Think About This

What engineering advancements have made these modes of ventilation possible?

Helpful Web Sites

- Dräger Medical AG & Co, "Auto Flow: 20 Questions — 20 Answers" — http://www.draeger-medical
- *Respiratory Care* journal, "The Role of Ventilator Graphics When Setting Dual-Control Modes," Richard D. Branson and Jay A. Johannigman — http://www.rcjournal.com

22. Contrast the three methods of minimum minute ventilation as achieved by current-generation ventilators.

22A. What is minimum minute ventilation?

_____

_____

_____

_____

_____

22B. In general, when the minimum minute volume is not met, what does the ventilator do?

_____

_____

22C. How does the Hamilton VEOLAR achieve minimum minute ventilation?

_____

_____

22D. How does the Bear 1000 achieve minimum minute ventilation?

_____

_____

22E. How does the Servo 300 achieve minimum minute ventilation?

_____

_____

Think About This

Where do ideas for new modes of ventilation originate?

Helpful Web Site

■ Nature Publishing Group, *Journal of Perinatology*, "A Crossover Analysis of Mandatory Minute Ventilation Compared to Synchronized Intermittent Mandatory Ventilation in Neonates," Scott O. Guthrie et al — http://www.nature.com

23. Define each of the following modes of ventilation: airway pressure-release ventilation (APRV), proportional assist ventilation (PAV), neurally adjusted ventilatory assist (NAVA), and adaptive support ventilation (ASV).

23A. What was the original use for APRV?

_____

_____

_____

_____

23B. Define *APRV* in terms of trigger, limit, and cycle.

_____

_____

23C. What makes APRV different from modes with similar trigger, limit, and cycle variables?

_____

_____

23D. What type of patient is APRV most frequently used to support?

_____

_____

23E. Draw the following APRV pressure waveform on Figure 11-21: a high CPAP level of 25 cm H_2O for 1.5 second and a low CPAP of 5 cm H_2O for 0.5 second, with spontaneous breathing at each level.

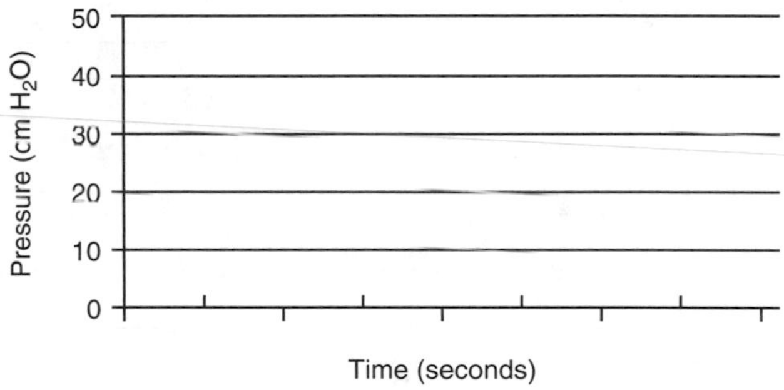

FIGURE 11-21

23F. What ventilators have APRV?

_____

_____

_____

23G. What does the practitioner adjust when using the PAV mode?

_____

_____

_____

_____

_____

_____

177

23H. What types of patient could benefit from the use of PAV?

_____

_____

_____

_____

23I. How does the ventilator respond to increasing effort during inspiration in the PAV mode?

_____

_____

23J. What is the purpose of the ventilator's response in the PAV mode?

_____

_____

23K. What type of mode is PAV?

_____

23L. What is NAVA?

_____

_____

_____

_____

23M. What is the trigger variable in NAVA?

_____

_____

_____

_____

_____

23N. What is the cycle variable in NAVA?

_____

_____

23O. How would NAVA be characterized using the Chatburn classification system?

_____

_____

23P. Which ventilator has NAVA?

_____

23Q. Why is ASV considered to be an optimal control mode of ventilation?

_____

_____

23R. How does ASV operate on the Hamilton GALILEO Gold model?

_____

_____

_____

_____

_____

_____

_____

23S. What settings does the operator set in the ASV mode?

_____

_____

_____

_____

_____

_____

23T. If a patient became apneic in the ASV mode, what would happen?

_____

_____

_____

_____

Think About This

Do these new modes reduce ventilator days?

Helpful Web Sites

■ Arrow Group Publishing, RPNmed, "Dräger APRV" [video and information] — http://www.rpnmed.com
■ Puritan Bennett, "Proportional Assist™ Ventilation Plus (PAV™ +) Software Option" — http://www.puritanbennett.com
■ Maquet, Inc; Information on NAVA — http://www.maquet.com
■ Hamilton Medical, Inc, "Adaptive Support Ventilation" — http://www.hamilton-medical.com

24. List the five common methods of delivering high-frequency ventilation.

24A. Define *high-frequency ventilation*.

_____

_____

24B. Define high-frequency positive-pressure ventilation.

_____

_____

_____

_____

24C. What rates does high-frequency jet ventilation use?

_____

24D. What is the operational principle of high-frequency jet ventilation?

_____

_____

_____

24E. The tidal volume in high-frequency jet ventilation depends on what four basic factors?

_____

_____

_____

_____

24F. What rates does high-frequency oscillatory ventilation (HFOV) use?

_____

_____

24G. How is gas moved during HFOV?

_____

_____

_____

_____

24H. How does high-frequency flow interuption differ from high-frequency jet ventilation?

_____

_____

_____

_____

24I. What are the rates for HFFI?

_____

24J. How does high-frequency percussive ventilation operate?

_____

_____

_____

Think About This

Is HFV more advantageous than conventional ventilation for adults in respiratory failure?

Helpful Web Sites

- University of Michigan Hospitals and Health Centers, Respiratory Care, High Frequency Ventilation — http://www.respcare.med.umich.edu
- "Management Strategies with High Frequency Jet Ventilation," Jonathan M. Klein — http://www.uihealthcare.com
- Auckland District Health Board, Newborn Services Clinical Guideline, "High Frequency Oscillatory Ventilation: SensorMedics High Frequency Oscillator" — http://www.adhb.govt.nz
- PubMed Central, *Annals of Surgery* journal, "Prophylactic Use of High-frequency Percussive Ventilation in Patients with Inhalation Injury," W. G. Cioffi Jr. et al — http://www.pubmedcentral.nih.gov

25. Analyze ventilator graphics to determine modes of ventilation and common problems occurring during ventilation.

Identify and label Figures 11-22 through 11-27 in Questions 25A through 25F with the appropriate mode.

25A.

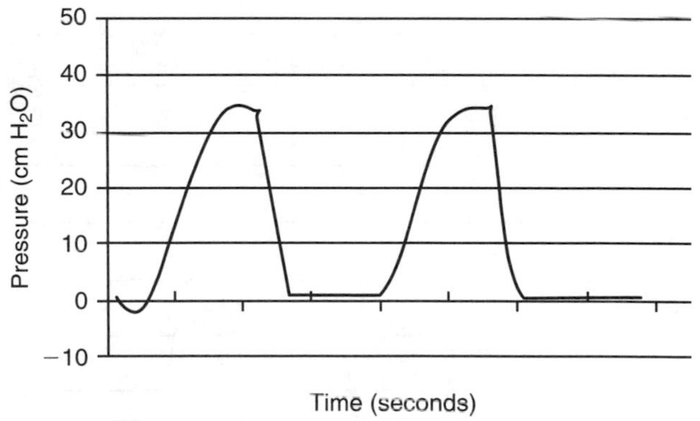

FIGURE 11-22

_____

_____

25B.

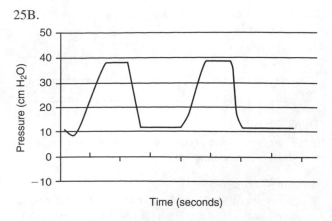

FIGURE 11-23

_____

_____

25C.

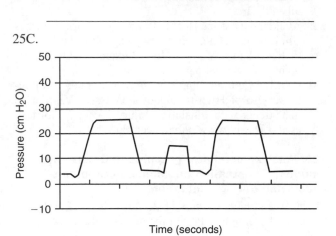

FIGURE 11-24

_____

_____

25D.

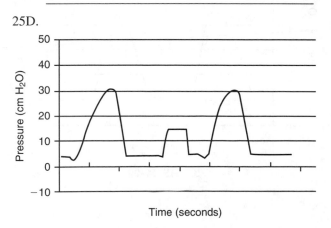

FIGURE 11-25

_____

_____

25E.

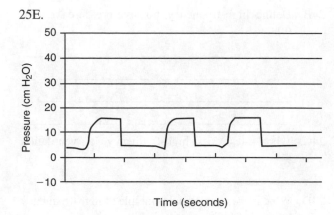

FIGURE 11-26

_____

_____

25F.

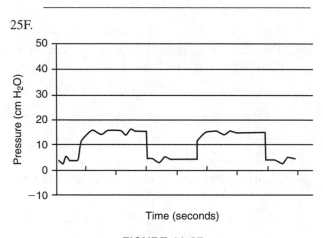

FIGURE 11-27

_____

_____

Questions 25G through 25I refer to Figure 11-28.

Questions 25J through 25L refer to Figure 11-29.

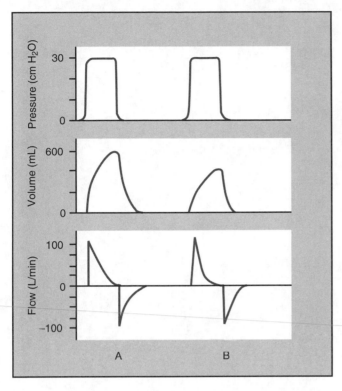

FIGURE 11-28

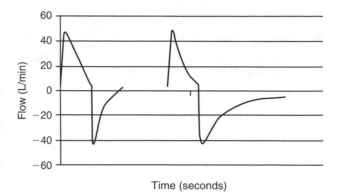

Time (seconds)

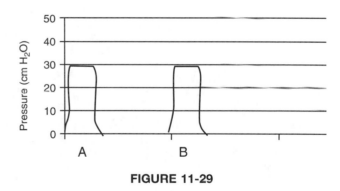

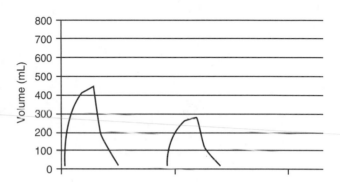

FIGURE 11-29

25G. What mode is shown in Figure 11-28?

_____

25H. What change has occurred between *A* and *B* in Figure 11-28?

_____

25I. What could cause the change shown in Figure 11-28?

_____

25J. What mode is shown in Figure 11-29?

_____

25K. What change has occurred between *A* and *B* in Figure 11-29?

_____

_____

25L. What could cause the change shown in Figure 11-29?

_____

_____

Think About This

Electrocardiogram waves are to cardiology as ventilator graphics are to ventilator management.

Helpful Web Site

- "Ventilator Graphics Made Easy," W. C. Pruitt — http://www.rtmagazine.com

- Auckland District Health Board — http://www.adhb.govt.nz

NATIONAL BOARD FOR RESPIRATORY CARE (NBRC)–TYPE QUESTIONS

1. Active expiration occurs in which ventilator mode?
   A. Proportional assist ventilation
   B. High-frequency jet ventilation
   C. Airway pressure-release ventilation
   D. High-frequency oscillatory ventilation

2. A patient receiving mask continuous positive airway pressure (CPAP) 7.5 cm H_2O via a freestanding system appears to be in distress. The patient is using accessory muscles and is diaphoretic. The manometer is fluctuating between –5 cm H_2O on inspiration and 7.5 cm H_2O on expiration. The most apparent cause of the patient's distress is which of the following?
   A. Leak in the system
   B. Improper mask fitting
   C. Inadequate flow rate
   D. Obstruction of the threshold resistor

3. The amount of time for a pressure-targeted ventilator breath to reach the set pressure is known as which of the following?
   A. *Rise time*
   B. *Inspiratory time*
   C. *Total cycle time*
   D. *Inspiratory hold*

4. After patient-triggering, the pressure rises to the set level, the ventilator monitors inspiratory flow, and volume cycles if necessary. What ventilator mode does this describe?
   A. Proportional assist ventilation
   B. Mandatory minute ventilation
   C. Airway pressure-release ventilation
   D. Pressure augmentation

5. What type of flow-time curve will be created by a spring-loaded bellows when working pressure is high and the patient's airway resistance is low?
   A. Ascending ramp
   B. Descending ramp
   C. Rectangular
   D. Sine wave

6. The baseline pressure is elevated but is periodically released to a lower level for a very brief period. This statement describes which ventilator mode?
   A. Bilevel positive airway pressure (BiPAP)
   B. Pressure-controlled inverse-ratio ventilation (PCIRV)
   C. Airway pressure-release ventilation (APRV)
   D. Mandatory minute ventilation (MMV)

7. Patient discomfort from rapid gas flow during pressure-targeted ventilation may be alleviated by which of the following adjustments to the ventilator?
   A. Increasing inspiratory time
   B. Increasing rise time
   C. Decreasing expiratory time
   D. Decreasing total cycle time

8. The flow cycle setting for a pressure-supported breath, with a peak flow of 30 L/min, that will allow enough time for a visible plateau on the pressure-time curve is which of the following?
   A. 5 L/min
   B. 5% of peak flow
   C. 20 L/min
   D. 20% of peak flow

9. A flow-time curve that does not return to 0 before the next mandatory breath indicates which of the following?
   A. Flow-triggering
   B. Auto-PEEP
   C. Flow-cycling
   D. A system leak

10. A ventilator mode used prophylactically in patients with thermal airway injury to help prevent pneumonia and atelectasis is:
    A. ARPV.
    B. High-frequency percussive ventilation.
    C. High-frequency jet ventilation.
    D. PCIRV.

12 Mechanical Ventilators: General-Use Devices

This chapter has been designed in a slightly different manner than other chapters in the workbook. The chapter is divided into ventilator manufacturer sections. Each of these sections has a crossword puzzle. The sections are then divided into the various ventilators with their own set of learning objectives, as identified in the textbook, short-answer questions, fill-in questions, and National Board for Respiratory Care (NBRC)–type multiple-choice questions. The "Think About This" and "Helpful Web Sites" appear at the end of each ventilator section.

OUTLINE

SECTION I: CARDINAL HEALTH VENTILATORS

Cardinal AVEA
Cardinal Bear 1000
Cardinal VELA

"The cardinal virtue of a teacher (is) to protect the pupil from his own influence."
Ralph Waldo Emerson

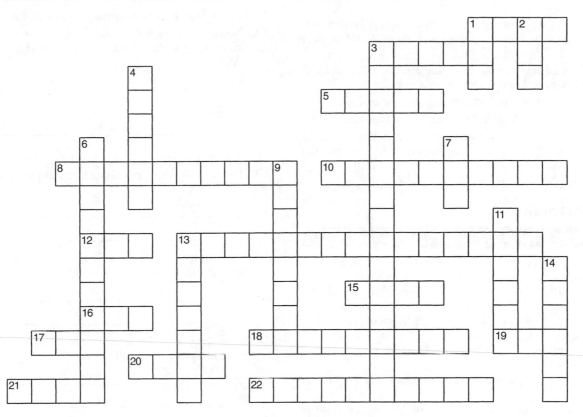

CROSSWORD PUZZLE 12-1

Use the clues to complete the crossword puzzle.

Across

1. A dual-control, closed-loop mode of ventilation on the Bear 1000 (*abbreviation*).
3. The AVEA has this type of rise feature.
5. The number of versions of the VELA ventilator.
8. This internal compressor on the AVEA was designed with technology similar to refrigerator compressors (*two words*).
10. A type of relief valve contained in the VELA that opens if the ventilator cannot provide adequate air during inspiratory demand.
12. A type of weaning mode available on the Bear 1000 (*abbreviation*).
13. Another name for the answer to **10 across**.
15. When activated, this type of breath is delivered every 100th mandatory breath in volume ventilation on the Bear 1000.
16. When turned on, the AVEA will adjust the pressure delivered to compensate for the pressure drop across the artificial airway (*abbreviation*).
17. From the beginning of inspiration to the end of expiration (*abbreviation*).

18. _____ control is used for the delivery of medication on the Bear 1000.
19. This can affect the operation of the Bear 1000 (*abbreviation*).
20. The Cardinal Health ventilator that can be used with neonatal patients.
21. From the flow-control valve on the Bear 1000, gas travels through this and out of the ventilator through the outlet check valve (*abbreviation*).
22. The patient is beginning the ventilator breath using pressure _____.

Down

1. The pressure mode on the Bear 1000 (*abbreviation*).
2. It contains all the AVEA's software and electronic control mechanisms (*abbreviation*).
3. The type of pneumotachometer used by the AVEA to measure tidal volume delivery at the patient Y-connector (*two words*).

185

4. The type of pressure manometer on the from panel of the Bear 1000.

6. Serves as an internal reservoir to supply flow on-demand to the patient who is using an AVEA or Bear 1000.

7. This emergency mode on the VELA will activate if no patient effort is detected (*abbreviation*).

9. One type of targeted ventilation on the AVEA.

11. One type of targeted ventilation on the Bear 1000.

13. _____ volume sets the minimum tidal volume for a pressure-targeted breath on the VELA.

14. The AVEA is able to deliver this type of gas.

Cardinal AVEA

LEARNING OBJECTIVES

Upon completion of this section, you will be able to:

1. Explain the power sources of the AVEA.
2. Describe the function of each of the membrane buttons.
3. Identify indicators located on the front of the ventilator.
4. Determine the current power source and battery status.
5. Outline the parameter setup when "New Patient" is selected.
6. Name the limit for the ratio of inspiratory time to expiratory time (I:E ratio) variable.
7. Compare the trigger, target (limit), and cycle variables for the available modes of ventilation.
8. Identify the icons and waveforms on the main screen.
9. Recognize visual and audio alarm signals in terms of level of priority.
10. Explain how to access the following: ventilator set-up, screen menu, main screen, advanced settings, alarm limits, and mode menu.
11. Describe the purpose of each of the advanced settings.
12. Explain how to access respiratory mechanics and the function of each of the respiratory mechanics.

ACHIEVING THE OBJECTIVES

1. Explain the power sources of the AVEA.

1A. Name four pneumatic power sources and their pressure ranges for appropriate operation of the AVEA.

_____

_____

_____

_____

1B. Describe the three possible electrical power sources for the AVEA.

_____

_____

1C. How long can the AVEA's internal battery power the ventilator?

_____

_____

1D. How long can the internal and external batteries together power the ventilator?

_____

_____

1E. How long can the internal and external batteries together power both the ventilator and the compressor?

_____

_____

1F. Where are the battery indicators located on the AVEA?

_____

_____

2. Describe the function of each of the membrane buttons.

Refer to Figure 12-1 to answer Questions 2A through 2T.

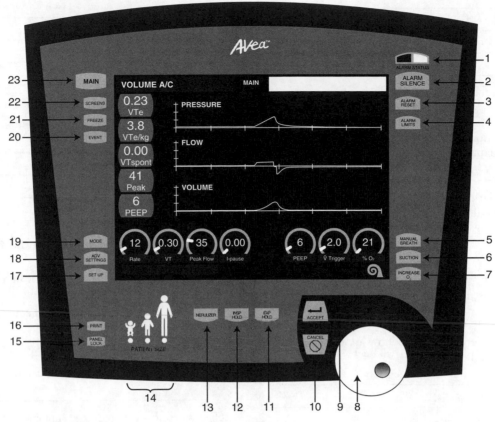

FIGURE 12-1

2A. Which membrane button on Figure 12-1 opens and closes the MODE menu?

_____

_____

2B. The button that opens and closes an advanced-settings window for future activation or parameter adjustment is identified on Figure 12-1 as number

_____.

2C. Which membrane button on Figure 12-1 opens and closes the VENTILATOR SETUP screen?

_____

_____

2D. The button that activates proposed changes to a highlighted field or controls on Figure 12-1 is

_____

_____.

2E. The button on Figure 12-1 that causes the AVEA to disregard proposed changes and revert to the previous settings, still in effect.

_____

2F. If a single breath with the current settings is needed, which button on Figure 12-1 should be pressed?

_____

_____

2G. Describe the function of the "alarm silence" button.

_____

_____

2H. When the button identified as 6 on Figure 12-1 is pressed, what will occur?

_____

_____

_____

_____

_____

_____

2I. Describe the function of the "Increase O_2" button (#7).

_____

_____

_____

_____

2J. Which button is used to determine plateau pressure?

_____

2K. Which button is used to determine automatic positive end-expiratory pressure (auto-PEEP)?

_____

2L. What is the name and location, in Figure 12-1, of the button that allows the operator to adjust the alarm settings?

_____

_____

2M. How long is the audible alarm silence?

_____

2N. Once a problem is resolved, how are visual indicator alarms cancelled?

_____

_____

2O. How is the SCREEN menu accessed?

_____

2P. How does the operator examine specific data points on the graphics being generated while ventilating a patient?

_____

_____

_____

_____

2Q. What is the function of the EVENT button?

_____

_____

_____

_____

2R. What is the function of the MAIN button?

_____

_____

2S. How does the NEBULIZER button operate?

_____

_____

_____

_____

_____

_____

2T. What does the PANEL LOCK button do?

_____

_____

_____

_____

3. Identify indicators located on the front of the ventilator.

Refer to Figure 12-1 to answer Questions 3A through 3C.

3A. Where are the patient size indicator light-emitting diodes (LEDs)?

_____

3B. Locate the alarm-priority indicator.

_____

3C. Where do alarm messages appear on the front of the AVEA?

_____

_____

4. Determine the current power source and battery status.

4A. Where are the power source indicators located on the AVEA?

_____

_____

4B. Where is the on/off switch located?

_____

4C. When alternating current (AC) power is connected and running the ventilator, what is displayed by the power-source indicators?

_____

_____

4D. How is it determined that there is an alternate power source being used?

_____

_____

_____

_____

_____

4E. How is the status of the alternate power source determined?

_____

_____

_____

_____

4F. What is the order of power consumption for the AVEA ventilator?

_____

_____

_____

_____

5. Outline the parameter set-up when "New Patient" is selected.

5A. Before you choose "New Patient" or "Resume Current," what needs to be done to the ventilator?

_____

_____

5B. What occurs when "New Patient" is selected?

_____

_____

_____

_____

5C. The ventilator will begin operation with which parameters following "New Patient" selection?

_____

_____

_____

_____

5D. What does the SETUP screen allow the operator to choose?

_____

_____

_____

_____

5E. What other information must be entered into the ventilation set-up window before beginning ventilation of the new patient?

_____

_____

_____

_____

_____

_____

_____

_____

5F. How are the aforementioned patient parameters (Question 5E) finalized?

_____

_____

6. Name the limit for the I:E variable.

6A. How does the high-pressure limit change the I:E ratio?

_____

_____

_____

_____

_____

6B. Explain *PSV Tmax*.

_____

_____

_____

_____

6C. What is the maximum I:E ratio allowed by the AVEA? _____

7. Compare the trigger, target (limit), and cycle variables for the available modes of ventilation.

	Mode of Ventilation	Trigger	Target (limit)	Cycle
7A.				
7B.				
7C.				
7D.				
7E.				
7F.				
7G.				
7H.				
7I.				
7J.				

8. Identify the icons and waveforms on the main screen.

8A. How is the screen digital display customized?

_____

_____

_____

_____

_____

_____

_____

_____

8B. What is the maximum number of waveforms that can be displayed on the main screen?

_____

_____

8C. Which waveform tracings can be displayed on the main screen?

_____

_____

_____

_____

8D. How many real-time loops can be displayed on the main screen? _____

8E. Where is the current mode displayed on the main screen? (*see Figure 12-1*)

_____

_____

8F. Where do the PEEP, flow trigger, and fractional inspired oxygen (F_IO_2) appear on the main screen? (*see Figure 12-1*)

_____

_____

9. Recognize visual and audio alarm signals in terms of level of priority.

9A. What is the location of ALARM INDICATOR on the main screen?

_____

_____

9B. What does the presence of a white triangle to the right of the alarm message indicate?

_____

_____

_____

_____

9C. A solid-yellow alarm indicator with single-tone audio indicates what priority of alarm?

_____

_____

9D. A flashing red alarm indicator with five tones repeated indicates what priority of alarm?

_____

_____

9E. A flashing yellow alarm indicator with three tones repeated indicates what priority of alarm?

_____

_____

9F. How is normal ventilator status identified?

_____

_____

10. Explain how to access the following: ventilator set-up, screen menu, main screen, advanced settings, alarm limits, and mode menu.

10A. How does the operator access ventilator set-up?

_____

_____

10B. The screen menu can be accessed by doing what?

_____

_____

10C. How is the main screen accessed?

_____

10D. How are the advanced settings accessed?

_____

10E. The operator accesses the ALARM LIMITS menu by doing what?

_____

_____

_____

_____

10F. How does a clinician change modes?

_____

_____

_____

_____

11. Describe the purpose of each of the advanced settings.

11A. What do the advanced settings allow the clinician to do?

_____

_____

11B. What is volume limit and why is it used?

_____

_____

_____

_____

_____

11C. During which modes of ventilation can volume limit be used?

_____

_____

11D. Describe machine volume ("Mach Vol") and its purpose.

_____

_____

_____

_____

_____

_____

_____

_____

11E. What is the purpose of "Inspiratory Rise"?

_____

_____

_____

_____

11F. What does the flow-cycle setting adjust?

_____

_____

_____

_____

11G. What does "PSV" Tmax limit?

_____

_____

_____

_____

11H. Describe the waveform feature.

_____

_____

_____

_____

11I. What is the "Sigh" control?

_____

_____

_____

11J. What is the default value and range for the bias flow?

_____

_____

11K. What is unique about patient-triggering on the AVEA?

_____

_____

_____

_____

_____

11L. What procedure does the ventilator follow when "Vsync" is turned on?

_____

_____

_____

_____

_____

_____

_____

11M. How does the AVEA respond to a change in volume delivery when using "Vsync"?

_____

_____

_____

_____

_____

11N. When "Vsync" is enabled, how is the slope of the inspiratory pressure adjusted?

_____

_____

12. Explain how to access respiratory mechanics and the function of each of the respiratory mechanics.

12A. How are the respiratory mechanics accessed on the AVEA?

_____

_____

12B. What additional equipment is necessary for the measurement of esophageal pressure?

_____

_____

12C. What is the purpose of esophageal pressure?

_____

_____

12D. What is the difference between maximum inspiratory pressure and pressure drop at 100 milliseconds?

_____

_____

_____

_____

_____

_____

_____

12E. What are the two points that the inflection point maneuver determines?

_____

_____

12F. What is the advantage of knowing the two Pflex points?

_____

_____

_____

_____

_____

_____

_____

12G. When the auto-PEEP maneuver is active, what values will the ventilator display?

_____

_____

_____

_____

Think About This

What are the advantages and disadvantages of having a panel lock?

Helpful Web Site

- Cardinal Health, AVEA Comprehensive Ventilator — http://www.viasyshealthcare.com

NBRC-TYPE QUESTIONS CARDINAL AVEA

1. *Apnea back-up ventilation* (ABV) is active on the AVEA ventilator during the use of which of the following modes of ventilation?
   I. Volume assist/control (A/C)
   II. Pressure synchronized intermittent mandatory ventilation (SIMV)
   III. Airway pressure-release ventilation (APRV)/BiPhasic
   IV. Pressure-regulated volume control (PRVC) A/C
   A. I and II only
   B. II and III only
   C. III and IV only
   D. I and IV only

2. Calculate the flow at which the ventilator will cycle when the AVEA ventilator is in the pressure A/C mode, the flow cycle is set at 40%, and the peak inspiratory flow is 45 L/min.
   A. 18 L/min
   B. 20 L/min
   C. 25 L/min
   D. Flow-cycling is available only during spontaneous breaths.

3. The battery-status indicator on the AVEA is yellow. The percentage of charge remaining in the external battery is equal to which of the following?
   A. 85%
   B. 60%
   C. 35%
   D. 20%

4. The AVEA is in the pressure-support ventilation (PSV) mode; the PSV cycle is set to 10%; and the peak inspiratory flow is measured at 35 L/min. The ventilator is continuously time-cycling at 2 seconds. The most-appropriate action to take at this time is which of the following?
   A. Increase the flow-rate setting.
   B. Increase the PSV cycle to 40%.
   C. Increase the PSV Tmax to 3 seconds.
   D. Change the mode to pressure-targeted SIMV.

5. Use of Vsync on the AVEA ventilator will change volume breaths into which of the following?
   A. Pressure-limited, volume-targeted breaths
   B. Volume-limited, pressure-targeted breaths
   C. Pressure-limited, flow-cycled breaths
   D. Volume-limited, time-cycled breaths

6. When pressure-targeted breaths are activated, triggering is based on which of the following?
   I. Flow
   II. Time
   III. Volume
   IV. Pressure
   A. II
   B. I and III
   C. III and IV
   D. I, II, and IV

7. An adult is being ventilated with the AVEA in the PRVC mode. The ventilator is not delivering the set volume. The ventilator will do which of the following?
   A. Initiate ABV.
   B. Change over to volume-targeted ventilation.
   C. Produce an audible and visual high-priority alarm.
   D. Increase pressure by 3 cm H_2O to achieve the minimum volume.

8. An neonate is being ventilated with the AVEA and is receiving 40% oxygen. Just before tracheal suctioning, the "Increase O_2" button is pressed. What F_IO_2 will the infant receive for 2 minutes?
   A. 100%
   B. 75%
   C. 48%
   D. 36%

Cardinal Bear 1000

Upon completion of this section, you will be able to:

1. Describe the major components of the internal mechanisms of the Bear 1000.
2. Identify the controls, and discuss the function of each.
3. Explain how the controls are set.
4. Discuss how the alarms are set.
5. Assess what alarm-activated LEDs and alarm messages indicate, and state possible causes for them.
6. Compare each of the modes of ventilation on the Bear 1000, including the trigger and cycle mechanisms and the target variables (pressure or volume).
7. Evaluate a graph or a description of a graphics display that shows pressure-sloping or pressure augmentation (PAug) to determine whether the ventilator is set appropriately.
8. Explain the function of the "compliance comp." control.
9. Identify a resource that can help you determine the cause(s) of a functional problem in the Bear 1000.

ACHIEVING THE OBJECTIVES

1. Describe the major components of the internal mechanisms of the Bear 1000.

1A. Where do oxygen and air mix within this ventilator?

_____

1B. How much gas is held in a reservoir for high-flow situations? _____

1C. What is the driving pressure of the gas held in reserve? _____

1D. What controls the output from the flow-control valve?

_____

_____

1E. Which device operates the flow-control valve, making rapid changes in flow possible?

_____

_____

1F. Trace the air and oxygen as they enter the Bear 1000 until they exit the ventilator toward the patient.

_____

_____

_____

_____

_____

_____

_____

_____

_____

_____

_____

2. Identify the controls and discuss the function of each.

Use Figure 12-2 to answer Questions 2A through 2N.

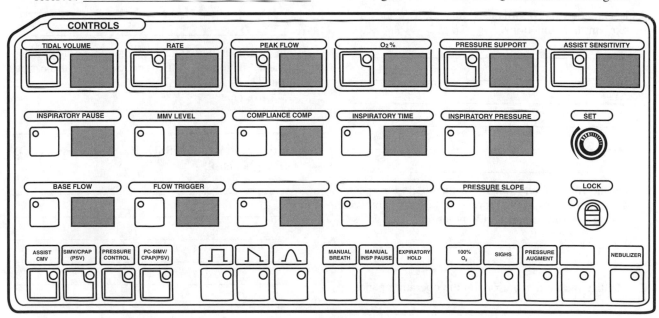

FIGURE 12-2

2A. Identify the six controls in the top row and give their ranges.

_____

_____

_____

_____

2B. How can tidal volumes and flows that are below the adult ranges be accessed to ventilate pediatric patients?

_____

_____

_____

_____

2C. Identify and explain the use of the five controls in the second row.

_____

_____

_____

_____

_____

_____

_____

_____

2D. Locate the two controls used to set flow trigger and explain their functions.

_____

_____

_____

_____

_____

2E. On the Bear 1000, the control that alters the speed at which the inspiratory pressure level is achieved during pressure-controlled ventilation is known as

_____

_____.

2F. Identify the mode controls on the operating panel.

_____

_____

2G. Explain the function of the flow waveform controls.

_____

_____

_____

_____

_____

_____

_____

_____

_____

_____

_____

_____

2H. What is the function of the MANUAL BREATH control?

_____

_____

2I. A single inspiratory pause, up to a maximum of 2 seconds, can be performed by using which control?

_____

_____

2J. Auto-PEEP can be measured by using which control on the front panel?

_____

_____

2K. In order to hyperoxygenate a patient before endotracheal suctioning, which control should be activated?

_____

_____

2L. Explain the PRESSURE AUGMENTATION (PAug) control.

_____

_____

_____

_____

_____

_____

_____

2M. Describe the function of the NEBULIZER control.

_____

_____

_____

_____

_____

2N. Where is the PEEP control located, and how is it set?

_____

_____

_____

_____

3. Explain how the controls are set.

_____

_____

_____

_____

4. Discuss how the alarms are set.

4A. Where are the adjustable alarms located?

_____

4B. Name the adjustable alarms.

_____

_____

4C. Describe the procedure for setting these alarms.

_____

_____

_____

_____

_____

_____

_____

_____

_____

_____

_____

_____

5. Assess what alarm-activated-LEDs and alarm messages indicate, and state possible causes for them.

5A. During operation the abbreviation "Pro" appears in the peak inspiratory pressure (PIP) alarm display window. What does this indicate, and what are the possible causes?

_____

_____

_____

_____

5B. During operation of a ventilator in the Assist CMV (continuous mandatory ventilation) mode, the TOTAL MINUTE VOLUME light to the right of the digital display begins to flash and an audible alarm sounds. Further investigation reveals it is the high TOTAL MINUTE VOLUME alarm that is active. What are the possible causes?

_____

_____

_____

_____

_____

5C. What is the most likely cause of a low BASELINE PRESSURE alarm?

_____

_____

5D. What does the activation of the GAS SUPPLY FAILURE alarm indicate?

_____

_____

5E. During operation of a ventilator, the RUN DIAGNOSTICS alarm is active; what does this indicate?

_____

_____

_____

_____

_____

5F. Describe the two possible causes for the activation of the TIME/I:E LIMIT alarm.

_____

_____

_____

_____

5G. What happens to the Bear 1000 if there is an internal or external condition that does not allow the ventilator to operate properly?

_____

_____

_____

6. Compare each of the modes of ventilation on the Bear 1000, including the trigger and cycle mechanisms and the target variables (pressure or volume).

	Mode of ventilation	Trigger	Target (limit)	Cycle
6A.	Assist CMV			
6B.	SIMV			
6C.	Continuous positive airway pressure (CPAP)			
6D.	PSV			
6E.	Pressure control			
6F.	Pressure-controlled SIMV (PC-SIMV)			
6G.	Pressure Augment (PAug)			
6H.	Mandatory minute volume (MMV) ventilation			

7. Evaluate a graph or a description of a graphics display that shows pressure-sloping or pressure augmentation (PAug) to determine whether the ventilator is set appropriately.

7A. An adult patient was just switched from CMV to PAug with a set pressure of 20 cm H_2O, a PEEP of 5 cm H_2O, and a tidal volume of 550 mL, with a constant flow pattern. Figure 12-3 shows a sample of the pressure, flow, and volume scalars following this change. Interpret this graphics display.

_____

_____

_____

_____

_____

_____

_____

_____

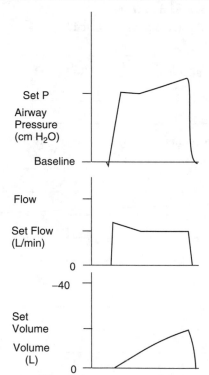

FIGURE 12-3

7B. The pressure waveform is taking about half of inspiratory time to reach the set airway pressure during pressure-supported breaths. What could be done to improve this situation?

_____

_____

_____

_____

7C. A patient is being ventilated in the PAug mode on the Bear 1000. Evaluate the pressure waveform in Figure 12-4. What action should be taken?

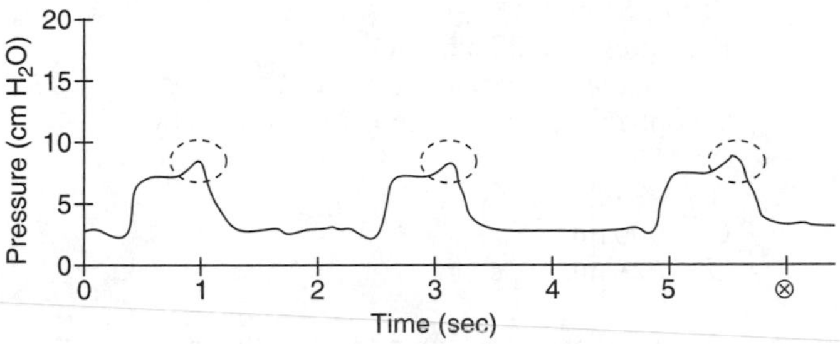

FIGURE 12-4

_____

_____

_____

_____

_____

7D. Explain the pressure waveform generated during PSV (Figure 12-5). What action should be taken?

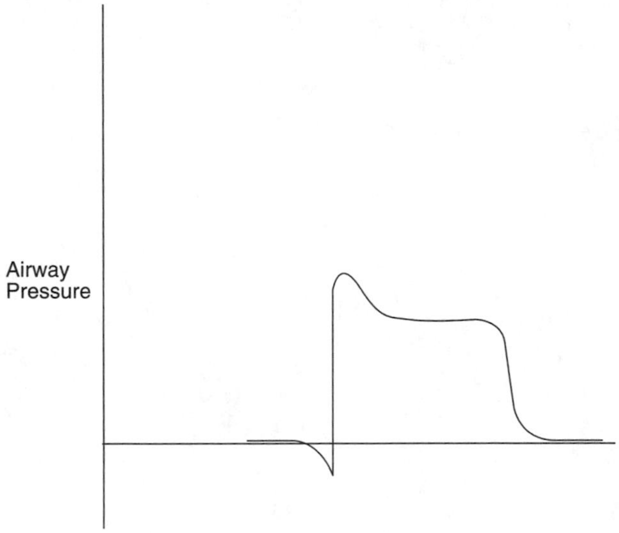

FIGURE 12-5

_____

_____

_____

_____

_____

_____

_____

8. Explain the function of the "compliance comp." control.

8A. How is tubing compliance obtained?

_____

8B. How does the Bear 1000 calculate the amount of volume that needs to be added to compensate for tubing compressibility?

_____

8C. What formula does the Bear 1000 use to calculate the volume output from the ventilator that is necessary to deliver the set tidal volume?

_____

_____

8D. Given tubing compliance of 2.5 mL/cm H_2O, calculate the total volume output from the Bear 1000 if the set tidal volume is 475 mL, the PIP is 15 cm H_2O, and the PEEP is 5 cm H_2O.

_____

_____

_____

_____

9. Identify a resource that can help you determine the cause(s) of a functional problem in the Bear 1000.

_____

_____

Think About This

Is it possible to shield ventilators from the effects of electromagnetic frequency interference?

Helpful Web Site

■ The University of Kansas, Respiratory Care Education, Bear 1000 Information — http://www.kumc.edu

199

NBRC-TYPE QUESTIONS CARDINAL BEAR 1000

1. Which of the following is the sigh volume and sigh pressure limit for a Bear 1000 ventilator set at a tidal volume of 475 mL and a pressure limit of 30 cm H_2O?
   A. 590 mL and 37 cm H_2O
   B. 712 mL and 45 cm H_2O
   C. 850 mL and 60 cm H_2O
   D. 950 mL and 55 cm H_2O

2. Mandatory breaths in the PC-SIMV mode can be triggered by which of the following?
   I. Time
   II. Flow
   III. Volume
   IV. Pressure
      A. II only
      B. I and II only
      C. III and IV only
      D. II, III, and IV only

3. In the PAug mode on the Bear 1000, the tidal volume has been delivered quickly, so inspiration will end when which of the following occurs?
   A. The set pressure is reached.
   B. The set volume is obtained.
   C. The inspiratory time setting is reached.
   D. The flow drops to 30% of the measured peak flow.

4. On the Bear 1000 the control that alters the speed at which the inspiratory pressure level is achieved during pressure-controlled ventilation is known as which of the following?
   A. Base Flow
   B. Smart Trigger
   C. Pressure Slope
   D. Pressure Augment

5. The PEAK INSP PRESSURE digital message display window is showing the abbreviation "Pro." Which of the following is the most-appropriate action to correct this?
   A. Suction and lavage the patient.
   B. Decrease the low PEEP alarm.
   C. Dry off the pressure transducer.
   D. Reconnect the proximal pressure line.

6. Calculate the volume output from a Bear 1000 ventilator by using the following data:
   PEEP: 8 cm H_2O
   Peak pressure: 28 cm H_2O
   Set tidal volume: 550 mL
   Compliance compensation: 2.8 mL/cm H_2O
   A. 56 mL
   B. 78 mL
   C. 606 mL
   D. 628 mL

7. During a pressure-supported breath, the patient's peak inspiratory flow rate is 60 L/min. At what flow rate will inspiration end?
   A. 18 L/min
   B. 30 L/min
   C. 45 L/min
   D. 55 L/min

8. What is the cycle mechanism for mandatory breaths in the PC-SIMV mode?
   A. Flow
   B. Time
   C. Pressure
   D. Volume

Cardinal VELA

Upon completion of this section, you will be able to:
1. Explain the function of the available oxygen sources for the VELA.
2. Discuss the function of the internal turbine.
3. Describe the leak-compensation function.
4. Compare ventilator controls on the VELA with those on the AVEA.
5. Perform a preuse test on the VELA.
6. Describe how and when to set up ABV.
7. Define the following: *assured volume, volume limit, Vsync,* and *flow-cycle.*
8. Explain the use of PSV during APRV/BiPhasic ventilation.

ACHIEVING THE OBJECTIVES

1. Explain the function of the available oxygen sources for the VELA.

1A. Describe the two different methods of adding supplemental oxygen to the VELA.

_____

_____

_____

_____

_____

1B. During which type of ventilation would the low-pressure oxygen source be most appropriate?

_____

_____

1C. When the low-pressure oxygen source is in use, how is F_IO_2 determined?

_____

_____

_____

2. Discuss the function of the internal turbine.

_____

_____

_____

_____

_____

_____

3. Describe the leak-compensation function.

3A. What is the purpose of leak compensation on the VELA?

_____

_____

3B. What is the maximum amount of leakage for which this function can compensate?

_____

_____

3C. How does the leak compensation operate?

_____

_____

_____

_____

_____

_____

4. Compare ventilator controls on the VELA with those on the AVEA.

_____

_____

_____

_____

_____

_____

_____

_____

_____

_____

_____

5. Perform a preuse test on the VELA.

5A. When should a preuse test be performed?

_____

_____

5B. What is the procedure for performing this test while a patient is using the VELA?

_____

_____

_____

_____

5C. Explain the procedure for setting up the preuse test.

_____

_____

_____

_____

_____

_____

5D. What types of tests are accessible from the preuse test menu?

_____

_____

6. Describe how and when to set up ABV.

6A. When should ABV be used?

_____

_____

6B. What parameters need to be set for ABV?

_____

_____

6C. What is the default breath rate for ABV?

_____

6D. When will ABV be initiated?

_____

_____

6E. What alarm priority level pertains to ABV?

_____

_____

7. Define the following: *assured volume, volume limit, Vsync,* and *flow-cycle.*

7A. Explain assured volume.

_____

_____

_____

_____

_____

_____

_____

_____

7B. Define *volume limit.*

_____

_____

_____

_____

_____

7C. What is Vsync?

_____

_____

_____

_____

7D. Explain flow-cycle.

_____

_____

_____

_____

8. Explain the use of PSV during APRV/BiPhasic ventilation.

_____

_____

_____

_____

_____

Think About This

What is the advantage of having a ventilator that can operate noninvasively as well as invasively?

Helpful Web Site

■ Cardinal Health, VELA Ventilator Series — http://www.viasyshealthcare.com

NBRC-TYPE QUESTIONS CARDINAL VELA

1. When this feature is set on the VELA, the machine delivers the set pressure and monitors volume delivery. If the set volume is not reached before the normal cycling mechanism, the ventilator delivers the minimum volume by continuous flow. This is known as which of the following?
   A. Vsync
   B. Volume limit
   C. Machine volume
   D. Inspiratory rise

2. On the VELA, inspiratory rise adjusts the rate of which of the following?
   A. Flow
   B. Pressure
   C. Volume
   D. Oxygen

3. ABV is active on the VELA ventilator during the use of which of the following modes of ventilation?
   I. SIMV
   II. Volume A/C
   III. CPAP/PSV
   IV. PRVC A/C
   A. I and II only
   B. I and III only
   C. II and IV only
   D. III and IV only

4. On the VELA ventilator, which of the following is the setting that will extend inspiratory time to ensure that a minimum volume has been delivered?
   A. Vsync
   B. Flow cycle
   C. Volume limit
   D. Assured volume

5. Auto-PEEP can be measured on the VELA by using which of the following?
   A. Freeze button
   B. Inspiratory hold
   C. Expiratory hold
   D. Manual breath

SECTION II: DRÄGER VENTILATORS

E-4 (Evita 4)
EvitaXL SW 6.0

"Every great advance in science has issued from a new audacity of the imagination."
John Dewey

KEY TERMS CROSSWORD PUZZLE

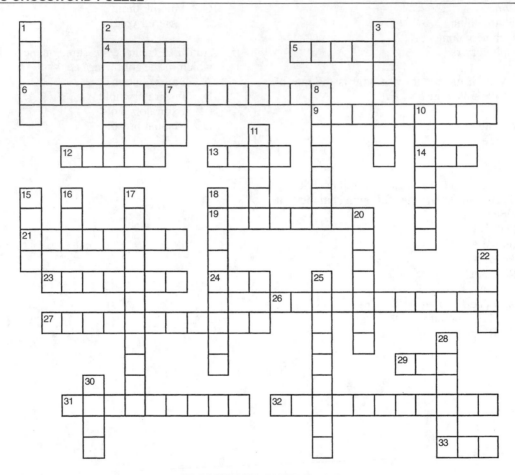

CROSSWORD PUZZLE 12-2

Use the clues to complete the crossword puzzle.

Across

4. A mode of ventilation that uses two levels of CPAP (*abbreviation*).
5. Another name for the answer to **27 across**.
6. The Evita 4 contains these types of servo valves.
9. A type of pressure used to evaluate neuromuscular drive.
12. This type of ventilation is initiated when a patient stops breathing.
13. A mode that allows the patient to breathe spontaneously between mandatory ventilator breaths (*abbreviation*).
14. A mode that provides a positive feedback system of respiration (*abbreviation*).
19. A dual mode of ventilation similar to PRVC and volume support (*two words*).
21. A low-priority alarm.
23. Something that watches and checks on performance.
24. Helps to compensate for the airway resistance associated with small artificial airways (*abbreviation*).
26. The setting that changes the ability of the patient to trigger the ventilator.
27. A hold used to establish static compliance.

29. A mode of ventilation that is patient-triggered, pressure-targeted, and flow-cycled (*abbreviation*).
31. A closed-loop form of ventilation designed to shorten weaning time (*two words*).
32. The use of **27 across** increases this time.
33. A supplementary function or safety feature that can be used in CMV, SIMV, and MMV ventilation (*abbreviation*).

Down

1. Soft knobs are also called _____ knobs.
2. A medium-priority alarm.
3. Allows the E-4 to be adapted for use with very small patients.
7. A closed-loop form of ventilation used with a patient who can perform part of the work of breathing (WOB) and who is progressing toward discontinuation of the ventilator (*abbreviation*).
8. The panel that contains touch pads and a dial knob.
10. Spontaneous breaths can be assisted with pressure _____.
11. A type of window on the E-4 that appears at the bottom left of the screen.
15. A type of ventilator mode that has the patient breathing spontaneously throughout the entire cycle (*abbreviation*).
16. A type of ventilator mode that provides full ventilatory support for the patient (*abbreviation*).
17. A type of patient trigger (*two words*).
18. Time-triggered breaths are _____.
20. A top-priority alarm.
22. The areas of the touch-sensitive screen that are touched are known as _____.
25. _____ PEEP or auto-PEEP.
28. A feature used to evaluate upper and lower inflection points (*abbreviation*).
30. A safety feature of the E-4 that exists to control pressure during the delivery of a volume breath in CMV, SIMV, and MMV ventilation (*abbreviation*).

Evita 4 (E-4)

LEARNING OBJECTIVES

Upon completion of this section, you will be able to:
1. Describe the front panel of the Dräger E-4.
2. Discuss the function of each control on the E-4 front panel.
3. Compare the set-up of a ventilator mode on the E-4 with that on another microprocessor-controlled intensive care unit (ICU) ventilator.
4. Assess an alarm situation, describe its priority level, and suggest a possible cause and solution.
5. Identify a pressure/time graph for a patient breathing spontaneously during pressure-controlled ventilation (PCV).

6. Compare the upper Paw alarm limit to the P_{max}.
7. Describe the method for setting PCV and APRV and compare the two modes of ventilation.
8. Discuss the similarities and differences between AutoFlow and PRVC on the Servo 300.
9. List the features available when NeoFlow™ is added as an upgrade to the Dräger E-4.
10. Explain the set-up and function of proportional pressure support.

ACHIEVING THE OBJECTIVES

1. Describe the front panel of the Dräger E-4.

1A. What type of technology does the computer screen use? _____
_____

1B. How do the images or icons appear on the computer screen? _____
_____

1C. What is located below the front operating panel?
_____
_____
_____
_____
_____
_____

2. Discuss the function of each control on the E-4 front panel.

2A. Explain the function of the controls located on the left side of the screen.
_____
_____
_____
_____
_____
_____
_____
_____
_____
_____
_____
_____
_____
_____

Chapter **12** **Mechanical Ventilators: General-Use Devices**

2B. Explain the function of the touch pads on the far right side of the front panel.

_____

_____

_____

_____

_____

_____

2C. What touch pads are located on the immediate right side of the computer screen, and what are their functions?

_____

_____

_____

_____

_____

_____

_____

_____

_____

_____

3. Compare the set-up of a ventilator mode on the E-4 with that on another microprocessor-controlled ICU ventilator.

3A. Explain the standard start-up configuration for the E-4.

_____

_____

_____

_____

_____

_____

_____

_____

_____

_____

3B. Explain how to change the start-up mode.

_____

_____

_____

_____

_____

_____

3C. How can the programmed values be changed?

_____

_____

_____

_____

4. Assess an alarm situation, describe its priority level, and suggest a possible cause and solution.

Fill in the blanks for the following table.

	Alarm situation	Priority	Cause	Solution
4A.	Airway pressure high			
4B.			Patient's breathing has stopped	
4C.			Faulty ventilator	
4D.	Malfunctioning fan			
4E.			Patient is breathing at a very high spontaneous respiratory rate	

5. Identify a pressure/time graph for a patient breathing spontaneously during PCV.

Identify the following pressure/time graphs.

5A. _____

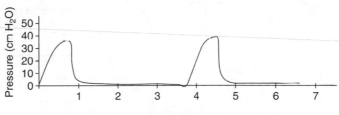

FIGURE 12-6

5B. _____

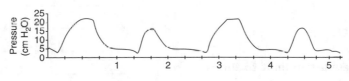

FIGURE 12-7

5C. _____

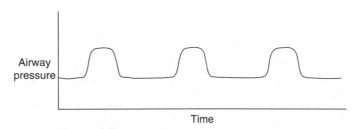

FIGURE 12-8

5D. _____

_____

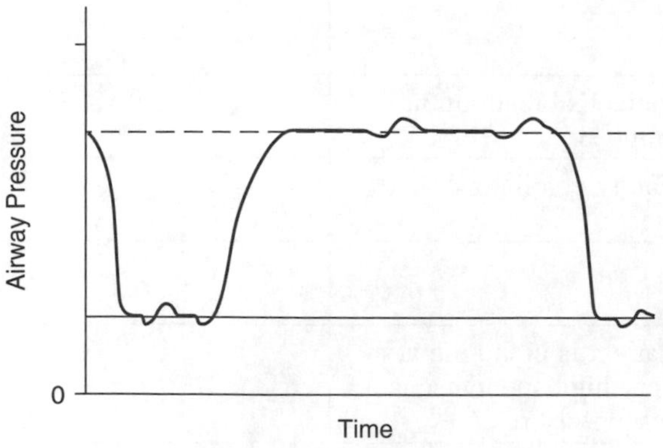

FIGURE 12-9

5E. _____

_____

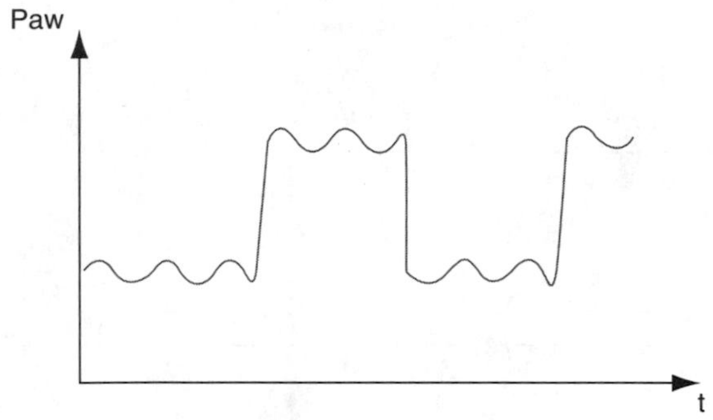

FIGURE 12-10

6. Compare the upper Paw alarm limit to the Pmax pressure limit.

6A. During volume-targeted ventilation on a generic ventilator, the PIP rises to the set upper Paw alarm limit, or maximum safety pressure. What happens to inspiration at this time?

_____

_____

6B. What is the cycle variable when the set upper Paw alarm limit is reached?

_____

_____

6C. What happens to flow when the set upper Paw alarm limit is reached?

_____

_____

6D. If the "Pmax Pressure-Limit Function" is used on the E-4, what happens to inspiration when the Pmax pressure setting is reached?

_____

_____

6E. What is the cycle variable when the Pmax pressure setting is reached?

_____

_____

6F. What happens to flow when the Pmax pressure setting is reached?

_____

_____

7. Describe the method for setting PCV and APRV and compare the two modes of ventilation.

7A. How is PCV+ set up on the E-4?

_____

_____

_____

_____

_____

_____

7B. What is the function of pressure rise time in PCV+?

_____

_____

_____

_____

7C. Explain the operation of PCV+.

_____

_____

_____

_____

_____

_____

_____

_____

_____

_____

7D. How is APRV set up on the E-4?

_____

_____

_____

_____

_____

_____

_____

7E. Explain the operation of APRV.

_____

_____

_____

8. Discuss the similarities and differences between AutoFlow and PRVC on the Servo 300.

8A. What is the difference in the first few breaths of AutoFlow and those of PRVC?

_____

_____

_____

_____

_____

_____

_____

_____

_____

8B. What similarities do these two modes have in their method for establishing the minimum pressure needed to deliver the set volume?

_____

_____

_____

8C. Which ventilator also calculates out resistance to aid in the establishment of minimum pressure for a set volume?

_____

8D. What is the major difference between AutoFlow on the E-4 and PRVC on the Servo 300?

_____

_____

_____

_____

_____

_____

_____

_____

_____

_____

_____

9. List the features available when NeoFlow™ is added as an upgrade to the Dräger E-4.

9A. What must be added to the E-4 to allow NeoFlow™ to operate?

_____

_____

9B. In the neonatal mode, what features are active?

_____

_____

_____

_____

9C. What measurements can be provided in the neonatal mode?

_____

_____

_____

10. Explain the set-up and function of proportional pressure support.

10A. Describe the set-up procedure for proportional pressure support (PPS) on the E-4.

_____

_____

_____

_____

_____

_____

_____

209

10B. What are the differences between pressure support and PPS?

_____

_____

_____

_____

10C. Why do safety limits need to be set when PPS is in use?

_____

_____

_____

_____

10D. What are the two components for which PPS is compensating?

_____

_____

10E. Which PPS settings help overcome these two components?

_____

_____

Think About This

What are the steps in the development of new ventilator modes?

Helpful Web Site

■ Dräger Medical AG & Co, Evita 4 — http://www.draeger.com

NBRC-TYPE QUESTIONS DRÄGER E-4 (EVITA 4)

1. Which of the following statements is true concerning Pmax?
   A. Pmax is a PIP alarm.
   B. Pmax sets the upper pressure during APRV.
   C. PCV+ uses Pmax to set the PIP.
   D. Pmax changes breath delivery during CMV, SIMV, and MMV ventilation.

2. Which of the following is the cycle variable during Pmax use?
   A. Flow
   B. Time
   C. Volume
   D. Pressure

3. A patient being mechanically ventilated with an E-4 has an occlusion pressure of -8 cm H_2O. Which of the following is the most-appropriate statement concerning this measurement?
   A. The patient is ready for extubation.
   B. The patient has respiratory muscle fatigue.
   C. This is a normal value for a ventilated patient.
   D. This value indicates that the patient has chronic obstructive pulmonary disease (COPD).

4. System compliance and resistance are calculated by the E-4 to establish the minimum pressure needed to deliver a set volume when which of the following modes is used?
   A. PPS
   B. PCV+
   C. AutoFlow
   D. MMV/PSV

5. If there is no inspiratory effort from the patient, there will be no support from the E-4 in which of the following modes?
   A. PPS
   B. PCV+
   C. MMV
   D. CMV

6. The circuit pressure rarely builds to the upper Paw alarm limit during ventilation with which of the following modes?
   A. PPS
   B. PCV+
   C. APRV
   D. AutoFlow

EvitaXL SW 6.0

Upon completion of this section, you will be able to:
1. Identify the specific areas of the EvitaXL front control panel.
2. Explain the procedure for selecting and setting parameters and modes.
3. Recognize the way to identify which electrical source is operating with the EvitaXL.
4. List the modes of ventilation available for the EvitaXL.
5. Describe the following modes or functions as they operate with the EvitaXL: APRV, Pmax (pressure-limit ventilation [PLV]), AutoFlow, and sigh.
6. Compare the difference between the operating screen of the E-4 and that of the EvitaXL.
7. Describe the measures obtained with the expiratory hold, inspiratory hold, and occlusion pressure controls.
8. Suggest one use for the reference loops available with the EvitaXL.
9. Explain the purpose of the low-flow pressure-volume loop feature.
10. Compare weaning through SmartCare with weaning through traditional methods.

ACHIEVING THE OBJECTIVES

1. Identify the specific areas of the EvitaXL front control panel.

1A. Name the peripheral control keys, from top to bottom, located on the right side of the screen.

_____

_____

_____

_____

1B. Where is the control knob located?

_____

_____

1C. Where are alarm messages located?

_____

_____

1D. Where are the set ventilation parameters for the active ventilation mode located?

_____

_____

2. Explain the procedure for selecting and setting parameters and modes.

2A. After the ventilator's self-tests are complete, what is displayed on the start-up screen?

_____

_____

2B. What is the procedure for setting up a new patient?

_____

_____

_____

2C. What are the default values for a new patient?

_____

_____

_____

_____

_____

_____

2D. How can the operator choose values other than those that have been preprogrammed (configured)?

_____

_____

_____

_____

_____

_____

_____

_____

2E. What are the steps to alter the unit's preprogrammed start-up mode?

_____

_____

_____

_____

_____

_____

_____

_____

3. Recognize the way to identify which electrical source is operating with the EvitaXL.

3A. What is the standard electrical source used to power the microprocessor and the electrical components of the unit?

_____

_____

3B. What are the two alternative electrical power sources?

_____

_____

3C. How does the operator know which power source is being used?

_____

_____

_____

3D. Describe the icons used to represent each power source.

_____

_____

_____

_____

4. List the modes of ventilation available for the EvitaXL.

_____

_____

_____

_____

5. Describe the following modes or functions as they operate with the EvitaXL: APRV, Pmax (PLV), AutoFlow, and sigh.

5A. How does APRV operate on the EvitaXL?

_____

_____

_____

_____

_____

_____

_____

_____

_____

_____

_____

_____

_____

_____

5B. What is PLV, or Pmax?

_____

_____

_____

_____

_____

_____

_____

_____

_____

_____

_____

_____

_____

5C. How does AutoFlow operate on the EvitaXL?

_____

_____

_____

_____

_____

_____

_____

_____

_____

_____

_____

_____

_____

5D. Describe the sigh function on the EvitaXL.

_____

_____

_____

_____

_____

_____

6. Compare the difference between the operating screen of the E-4 and that of the EvitaXL.

6A. Compare the location of the monitored parameters of both ventilators.

_____

_____

_____

_____

6B. Where are the graphics located on both ventilators?

_____

_____

6C. What are the differences between the E-4 and XL VALUES screen that displays values being measured or calculated?

_____

_____

_____

_____

_____

6D. What differences are there in the graphic displays?

_____

_____

_____

_____

_____

7. Describe the measures obtained with the expiratory hold, inspiratory hold, and occlusion pressure controls.

7A. How does expiratory hold determine the amount of trapped air?

_____

_____

_____

_____

7B. Expiratory hold can be used for what other measurement?

_____

_____

_____

_____

_____

7C. Inspiratory hold is traditionally used for what?

_____

_____

7D. Occlusion pressure is used for what function?

_____

_____

_____

_____

_____

_____

_____

8. Suggest one use for the reference loops available with the EvitaXL.

_____

_____

_____

_____

_____

9. Explain the purpose of the low-flow pressure-volume loop feature.

_____

_____

_____

_____

_____

10. Compare weaning through SmartCare with weaning through traditional methods.

10A. What is the goal of SmartCare?

_____

_____

_____

_____

_____

_____

10B. How does SmartCare maintain a patient's tidal volume?

_____

_____

_____

_____

_____

_____

_____

10C. How do the criteria for traditional weaning compare with those for SmartCare?

_____

_____

_____

_____

_____

10D. In SmartCare, pressure support is adjusted to maintain respiratory rate, tidal volume, and end-tidal CO_2 within what ranges?

_____

_____

_____

_____

_____

_____

Think About This

How long does it take for a new ventilator to go from the research and design stage to operation in the clinical setting?

Helpful Web Sites

- The Chinese University of Hong Kong, EvitaXL, Charles Gomersall — http://www.aic.cuhk.edu.hk
- The Chinese University of Hong Kong, SmartCare, Charles Gomersall — http://www.aic.cuhk.edu.hk
- Dräger Medical AG & Co, EvitaXL — http://www.draeger.com

NBRC-TYPE QUESTIONS DRÄGER EVITAXL SW 6.0

1. How long does the internal battery on the EvitaXL last?
   A. 5 minutes
   B. 10 minutes
   C. 30 minutes
   D. 60 minutes

2. Which of the following functions automatically increases the level of PEEP for two consecutive breaths while the ventilator is in the CMV mode?
   A. Sigh
   B. Automatic tube compensation (ATC)
   C. Occlusion pressure
   D. Low-flow PV-loop

3. Which of the following is used to measure auto-PEEP on the EvitaXL?
   A. Inspiratory hold
   B. Expiratory hold
   C. Occlusion pressure
   D. Manual inspiration

4. During SmartCare a patient's spontaneous respiratory rate increases from 20 to 35 breaths/min. The EvitaXL will respond by doing which of the following?
   A. Switching to SIMV
   B. Increasing tidal volume
   C. Sounding an alarm for high respiratory rate
   D. Increasing pressure by 4 mbar

5. On the EvitaXL, apnea ventilation is operational during the use of which of the following modes?
   I. PLV
   II. CMV
   III. PCV+
   IV. APRV
      A. I and II only
      B. III and IV only
      C. I and IV only
      D. II and III only

6. Which of the following is a pressure-limited, volume-targeted dual-control mode of ventilation in which the EvitaXL can adjust pressure to achieve the set volume?
   A. PLV
   B. PCV+
   C. APRV
   D. AutoFlow

7. In the PCV+ (BiPAP) mode, which of the following is the control that is used to set the length of time at the different pressure levels?
   I. Rate
   II. T_{high}
   III. T_{low}
   IV. Rise time
      A. I only
      B. II and III only
      C. I and IV only
      D. II and IV only

8. During PSV with an EvitaXL an adult patient's spontaneous PIP is 46 L/min. At what flow rate will flow-cycling occur?
   A. 3 L/min
   B. 9.2 L/min
   C. 11.5 L/min
   D. Can vary depending on the operator-selected value.

9. During PSV the EvitaXL begins to time-cycle. The most likely cause of the time cycle is which of the following?
   A. Leak
   B. Secretions
   C. Bronchospasm
   D. Weaning failure

10. Which of the following is a closed-loop form of ventilation that is supposed to decrease weaning time?
   A. APRV
   B. BiPAP
   C. SmartCare
   D. SIMV with PSV

SECTION III: HAMILTON VENTILATORS

Hamilton GALILEO Gold
Hamilton RAPHAEL

"All truths are easy to understand once they are discovered; the point is to discover them."
Galileo Galilei

KEY TERMS CROSSWORD PUZZLE

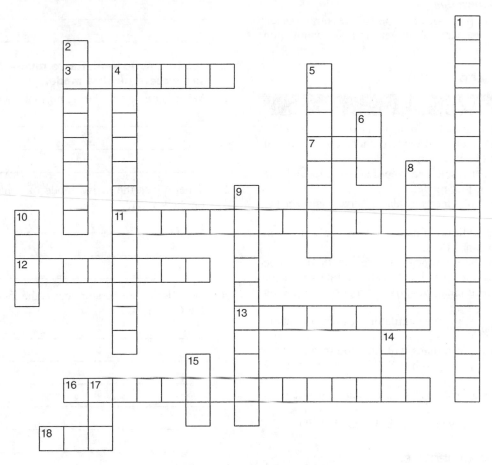

CROSSWORD PUZZLE 12-3

Use the clues to complete the crossword puzzle.

Across

3. The name of the nomogram that aids in the determination of anatomic dead space.

7. It is the flow-cycle setting for PSV (*abbreviation*).

11. This flow-control valve governs the pattern of gas delivery to the patient and is under the control of the microprocessor unit.

12. _____ tidal volume support.

13. A mode that is similar to APRV (*abbreviation*).

16. _____ expiratory threshold resistor (*two words*).

18. If the set apnea time is exceeded, this form of ventilation becomes active (*abbreviation*).

Down

1. The pressure transducer is a variable-orifice _____ _____.

2. A word for "close to."

4. The patient circuit has a proximal airway sensor that uses a variable-orifice _____ pressure transducer.

5. This reservoir tank holds up to 8 L under pressures of up to 350 cm H_2O.

6. A spontaneous mode (*abbreviation*).

8. An external power source.

9. A device that translates pressure to an electrical signal.

10. Upper pressure limit (*abbreviation*).

14. Reduces the patient's WOB (*abbreviation*).

15. Is used to determine the anatomic dead space of a patient (*abbreviation*).

17. A closed-loop mode that uses pressure-targeted breaths to ensure a target minute ventilation (*abbreviation*).

Hamilton GALILEO Gold

LEARNING OBJECTIVES

Upon completion of this section, you will be able to:

1. Describe the function of the two knobs on the front of the GALILEO ventilator.

2. Explain how to select a ventilator mode and the parameters for that mode.

3. Explain how to select the alarm screen and set the alarms.

4. Compare the addition of adaptive pressure ventilation (APV) to standard PCV.

5. Discuss how the microprocessor selects tidal volume (V_T), expired minute volume ($\dot{V}_E$), and rate values for a patient receiving adaptive support ventilation (ASV).

6. Describe the method the ventilator uses when a patient is first placed on ASV.

7. Predict how the ventilator will function in one of the three scenarios in which ASV is most commonly used.

8. Troubleshoot a problem when an alarm indicator is activated.

9. Describe back-up ventilation in the GALILEO.

ACHIEVING THE OBJECTIVES

1. Describe the function of the two knobs on the front of the GALILEO ventilator.

1A. What is the function of the right knob?

_____

_____

_____

_____

_____

_____

1B. What is the function of the left knob?

_____

_____

_____

_____

_____

_____

_____

_____

_____

2. Explain how to select a ventilator mode and the parameters for that mode.

2A. What is on-screen during normal operation?

_____

_____

_____

2B. Where does the active mode of ventilation appear on the screen?

_____

_____

_____

2C. How does the operator access the mode options for the GALILEO?

_____

_____

_____

_____

_____

_____

2D. What is the procedure for changing a mode?

_____

_____

_____

_____

_____

_____

_____

_____

_____

2E. How does the operator change parameters for a mode?

_____
_____
_____
_____
_____
_____
_____
_____
_____
_____
_____
_____
_____

2F. How does the mode or parameter change become active?

_____
_____
_____
_____

3. Explain how to select the alarm screen and set the alarms.

3A. How is the alarm screen activated?

_____
_____
_____

3B. What are the two options for setting alarms?

_____
_____
_____
_____

3C. How are the alarms manually adjusted?

_____
_____
_____
_____
_____
_____
_____
_____
_____
_____

4. Compare the addition of APV to standard PCV.

4A. Describe PCV in terms of trigger, target, and cycle.

_____
_____
_____
_____

4B. What type of mode is APV?

_____
_____

4C. How does PCV differ when APV is added? (P-A/C + APV)

_____
_____
_____
_____
_____
_____
_____
_____
_____
_____

4D. Explain the maximum pressure setting when P-A/C + APV is used on the GALILEO.

_____

_____

_____

_____

_____

4E. In the P-A/C + APV mode the Pmax is set at 25 cm H_2O. What is the maximum pressure that the GALILEO can use to deliver the targeted volume?

_____

_____

4F. During ventilation in the P-A/C + APV mode, there are audible and visible alarms and the screen shows "pressure limitations." What is occurring? What should be done?

_____

_____

_____

_____

5. Discuss how the microprocessor selects V_T, $\dot{V}_E$, and rate values for a patient receiving ASV.

5A. Define ASV in terms of trigger, target, and cycle.

_____

_____

_____

_____

_____

5B. Describe ASV.

_____

_____

_____

_____

5C. What is the goal of ASV?

_____

_____

_____

_____

5D. Which equations are used by the GALILEO to select minute ventilation for adult and pediatric patients?

_____

_____

_____

5E. How does the microprocessor determine the rate and V_T?

_____

_____

_____

_____

_____

_____

_____

_____

_____

_____

_____

6. Describe the method the ventilator uses when starting ASV.

6A. How does the GALILEO enable assessment of a patient who is just beginning ASV?

_____

_____

_____

6B. What measurements and calculations are occurring during the assessment?

_____

_____

_____

_____

_____

6C. How does the ventilator prevent complications associated with mechanical ventilation?

_____

_____

6D. How does the GALILEO show the targeted volume and rate to the operator?

_____

_____

7. Assess a patient case representing one of the three common scenarios that describes the function of ASV to determine how the ventilator will function.

The questions in learning objective 7 refer to the following scenario:

A patient is placed on a GALILEO in the ASV mode that is set with the following parameters: Pmax = 45 cm H_2O; ideal body weight (IBW) = 78 kg; % Min Vol = 100%; trigger = 2 L/min; PEEP = +6 cm H_2O; $F_IO_2 = 0.5$; and expiratory trigger sensitivity (ETS) = 25%.

7A. What target $\dot{V}_E$ will the ventilator set?

_____

_____

7B. This patient has no spontaneous efforts. What kind of breaths will the ventilator be providing?

_____

_____

7C. If lung compliance decreased, what would happen to pressure?

_____

_____

_____

_____

7D. The patient begins having inspiratory efforts. What type of breaths will the ventilator now deliver?

_____

_____

7E. The patient's spontaneous rate is now 6 breaths/min with a volume delivery of 600 mL. How is the targeted $\dot{V}_E$ going to be achieved?

_____

_____

_____

_____

_____

_____

7F. A graphic representation showing rate on the x-axis and volume on the y-axis shows each breath consistently in the lower left quadrant (IV). What is the problem, and how will the GALILEO respond?

_____

_____

_____

_____

7G. This patient is now spontaneously breathing and triggering all breaths. How does ASV respond?

_____

_____

8. Troubleshoot a problem when an alarm indicator is activated.

8A. Which audible alarms are not able to be silenced?

_____

_____

8B. The AIR TRAPPING alarm is the only alarm that is currently active. Name two patient-related problems that can cause this.

_____

_____

_____

_____

8C. In the PSV-CPAP mode, the high respiratory rate and low V_T alarms are active. What is the likely cause of this problem, and what can be done to alleviate it?

_____

_____

_____

_____

_____

_____

_____

9. Describe back-up ventilation in the GALILEO.

9A. When is it recommended that back-up ventilation be used?

_____

_____

9B. How does back-up ventilation become active?

_____

_____

9C. What priority is the back-up ventilation alarm? ___

_____

9D. During the use of back-up ventilation, what does the screen display?

_____

_____

9E. How can the operator check and alter the back-up ventilation parameters?

_____

_____

_____

_____

_____

_____

Think About This

Can ASV reduce medical errors?

Helpful Web Sites

■ Hamilton Medical, Inc, GALILEO — http://www.hamilton-medical.com/GALILEO-ventilators.37.0.html

■ Hamilton Medical, Inc, Adaptive Support Ventilation — http://www.hamilton-medical.com/Adaptive-Support-Ventilation.31.1.html

■ Hamilton Medical, Inc, Intelligent Ventilation — http://www.intelligentventilation.org

NBRC-TYPE QUESTIONS HAMILTON GALILEO GOLD

1. Which of the following are audible alarms that cannot be silenced on the GALILEO?
   I.   Air supply lost
   II. Exhalation obstruction
   III. Loss of battery power
   IV. Oxygen concentration high
      A. I and II only
      B. I and III only
      C. II and IV only
      D. III and IV only

2. A patient with COPD is being ventilated in the PSV mode on the GALILEO; the default ETS setting and a PIP of 48 L/min are being used. The air-trapping alarm becomes active. Which of the following is the most appropriate action to take at this time?
   A. Increase the ETS setting
   B. Change to the SIMV mode
   C. Change to the S(CMV) mode
   D. Increase the pressure-support level

3. In the P-A/C + APV mode, the Pmax is set at 32 cm H_2O. Which of the following is the maximum pressure that the GALILEO can use to deliver the targeted volume?
   A. 17 cm H_2O
   B. 22 cm H_2O
   C. 27 cm H_2O
   D. 32 cm H_2O

4. A 70-kg patient is being set up in the P-A/C + APV mode on the GALILEO; the Pmax setting is 30 cm H_2O and the volume target is 0.5 L. The "Pressure Limitation" message is immediately displayed with an audible alarm. Which of the following is the most-appropriate action to take?
   I.   Remove patient from the ventilator and suction the artificial airway.
   II. Increase Pmax to 35 cm H_2O.
   III. Decrease target volume.
   IV. Switch to S(CMV).
      A. IV only
      B. I and IV only
      C. II and III only
      D. I, II, and III only

5. A patient is being ventilated in the ASV mode on the GALILEO. The % Min Vol is 100%; PEEP is 6 cm H_2O; and the spontaneous respiratory rate is 10 breaths/min. An arterial blood gas analysis reveals a pH of 7.28 and a partial pressure of arterial carbon dioxide ($PaCO_2$) of 58. Which of the following changes to ASV could correct this problem?
   A. Increase the % Min Vol.
   B. Decrease the % Min Vol.
   C. Decrease PEEP setting.
   D. Increase the set frequency.

6. A patient is being ventilated with the GALILEO at the following settings: S(CMV) frequency, 14 breaths/min; tidal volume, 450 mL; PEEP, 8 cm H_2O. The respiratory therapist activates the sigh function. What is the sigh V_T and rate?
   A. Twice every 50 breaths with 900 mL
   B. Once every 100 breaths with 675 mL
   C. Once every 100 breaths with 900 mL
   D. Twice every 100 breaths at the volume generated by doubling PEEP

7. APRV is similar to which of the following modes on the GALILEO?
   A. ASV
   B. DuoPAP
   C. APVcmv
   D. S(CMV)

8. Which of the following is untrue concerning non-invasive ventilation with the GALILEO?
   A. It is more comfortable to flow-cycle.
   B. The suggested starting point for ETS is 25%.
   C. Maximum inspiratory time (T_I max) should be used as a back-up cycle mechanism.
   D. PIP should not exceed 28 cm H_2O.

Hamilton RAPHAEL

LEARNING OBJECTIVES

Upon completion of this section, you will be able to:

1. Describe the appropriate size of patient to ventilate with the RAPHAEL.
2. Name the power sources required to use the RAPHAEL.
3. Explain the operation of the internal battery in the event of an AC power failure.
4. Discuss how the nebulizer that comes installed with the RAPHAEL affects V_T and F_IO_2.
5. Review the function of the MODE control.
6. Explain how a control parameter can be adjusted or changed.
7. Describe how to identify an alarm when an alarm event occurs.
8. Compare the Pmax alarm available during the use of (S)CMV+ or SIMV+ to the high-pressure alarm used during other modes of ventilation.
9. Name the function of the touch pad identified with the lung icon.
10. Discuss what will occur if the "stand-by" control is activated while a patient is still connected to the RAPHAEL ventilator.

ACHIEVING THE OBJECTIVES

1. Describe the appropriate size of patient to ventilate with the RAPHAEL.

_____

_____

2. Name the power sources required to use the RAPHAEL.

2A. What is the required range of gas pressure necessary for normal operation?

_____

_____

2B. If no gas power source is available, how can the RAPHAEL operate?

_____

_____

2C. What type of AC is necessary to operate the RAPHAEL?

_____

_____

3. Explain the operation of the internal battery in the event of an AC power failure.

3A. How long can the internal battery power the RAPHAEL? _____

3B. How much time is left on the battery power when the low-battery alarm is active?

_____

_____

3C. What happens when internal battery power is completely lost?

_____

_____

4. Discuss how the nebulizer that comes installed with the RAPHAEL affects V_T and F_IO_2.

4A. What is the effect of nebulizer use on tidal volume?

_____

_____

4B. What effect does nebulizer use have on the delivered F_IO_2?

_____

_____

5. Review the function of the MODE control.

5A. What is the location of the control labeled *MODE*?

_____

_____

5B. How does the operator change modes?

_____

_____

_____

_____

_____

_____

_____

_____

6. Explain how a control parameter can be adjusted or changed.

6A. How can you access a control setting?

_____

_____

6B. Once they are accessed, how are settings adjusted?

_____

_____

_____

_____

_____

_____

_____

_____

_____

_____

7. Describe how to identify an alarm when an alarm event occurs.

7A. What happens to the ventilator when an alarm becomes active?

_____

_____

_____

7B. If more than one alarm is active at the same time, what is displayed on the screen?

_____

_____

7C. What happens to the screen when there are multiple alarms of the same priority?

_____

_____

7D. How can the operator track previously activated alarms?

_____

_____

_____

7E. How can the practitioner distinguish among alarm priorities without checking the ventilator's screen?

_____

_____

8. Compare the Pmax alarm available during the use of (S)CMV+ or SIMV+ to the high-pressure alarm used during other modes of ventilation.

8A. How does a high-pressure alarm function in most volume-targeted modes of ventilation?

_____

_____

_____

8B. What is the maximum pressure that the RAPHAEL will deliver during the use of (S)CMV+ or SIMV+?

_____

_____

8C. During the use of S(CMV)+ or SIMV+, what happens to breath delivery when the maximum pressure is reached?

_____

_____

8D. What advantage does Pmax have over a traditional high-pressure alarm?

_____

_____

9. Name the function of the touch pad identified with the lung icon.

9A. What functions are associated with the lung icon?

_____

9B. How are these functions accomplished?

_____

_____

_____

_____

_____

_____

_____

_____

10. Discuss what will occur if the "stand-by" control is activated while a patient is still connected to the RAPHAEL ventilator.

10A. When is "stand-by" useful?

_____

_____

10B. What happens if the "stand-by" feature is activated while a patient is connected to the ventilator?

_____

_____

_____

_____

_____

Think About This

Why do ventilators have names?

Helpful Web Site

■ Hamilton Medical, Inc, RAPHAEL Ventilator — http://www.hamilton-medical.com/Product-documentation.467.0.html?&L=

NBRC-TYPE QUESTIONS HAMILTION RAPHAEL

1. Which of the following represents the maximum pressure that the RAPHAEL will deliver during the use of (S)CMV+ or SIMV+?
   A. Pmax
   B. Pmax ± 2 cm H_2O
   C. Pmax − 10 cm H_2O
   D. Peak ventilating pressure + 10 cm H_2O

2. A patient is being ventilated in the SIMV+ mode on a RAPHAEL. The respiratory therapist notices a pressure-limitation alarm is active. Which of the following statements is true concerning this situation?
   A. Inspiration continues, but the volume might not be delivered.
   B. The ventilator is malfunctioning and will need to be replaced.
   C. The ventilator discontinues inspiration at the pressure limitation.
   D. Inspiration will continue with that pressure until the volume is delivered.

3. A respiratory therapist responds to a call to an ICU room where an intubated patient is being ventilated by a RAPHAEL ventilator. A buzzing sound is being generated by the ventilator. Which of the following actions should the respiratory therapist take?
   I. Manually ventilate the patient.
   II. Reconnect the power cord to the wall outlet.
   III. Switch out the ventilator for another.
   IV. Suction the patient's artificial airway.
   A. I and II only
   B. III only
   C. I and III only
   D. II and IV only

4. The RAPHAEL is set to S(CMV+) at a rate of 12; a V_T of 400 mL; and a PEEP of +8 cm H_2O. The PIP is 26 cm H_2O. The disconnect alarm will become active in which of the following situations?
   A. The PEEP drops to 4 cm H_2O.
   B. The volume delivered is 45 mL.
   C. The ventilator senses no patient activity.
   D. The PIP falls to 18 cm H_2O.

5. The apnea alarm trigger time for an adult on the RAPHAEL ventilator is which of the following?
   A. 10 seconds
   B. 15 seconds
   C. 20 seconds
   D. Operator-selected

6. Which of the following statements is true concerning the RAPHAEL ventilator?
   A. Nebulizer use will increase the delivered F_IO_2.
   B. The ABV parameters are nonadjustable.
   C. The ventilator can operate for 2 hours on an internal battery.
   D. The lung icon touch pad allows access to tube-resistance compensation.

SECTION IV: MAQUET VENTILATORS

Maquet Servo 300
Maquet Servo^i Ventilator System
Maquet Servo^s Ventilator

"Thought is the wind, knowledge the sail, and mankind the vessel."
Augustus W. Hare, British writer and cleric

KEY TERMS CROSSWORD PUZZLE

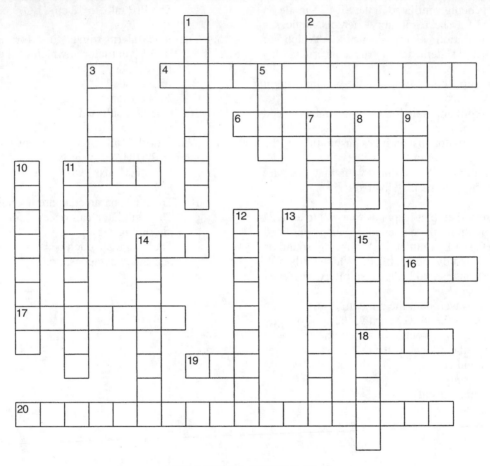

CROSSWORD PUZZLE 12-4

Use the clues to complete the crossword puzzle.

Across

4. Another term for *front panel* (*two words*).
6. The type of O_2 cell used by the Servo^i.
11. Not volume-regulated, not pressure-controlled (*abbreviation*).
13. Measurement of particle size (*abbreviation*).
14. Cellular phones can cause this (*abbreviation*).
16. The ventilator off-battery charging audible alert was turned off by this in older models (*abbreviation*).
17. These flash on the airway pressure bar graph.
18. Caused by overdistention, collapsing, and reexpansion of the lungs (*abbreviation*).
19. A similar problem to that described in **14 across** (*abbreviation*).
20. The control that allows adjustment of the ventilator's response to the patient (*two words*).

Down

1. Where gas flow is measured by ultrasonic transducers.
2. One breathing cycle time (*abbreviation*).
3. High or _____ pressure limit.
5. "PS above PEEP" (abbreviation).
7. A servo-controlled mode that might be considered the weaning counterpart to **11 across** and volume control (*two words*).
8. Requires a special nasogastric (NG) tube with an array of miniaturized sensors (*abbreviation*).
9. Inspiratory _____ _____ is used to set flow cycle (*two words*).

10. Switches from a control mode to a support mode when the patient triggers.
11. The control that is used to check plateau pressure (*two words*).
12. The mouth pressure 100 milliseconds after the start of a patient's inspiratory effort.
14. Adjusts the rate of rise to full inspiratory flow (*two words*).
15. Another term for *expiratory valve* (*two words*).

Maquet Servo 300

LEARNING OBJECTIVES

Upon completion of this section, you will be able to:

1. Label a diagram of the control panel of the Servo 300.
2. Explain the function of the controls on the operating panel of the Servo 300 and compare measured display values with set digital display values.
3. Recommend a safe method for changing rate and V_T settings on the Servo 300.
4. Assess an alarm situation, and recommend an action to correct the problem.
5. Compare each of the modes of ventilation on the Servo 300, including triggering and cycling mechanisms and breath delivery (volume versus pressure).
6. Explain the use of the set parameter guide (SPG) for setting up controls when switching to a new mode of ventilation.
7. Describe the function of volume support (PRVC mode) and "Automode, Subambient."

1. Label a diagram of the control panel of the Servo 300.

Refer to Figure 12-11 for Questions 1A through 1K.

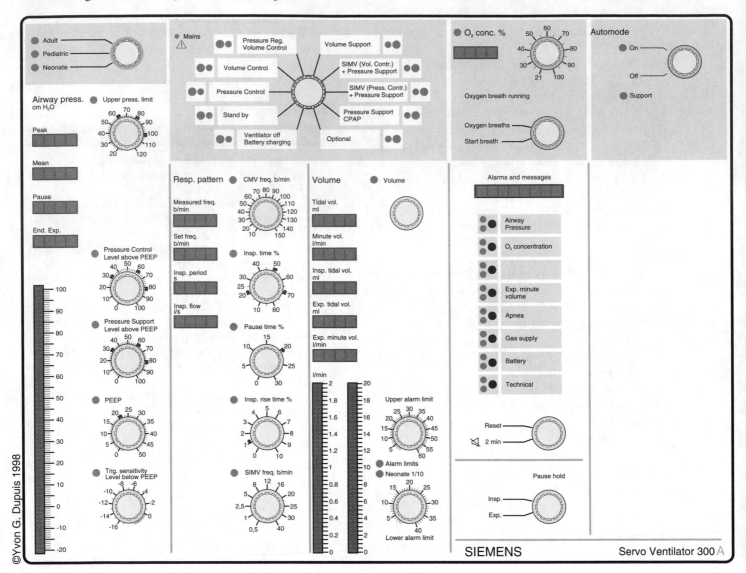

FIGURE 12-11

1A. Locate, circle, and label the PATIENT RANGE section on Figure 12-11.

1B. Locate, circle, and label the MODE SELECTION section on Figure 12-11.

1C. Locate, circle, and label the RESPIRATORY PATTERN section on Figure 12-11.

1D. Locate, circle, and label the VOLUMES (setting) section on Figure 12-11.

1E. Locate, circle, and label the VOLUMES ALARM area on Figure 12-11

1F. Locate, circle, and label the AIRWAY PRESSURES section on Figure 12-11.

1G. Locate, circle, and label the OXYGEN CONCENTRATION section on Figure 12-11.

1H. Locate, circle, and label the ALARMS AND MESSAGES section on Figure 12-11.

1I. Locate, circle, and label the ALARM SILENCE/RESET control on Figure 12-11.

1J. Locate, circle, and label the PAUSE HOLD control on Figure 12-11.

1K. Locate, circle, and label the AUTOMODE control on Figure 12-11.

2. Explain the function of the controls on the operating panel of the Servo 300 and compare measured display values with set digital display values.

2A. How does the PATIENT RANGE SELECTION affect the operation of the ventilator?

_____

_____

_____

_____

_____

2B. How is the Servo 300 turned off?

_____

_____

2C. What modes are available on the Servo 300?

_____

_____

_____

_____

2D. Explain the function of the five controls in the RESPIRATORY PATTERN section.

_____

_____

_____

_____

_____

_____

_____

_____

_____

_____

_____

_____

_____

2E. The volume control is active during which modes?

_____

_____

2F. What is the function of the two bar graphs in the VOLUME SECTION of the front panel?

_____

_____

_____

_____

_____

_____

_____

_____

_____

2G. What is the function of the UPPER PRESS. LIMIT control, and when should it be used?

_____

_____

_____

_____

2H. When is the PRESS. CONTROL knob active?

_____

_____

2I. When is the PRESS. SUPPORT knob active?

_____

_____

2J. What is the function of the TRIG. SENSITIVITY control?

_____

_____

_____

_____

2K. How are the upper and lower F_1O_2 alarms set?

_____

_____

_____

_____

_____

_____

2L. How does the OXYGEN BREATHS/START BREATH knob function?

_____

_____

_____

_____

_____

_____

_____

_____

_____

2M. What measurements can be obtained from the use of the PAUSE HOLD control?

_____

_____

2N. How does the control panel display the difference between selected and measured parameters?

_____

_____

_____

_____

3. Recommend a safe method for changing rate and V$_T$ settings on the Servo 300.

3A. Why should the CMV FREQ. B/MIN knob be set appropriately even if the ventilator is in a spontaneous mode?

_____

_____

3B. What are the effects of changing the CMV FREQ. B/MIN setting on SIMV?

_____

_____

_____

_____

_____

_____

3C. In the volume-control (VC mode) what happens when the mandatory breath rate is reduced? How can this be prevented?

_____

_____

_____

_____

_____

_____

4. Assess an alarm situation and recommend an action to correct the problem.

4A. Which alarm is displayed when more than one alarm is active at a time?

_____

_____

_____

_____

4B. What do constantly illuminated yellow lights mean?

_____

_____

4C. What does a flashing yellow light indicate?

_____

_____

4D. In the PRVC mode the message window reads "LIMITED PRESSURE" and an alarm is sounding. What is the problem, and what action will correct it?

_____

_____

_____

_____

_____

_____

_____

_____

_____

_____

_____

4E. The message window reads "HIGH CONTINUOUS PRESSURE," and a high-priority alarm is sounding. What causes this, and what action should be taken?

_____

_____

_____

_____

_____

_____

_____

_____

_____

_____

4F. There is a red flashing light next to the EXP. MINUTE volume, and the message window reads "EXP. MINUTE VOLUME TOO HIGH." What could cause this, and what action(s) should be taken?

_____

_____

_____

_____

_____

_____

_____

_____

4G. Name three problems that would cause a low exhaled minute volume alarm to become active, and provide solutions to these problems.

_____

_____

_____

_____

_____

_____

_____

_____

_____

_____

_____

_____

_____

_____

_____

4H. What action should be taken when there are any technical errors on the Servo 300?

_____

_____

_____

4I. What causes the internal safety valve and expiratory valve to open?

_____

_____

_____

5. Compare each of the modes of ventilation on the Servo 300, including triggering and cycling mechanisms and breath delivery (volume versus pressure).

Complete the following table.

	Mode	Trigger	Cycle	Breath-delivery type
5A.	VC			
5B.	PC			
5C.	VC-SIMV			
5D.	PC-SIMV			
5E.	PRVC			
5F.	PS/CPAP			
5G.	Volume Support (VS)			

6. Explain the use of the SPG for setting up controls when switching to a new mode of ventilation.

6A. Before connecting a patient to the 300, what is the first step when SPG is in use?

_____

_____

6B. What is the next step when the SPG is used for a new patient?

_____

_____

_____

_____

6C. How does the operator illuminate the first parameter to set?

_____

_____

_____

6D. How does the operator illuminate the rest of the parameters to set?

_____

_____

_____

_____

6E. What signal does the ventilator give on completion of the SPG?

_____

_____

_____

_____

6F. How does SPG use differ when there is a patient already connected to the ventilator?

_____

_____

_____

_____

_____

7. Describe the function of volume support (PRVC mode) and "Automode, Subambient."

7A. Why is VS considered a weaning mode?

_____

_____

7B. What are the differences between VS and PS?

_____

_____

_____

_____

7C. In the VS mode, what happens if the patient becomes apneic?

_____

_____

_____

_____

7D. What is the AUTOMODE designed to do?

_____

_____

_____

_____

_____

_____

7E. What are the control and support modes that are operational in the AUTOMODE?

_____

_____

7F. In PC with the AUTOMODE operational, the patient triggers two breaths. What will the ventilator do?

_____

_____

7G. What is the purpose of the AUTOMODE?

_____

_____

_____

_____

Think About This

What makes a ventilator obsolete?

Helpful Web Site

- VentWorld, Interactive Product Viewer for the Siemens Servo 300/300A — http://www.ventworld.com/equipment/viewer/

Chapter **12** **Mechanical Ventilators: General-Use Devices**

NBRC-TYPE QUESTIONS MAQUET SERVO 300

1. On the Servo 300, VC is active during which of the following modes?
   - I. VS
   - II. PRVC
   - III. APRV
   - IV. PC-SIMV
     - A. I and II only
     - B. II and III only
     - C. III and IV only
     - D. I and IV only

2. When the SIMV frequency is 8 breaths/min and the CMV frequency is 14 breaths/min, what is the spontaneous period?
   - A. 1.8 seconds
   - B. 3.2 seconds
   - C. 6.0 seconds
   - D. 7.5 seconds

3. An unconscious patient needs to be hyperventilated because of an increase in intracranial pressure from closed-head trauma. What is the most-appropriate mode with which to accomplish this?
   - I. VS
   - II. VC
   - III. PRVC
   - IV. PS/CPAP
     - A. I and II only
     - B. II and III only
     - C. III and IV only
     - D. I and IV only

4. Calculate the inspiratory and expiratory times when the set CMV frequency is 20 breaths/min; the set inspiratory time % is 20%; and the set pause time is 5%.
   - A. T_I = 1.63 second. T_E = 3 seconds.
   - B. T_I = 0.75 second. T_E = 2.25 seconds.
   - C. T_I = 0.6 seconds. T_E = 2.4 seconds.
   - D. T_I = 0.25 second. T_E = 0.75 second.

5. A patient is being ventilated in the PC mode on a Servo 300. The expiratory minute volume alarm is active, and the alarm message display shows "EXP MINUTE VOLUME TOO LOW." Which of the following is the most-appropriate action to take at this time?
   - I. Troubleshoot for a leak.
   - II. Increase the respiratory rate.
   - III. Increase the volume setting.
   - IV. Administer a bronchodilator.
     - A. I only
     - B. I and IV only
     - C. II and III
     - D. III only

6. Which of the following is the mode on the Servo 300 that will provide a patient low support pressure with a ventilation guarantee; automatic regulation of pressure if mechanical properties or patient effort changes; and controlled back-up in case of apnea?
   - A. VC
   - B. VS
   - C. PRVC
   - D. PC-SIMV+ PS

7. If the internal safety valve and exhalation valve both open on the Servo 300, the most-appropriate immediate action for the respiratory therapist to take is to:
   - A. Replace the exhalation valve.
   - B. Replace the oxygen and air gas sources.
   - C. Provide an alternative means of ventilation.
   - D. Troubleshoot for an obstruction in the circuit.

8. A patient is being mechanically ventilated with a Servo 300. The respiratory therapists hears a ticking sound as she walks by the patient's room. Which of the following actions could resolve the ticking sound?
   - I. Reconnect the oxygen cell.
   - II. Look for an unplugged power cord, then plug it in.
   - III. Replace one of the high-pressure gas sources.
   - IV. Suction the patient's endotracheal tube.
     - A. IV only
     - B. I and III only
     - C. I, II, and III only
     - D. II and IV only

Maquet Servo[i] Ventilator System

Upon completion of this section, you will be able to:

1. Identify the power source being used by the Servo[i].
2. Recognize the amount of time available on the batteries.
3. Describe the function of the modes available on the Servo[i]: VC, PC, PRVC, PS/CPAP, SIMV-VC, SIMV-PC, SIMV-PRVC, BiVent, and AUTOMODE.
4. Explain the function of the ultrasonic nebulizer available on the Servo[i].
5. Compare the two methods of setting ventilator parameters on the Servo[i], including use of the direct-access knobs and use of the touch screen.
6. Describe the alarm-profile screen and the alarms available on the Servo[i].
7. Identify the cause of a given alarm situation.
8. Explain the control settings for PSV.
9. Recognize an increase in patient flow demand during VC.
10. Discuss the accessing of trended data, alarm history, and the event log.
11. List the modes of ventilation available in conjunction with noninvasive ventilation (NIV) for adults and for infants.
12. Name the parameters graphed on the OPEN LUNG TOOL.

ACHIEVING THE OBJECTIVES

1. Identify the power source being used by the Servo[i].

1A. What type of power sources does the Servo[i] routinely use? _____

_____

_____

1B. How can the operator identify the power source being used?

_____

_____

2. Recognize the amount of time available on the batteries.

2A. What type of batteries are available for the Servo[i] for use during patient transport?

_____

_____

_____

_____

_____

_____

2B. Each battery can supply how many minutes of power? _____

2C. How can the operator check the amount of time available on the batteries?

_____

_____

3. Describe the function of the modes available on the Servo[i]: VC, PC, PRVC, PS/CPAP, SIMV-VC, SIMV-PC, SIMV-PRVC, BiVent, and AUTOMODE.

3A. Which modes available on the Servo[i] are controlled ventilation modes and offer full ventilatory support?

_____

_____

3B. Which modes available on the Servo[i] are considered supported ventilation modes?

_____

_____

3C. Which modes available on the Servo[i] are considered spontaneous ventilation modes?

_____

_____

3D. Which modes available on the Servo[i] are considered combined ventilation modes?

_____

_____

3E. Which full support mode delivers a preset tidal volume with a constant flow during the preset inspiratory time at the preset respiratory rate?

_____

_____

3F. In which mode does the ventilator deliver a supported breath in proportion to the inspiratory effort of the patient and the targeted volume? _____

_____

_____

_____

3G. Classify the following modes in terms of their trigger, limit, and breath type.

Mode	Trigger	Limit	Breath-delivery type
VC			
PC			
PRVC			
SIMV-VC			
SIMV-PC			
SIMV-PRVC			
PS/CPAP			

3H. How does VC on the Servo^i differ from VC on the Servo 300?

_____

_____

_____

_____

_____

_____

3I. How does the initiation of PRVC on the Servo^i differ from that on the Servo 300?

_____

_____

_____

_____

_____

_____

_____

_____

3J. Which mode on the Servo^i allows the patient to breathe spontaneously at two alternating levels of CPAP?

_____

_____

3K. What type of support ventilation is provided when the AUTOMODE is used with VC, PC, and PRVC?

_____

_____

3L. How many patient-triggered breaths are required to initiate supported ventilation in the AUTOMODE on the Servo^i?

_____

_____

4. Explain the function of the ultrasonic nebulizer available on the Servo^i.

4A. What type of power source must the Servo^i have to operate the ultrasonic nebulizer?

_____

_____

4B. How long will the ultrasonic nebulizer operate when activated?

_____

_____

4C. During which ventilator modes will the ultrasonic nebulizer operate?

_____

_____

4D. How does use of the ventilator's nebulizer differ from use of a separate nebulizer?

_____

_____

_____

_____

4E. How are medications placed into the ultrasonic nebulizer?

_____

_____

4F. What size of particles are produced by the ultrasonic nebulizer? _____

4G. Which other nebulizer can be used with the Servo[i] and not add to the volume delivery or change the F_IO_2?

_____

5. Compare the two methods of setting ventilator parameters on the Servo[i], including use of the direct-access knobs and use of the touch screen.

5A. Name the four ways of accessing functions on the Servo[i].

_____

_____

5B. Describe how the touch screen is used to change ventilator parameters.

_____

_____

_____

_____

_____

_____

_____

_____

_____

_____

5C. How are direct-access knobs used to change ventilator parameters?

_____

_____

_____

_____

_____

5D. Describe the safety mechanism on the Servo[i] that advises the operator of parameter limits during changes with the direct-access knobs.

_____

_____

_____

_____

_____

_____

_____

_____

_____

5E. Explain the process of selecting a different mode during operation.

_____

_____

_____

_____

_____

_____

_____

_____

6. Describe the alarm-profile screen and the alarms available on the Servo[i].

6A. What are the three categories of alarms on the Servo[i]?

_____

_____

6B. How do the different categories of alarms appear on the screen?

_____

_____

_____

_____

_____

_____

6C. What alarms are available on the Servo^i?

_____

_____

_____

_____

_____

6D. Describe the manual method for setting or adjusting alarm limits.

_____

_____

_____

_____

_____

_____

_____

_____

6E. The alarm AUTOSET can be used with which ventilator modes?

_____

_____

6F. How does the AUTOSET determine the alarm limits?

_____

_____

_____

_____

6G. Which alarms can be set using AUTOSET?

_____

_____

_____

_____

7. Identify the cause of a given alarm situation.

7A. The respiratory therapist is called to the room of a patient who is receiving mechanical ventilation through a Servo^i. At the time of the last check, the patient was ventilated in the VS mode. The ventilator is now sounding an alarm, and the patient is being ventilated in the VC mode at a rate of 15 breaths/min with an I:E ratio of 1:2. What is the most likely cause for this?

_____

_____

7B. An intubated patient is receiving ventilatory support via a Servo^i in the PRVC mode. The upper pressure limit and low minute volume alarms are active. What is the cause of this situation?

_____

_____

_____

_____

7C. The low minute volume alarm is active during PCV. The patient assessment reveals bilateral inspiratory and expiratory wheezing. What is the most-appropriate action for the respiratory therapist to take?

_____

_____

_____

_____

_____

_____

7D. What situation would cause the safety and the expiratory valves to open on the Servo^i?

_____

_____

8. Explain the control settings for PSV.

8A. Describe PS breaths in terms of trigger, limit, and cycle.

_____

_____

8B. What is the difference between flow-cycling on the Servo^i and that on the Servo 300?

_____

_____

_____

_____

8C. Which control adjusts flow-cycling on the Servo[i]?

_____

_____

8D. The patient's peak inspiratory flow is 45 L/min, and the flow cycle is set to 20%. At what flow rate will the inspiration end?

_____

_____

8E. How can inspiratory time be adjusted during PSV? Use the parameters from Question 8D as an example.

_____

_____

_____

_____

_____

_____

_____

_____

9. Recognize an increase in patient flow demand during VC.

9A. When there is no patient breathing activity in the VC mode, what type of flow pattern is delivered to the patient?

_____

_____

_____

_____.

9B. What happens to the Servo[i] ventilator when a patient in VC has spontaneous efforts?

_____

_____

_____

_____

10. Discuss the accessing of trended data, alarm history, and the event log.

10A. How many different ventilator parameters can be trended? _____

10B. Name 8 different parameters that can be trended on the Servo[i]. _____

_____

_____

_____

10C. How are the trended data accessed?

_____

_____

10D. How is the recorded information documented?

_____

_____

11. List the modes of ventilation available in conjunction with NIV for adults and for infants.

_____

_____

_____

_____

12. Name the parameters graphed by using the OPEN LUNG TOOL.

12A. What two types of patients have an increased risk of developing ventilator-induced lung injury?

_____

_____

12B. What causes ventilator-induced lung injury?

_____

_____

_____

_____

12C. How can ventilator-induced lung injury be minimized?

_____

_____

_____

12D. What parameters appear on the screen when the OPEN LUNG TOOL is accessed?

_____

_____

_____

_____

Think About This

What are the advantages of having a ventilator that does both NIV and invasive ventilation?

Helpful Web Sites

■ The Chinese University of Hong Kong, Maquet Servo[i] Ventilator [Tutorials and Lectures], Charles Gomersall — http://www.aic.cuhk.edu.hk

■ Maquet, Inc, Ventilation Products — http://www.maquet.com

NBRC-TYPE QUESTIONS MAQUET SERVO^i

1. During which circumstances should the TUBING COMPLIANCE FUNCTION on the Servo^i be turned off?
   I.   PRVC
   II. PS
   III. NIV
   IV. Use of uncuffed endotracheal tubes
   A. I and II only
   B. II and III only
   C. I and IV only
   D. III and IV only

2. Which type of oxygen sensor is used by the Servo^i? This sensor does not require frequent calibration and has a very long life.
   A. Galvanic cell
   B. Ultrasonic cell
   C. Polarographic cell
   D. Paramagnetic cell

3. The operator can tell how much time is available in the batteries of the Servo^i by doing which of the following?
   A. Looking at the lower-right corner of the screen.
   B. Looking for the green indicator light, which means full charge.
   C. Opening the utilities window while the ventilator is operating.
   D. Pressing "Status" on the upper right-hand corner of the screen.

4. On the Servo^i, the SUCTION SUPPORT function does which of the following?
   A. It automatically gives 2 minutes of 100% oxygen.
   B. It delivers 1 minute of 100% oxygen, then reduces PEEP automatically.
   C. It puts the ventilator in a pause mode without alarms and gas flow.
   D. It provides 4 cm H_2O of automatic PEEP so a disconnect can be sensed.

5. Which of the following statements is true concerning the Servo^i ventilator?
   A. The Servo^i can be adapted to use helium-oxygen (heliox).
   B. The ventilator can be adapted to be compatible with magnetic resonance imaging (MRI).
   C. Upgrading the unit requires a new central processing unit.
   D. AutoFlow facilitates weaning by allowing patient breath control.

6. During a patient-ventilator system check, the respiratory therapist wants to check whether or not there were any alarm situations since the last time check. The respiratory therapist can get this information by doing which of the following?
   A. Observing the text-message box located on the top-left side of the screen.
   B. Touching the "Menu" key, and then selecting "Alarm" and "Alarm History."
   C. Use the "Alarm Info" screen to view the alarms that were previously activated.
   D. Touch the "Alarm Summary Display" to view all of the alarms that were active since the last reset.

7. While a Servo^i is operating in the PC mode, the low minute volume alarm becomes active. A patient assessment reveals bilateral inspiratory and expiratory wheezing. Which of the following represents the most-appropriate action for the respiratory therapist to take?
   A. Change to the VC mode.
   B. Increase the inspiratory cycle off setting.
   C. Decrease the low minute volume alarm.
   D. Administer a beta adrenergic bronchodilator.

8. The patient's peak expiratory flow rate is 46 L/min with the VS mode on the Servo^i. If flow-cycling occurs at 11.5 L/min, what is the inspiratory cycle-off setting?
   A. 25%
   B. 40%
   C. 11.5 L/min
   D. 46 L/min

9. A patient being ventilated in the VC mode on the Servo^i ventilator begins to have spontaneous efforts. The ventilator will do which of the following?
   A. Switch to SIMV-VC.
   B. Provide additional flow from a demand valve.
   C. Provide assisted breaths with the set tidal volume.
   D. Switch to PS to satisfy the patient's flow demand.

10. When neurally adjusted ventilatory assist is in use, how/when is inspiration triggered?
    A. When the bias flow is reduced by 0.01 L/s.
    B. When pressure is reduced by 0.04 cm H_2O.
    C. By setting the cm H_2O/microvolts from 1 to 30.
    D. By setting the volume trigger to minimum.

Maquet Servo^s Ventilator

Upon completion of this section, you will be able to:
1. Indicate the appropriate size of patient to ventilate with the Servo^s.
2. List the primary differences between the Servo^s and the Servo^i.
3. Discuss the battery operation and battery alarms on the Servo^s.
4. Explain how parameters are set and activated on the Servo^s.
5. Describe how to perform a preuse test on the Servo^s.
6. Name the power sources required for operation of the Servo^s.

ACHIEVING THE OBJECTIVES

1. Indicate the appropriate size of patient to ventilate with the Servo^s.

_____

_____

2. List the primary differences between the Servo^s and the Servo^i.

_____

_____

_____

_____

_____

3. Discuss the battery operation and battery alarms on the Servo^s.

3A. How many minutes are left in the internal battery when the LIMITED BATTERY CAPACITY alarm is activated?

_____

3B. How many minutes are left in the internal battery when the NO BATTERY CAPACITY alarm is activated?

_____

3C. How much operating time can the internal batteries provide? _____

4. Explain how parameters are set and activated on the Servo^s.

4A How can the most commonly used parameters be altered?

_____

_____

4B. Describe the way the mode and parameters can be set.

_____

_____

_____

4C. How are new settings or altered parameters activated?

_____

_____

_____

5. Describe how to perform a preuse test on the Servo^s.

5A. How long does the preuse test last?

_____

_____

5B. What needs to be connected to perform this test?

_____

_____

5C. What functions are evaluated during the preuse test?

_____

_____

6. Name the power sources required for operation of the Servo^s.

6A. How many gas sources does the Servo^s require to operate?

_____

_____

6B. What type of electrical power is required to operate the Servo^s?

_____

_____

Think About This

Purchasing a ventilator is like purchasing an automobile.

Helpful Web Site

- Maquet, Inc, Ventilation Products — http://www.maquet.com

NBRC-TYPE QUESTIONS MAQUET SERVO[s]

1. How long can the Servo[s] operate on its internal battery?
   A. 30 minutes
   B. 60 minutes
   C. 90 minutes
   D. 120 minutes

2. Which of the following statements about the Servo[s] is **FALSE**?
   A. It cannot be used in an MRI suite.
   B. It can ventilate adult, pediatric, and neonatal patients.
   C. It uses an expiratory cassette to measure expired gas flow.
   D. The monitored and displayed data are the same as those on the Servo[i].

3. What functions are evaluated during the preuse test?
   A. Safety valve
   B. User interface
   C. Flow transducers
   D. Tubing compliance

4. The Servo[s] can ventilate all of the following populations **EXCEPT**:
   A. Geriatric
   B. Adult
   C. Pediatric
   D. Neonatal

5. The Servo[s] can operate in all of the following hospital areas or situations **EXCEPT**:
   I. Neonatal Intensive Care Unit
   II. During in-hospital transfers
   III. During MRI
   IV. Pediatric Intensive Care Unit
   A. I only
   B. I and III only
   C. II and IV only
   D. III and IV only

SECTION V: NEWPORT VENTILATORS

Newport Wave E200
Newport e500

"The winds and waves are always on the side of the ablest navigators."
Edward Gibbon

KEY TERMS CROSSWORD PUZZLE

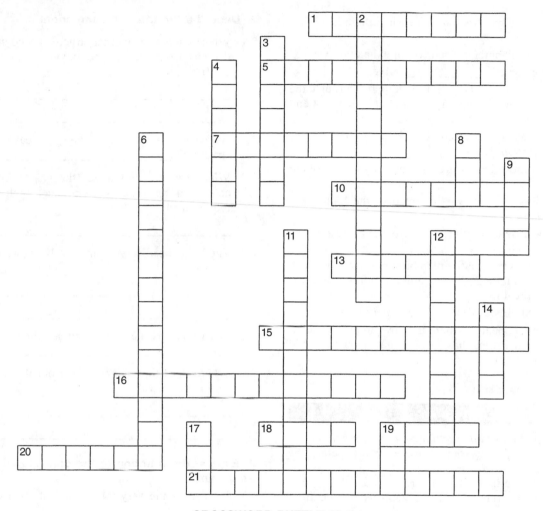

CROSSWORD PUZZLE 12-5

Use the clues to complete the crossword puzzle.

Across

1. A type of infant endotracheal tube.
5. A button that clears visual indicators and messages of alarms that are no longer active (*two words*).
7. This alarm rings when the ventilator outlet pressure is higher than the measured proximal pressure (*two words*).
10. Another name for *PEEP/CPAP*.

13. The expiratory monitor that can be added to enhance the E200's capabilities.
15. Just below the main inspiratory line connector.
16. Mutes audible alarms for 1 minute (*two words*).
18. A mode on the e500 that is similar to PRVC (*abbreviation*).

19. The type of flow used to wash out any exhaled carbon dioxide and reduce the ventilator's response time for triggering.

20. The _____ pressure should be approximately 10 cm H_2O above the high-pressure alarm setting.

21. Another name for the *high-speed servo-control valve* (*two words*).

Down

2. Automatic leak _____ is used to stabilize the baseline pressure when there is a small leak.

3. A type of diaphragm used for an exhalation valve.

4. Electromagnetic _____ valve.

6. A valve that limits pressure delivery through the patient circuit during any mode, but it does not end inspiration (*two words*).

8. Sixty seconds divided by the set breath rate (*abbreviation*).

9. A type of test that ensures the integrity of the patient circuit.

11. From this tank, flow is directed to the high-speed servo-control valve.

12. An alarm that rings when the patient's respiratory rate is too high.

14. If you press the small, green button next to the mode selector on the E200, the ventilator will provide this type of breath.

17. The e500 uses this monitor (*abbreviation*).

19. This mode begins when the low minute ventilation alarm setting has been violated on the e500 (*abbreviation*).

Newport Wave E200

LEARNING OBJECTIVES

Upon completion of this section, you will be able to:

1. Name the power sources required to operate the ventilator.
2. Describe the internal components.
3. Explain the function of the controls on the front panel.
4. Identify an alarm situation, and suggest a possible cause and solution.
5. Assess a problem associated with bias flow and trigger sensitivity during spontaneous ventilation; then recommend a solution.
6. Solve a problem related to use of the low-pressure alarm.
7. Describe the available modes of ventilation.
8. Explain the function of the NEBULIZER control.
9. Compare the setting of pressure-targeted modes with the setting of volume-targeted modes.
10. Identify a situation in which the pressure-relief valve is operating.

ACHIEVING THE OBJECTIVES

1. Name the power sources required to operate the ventilator.

1A. What pneumatic power does the E200 require?

_____

_____

1B. What amount of electrical power is required by the E200? _____

2. Describe the internal components.

2A. What is the first internal structure encountered by the gas from the air and oxygen sources in the E200?

_____

_____

2B. At what pressure does the gas leave the first structure? _____

2C. What structure pressurizes the gas to 2 atm and acts as a reservoir to help meet high gas-flow requirements?

_____

2D. The high-speed servo-control valve is what type of valve?

_____

_____

2E. What controls the high-speed servo-control valve?

_____

2F. Where does the gas move to from the high-speed servo-control valve?

_____

_____

3. Explain the function of the controls on the front panel.

3A. What does the very top portion of the front panel contain?

_____

_____

3B. What controls are used to set tidal volume on the E200?

_____

_____

3C. What is BIAS FLOW, and how does it work?

_____

_____

_____

_____

_____

_____

_____

3D. What should the BIAS FLOW be set at for adults and for pediatric and neonatal patients?

_____

_____

3E. What are the two functions of the SENSITIVITY setting?

_____

_____

_____

3F. When the PEEP/CPAP control is used, why is it important to watch the pressure displayed in the monitor window?

_____

_____

_____

_____

3G. What is the function of the PRESS. CONTROL (PC) knob?

_____

_____

_____

_____

3H. How does the INSP. MIN. VOL. ALARM operate?

_____

_____

_____

_____

_____

3I. How are the high- and low-pressure alarms set?

_____

_____

_____

_____

_____

4. Identify an alarm situation, and suggest a possible cause and solution.

4A. While the PCV mode is in use, the high-pressure alarm becomes active. What is the possible cause of this situation?

_____

_____

_____

4B. The low minute volume alarm has become active while the patient is being ventilated in the PCV mode.

(1.) What are the possible causes of this situation?

_____

(2.) What are the possible solutions to this situation?

_____

_____

_____

_____

5. Assess a problem associated with bias flow and trigger sensitivity during spontaneous ventilation; then recommend a solution.

5A. A patient is being ventilated in the PS mode on the E200. The bias flow setting is 8 L/min, and the sensitivity setting is −1 cm H_2O. The rate monitor is showing 4 breaths/min.

(1.) What is the problem?

_____

_____

(2.) How can this problem be alleviated?

_____

_____

5B. A patient is being ventilated in the PSV mode. While assessing the patient, the respiratory therapist notices that the patient is diaphoretic and is using accessory muscles. The respiratory therapist measures the patient's respiratory rate, which is 28 breaths/min. However, the respiratory rate monitor is displaying 6 breaths/min.

(1.) Why is there a discrepancy between the measured respiratory rate and the ventilator's respiratory rate monitor?

_____

_____

(2.) What can be done to reduce this patient's increased WOB?

_____

_____

6. Solve a problem related to use of the low-pressure alarm.

6A. In volume-targeted SIMV, the set rate is 10 breaths/min; T_I (or inspiratory time) is 1.0 second; flow rate is 40 L/min; PEEP is 8 cm H_2O; and sensitivity is set at 0.5 cm H_2O. The peak pressure is 20 cm H_2O; the high-pressure alarm is 30 cm H_2O; and the low-pressure alarm is 25 cm H_2O. The low-pressure alarm is active, and the pressure manometer reads 6 cm H_2O on exhalation and 18 cm H_2O on inspiration.

(1.) What has activated the low-pressure alarm?

_____

_____

_____

_____

(2.) Name two possible causes of this problem.

_____

_____

(3.) Suggest two corrective measures.

_____

_____

6B. A ventilator is operating in the PCV mode with a setting of 25 cm H_2O, and the low-pressure alarm becomes active. What action should the respiratory therapist take?

_____

_____

_____

7. Describe the available modes of ventilation.

7A. Which modes are available with volume-targeted breath types?

_____

7B. Which modes are available with pressure-targeted breath types?

_____

7C. Which spontaneous modes are available?

_____

8. Explain the function of the NEBULIZER control.

8A. Where is the NEBULIZER ON/OFF control located?

_____

_____

8B. When does the nebulizer function?

_____

_____

8C. How does the nebulizer keep the actual tidal volume and minute volume delivery constant?

_____

_____

9. Compare the setting of pressure-targeted modes with the setting of volume-targeted modes.

9A. In the volume-targeted modes, the E200 uses inspiratory time to determine what two variables?

_____

_____

9B. What function does inspiratory time have during PCV?

_____

_____

9C. Calculate the tidal volume and expiratory time for the following settings: A/C VOLUME control; RESP. RATE = 15; INSP. TIME = 1.0 second; and FLOW = 45 L/min.

_____

_____

_____

_____

9D. Calculate the tidal volume and expiratory time for the following settings: A/C VOLUME control; RESP. RATE = 15; INSP. TIME = 1.5 second; and FLOW = 45 L/min.

_____

_____

_____

_____

9E. Explain why there are different effects when changing the inspiratory time in the PC mode than in the VC mode.

_____

_____

_____

_____

_____

_____

_____

_____

_____

_____

_____

10. Identify a situation in which the pressure-relief valve is operating.

10A. How should the pressure-relief valve be set?

_____

_____

_____

_____

10B. If the pressure-relief valve is set below the high-pressure alarm setting, what will happen when the pressure-relief setting is reached?

_____

_____

_____

_____

10C. A patient is being ventilated by the E200 with a high-pressure alarm setting of 30 cm H_2O. The respiratory therapist notes that although the patient is being ventilated in the VC mode, the pressure-time scalar on the graphics display screen has the appearance of PCV. What is causing this to happen?

_____

_____

_____

_____

Think About This

What type of ventilator is used for large animals such as elephants?

Helpful Web Site

■ VentWorld, Newport Wave E200 information — http://www.ventworld.com/Booths/NewPort/wave_e200.asp

249

NBRC-TYPE QUESTIONS NEWPORT WAVE E200

1. During VC ventilation with the E200, increasing the inspiratory time will do which of the following?
   A. Decrease tidal volume
   B. Increase tidal volume
   C. Improve oxygenation
   D. Decrease the respiratory rate

2. A new order for a bronchodilator in the form of a small-volume nebulizer has been written for a patient using the E200 ventilator. Which of the following represents the most-appropriate action for the respiratory therapist to take?
   A. Connect the small-volume nebulizer to the ventilator's nebulizer outlet, and turn it on.
   B. Switch the patient to the VC A/C mode, and use the ventilator's nebulizer.
   C. Consult with the physician to change the small-volume nebulizer to a metered-dose inhaler with a ventilator adapter.
   D. Wait until the patient is extubated to do the small-volume nebulizer treatment.

3. In the VC A/C mode on the E200, the respiratory therapist needs to set a tidal volume of 450 mL, a respiratory rate of 12 breaths/min, and an I:E ratio of 1:4. Which of the following parameters will provide these settings?
   A. Flow rate = 27 L/min, and T_I = 1 second
   B. Flow rate = 33.75 L/min, and T_I = 1.25 second
   C. Flow rate = 40 L/min, and T_I 0.75 second
   D. Flow rate = 60 L/min, and T_I = 0.5 second

4. During ventilation with the E200 in the PSV mode, the actual patient respiratory rate is 20 breaths/min, but the rate monitor is showing 4 breaths/min. Which of the following statements are true?
   I. BIAS FLOW is too high.
   II. SENSITIVITY is set at a value that is too negative.
   III. FLOW TRIGGER is not set properly.
   IV. PRESS. SUPPORT is not set properly.
   A. I and II only
   B. II and III only
   C. III and IV only
   D. I and IV only

5. On the E200, which of the following can cause autotriggering?
   A. An obstruction in the airway
   B. A small airway leak
   C. SENSITIVITY is set at a value that is too negative
   D. BIAS FLOW is set too low

Newport e500

Upon completion of this section, you will be able to:

1. Describe the power sources and power indicators for the Newport e500.
2. Explain the function of the controls on the front panel of the Newport e500.
3. Compare flow delivery during pressure control, volume control, and automatic flow adjustment by the ventilator during inspiration.
4. Discuss the ventilator parameters that are activated when the ventilator is turned on.
5. List the conditions that will cause the F_IO_2 display in the monitored-data section of the e500 to show "- -".
6. Describe the function of the PRESET VENT SETTINGS control on the e500.
7. Review the adjustable and nonadjustable alarms and messages available on the Newport e500.
8. Explain the corrective actions needed to remedy situations that can result in ventilator messages and alarms.

ACHIEVING THE OBJECTIVES

1. Describe the power sources and power indicators for the Newport e500.

1A. What type of pneumatic power does the e500 require?

_____

_____

1B. What sources of electrical power can the e500 use?

_____

_____

1C. How long will the internal battery provide power?

_____

1D. When do the internal batteries charge?

_____

_____

1E. How does the operator know the unit is being powered by its internal battery?

_____

_____

_____

_____

1F. How can the respiratory therapist tell how much power is left in the internal battery?

_____

_____

2. Explain the function of the controls on the front panel of the Newport e500.

2A. Where is the on/standby control switch located?

_____

_____

2B. The front panel is broken down into how many areas?

_____

_____

_____

_____

_____

2C. What does the "mode control" box contain?

_____

_____

_____

2D. How is a VC mode selected?

_____

_____

2E. How is a PC mode selected?

_____

_____

2F. How does the VOL TARGETED PRESSURE CONTROL button operate?

_____

_____

2G. Match the following controls in the first column with their function in the second column.

1. __	Pause button	A.	Delivers a breath with a target pressure of PEEP/CPAP +15 cm H_2O.
2. __	Sigh button	B.	Allows selection of different settings without affecting current ventilator settings.
3. __	V̇ button	C.	3 minutes of 100% oxygen
4. __	Manual inflation	D.	This knob adjusts the sensitivity value for either trigger variable.
5. __	Inspiratory hold	E.	Causes 1.5 the set tidal volume every 100 breaths.
6. __	Expiratory hold	F.	Selects square or constant flow or descending ramp flow waveforms during volume-targeted breath delivery.
7. __	100% oxygen delivery	G.	Holds breath at end of expiration for up to 20 s.
8. __	PS	H.	Sets inspiratory pause during volume-targeted breaths.
9. __	V̇ or PTRIG	I.	Controls PS levels above PEEP/CPAP.
10. __	Preset ventilator settings	J.	Holds inspiration for up to 5 s.

2H. How are the basic ventilator parameter controls adjusted?

_____

_____

_____

_____

2I. What happens to the ventilator settings when the ventilator is turned off?

_____

_____

2J. What three things occur if a chosen parameter value is outside the available range?

_____

_____

2K. What breath types are available on the e500?

_____

_____

_____

_____

2L. What modes are available on the e500 ventilator?

_____

_____

3. Compare flow delivery during pressure control, volume control, and automatic flow adjustment by the ventilator during inspiration.

3A. What is the automatic slope/rise adjustment?

_____

_____

_____

3B. What two ways can flow be controlled during pressure-targeted modes?

_____

_____

3C. How is flow adjusted by the ventilator in PC modes?

_____

_____

_____

_____

_____

_____

_____

3D. How is flow controlled during volume or **VC** breaths?

_____

_____

3E. What types of flow patterns are available during volume **or VC** breaths?

_____

_____

_____

_____

_____

_____

_____

4. Discuss the ventilator parameters that are activated when the ventilator is turned on.

4A. What does the E500 do immediately after being turned on?

_____

_____

4B. What parameters will be activated when the E500 is powered up again after being in standby?

_____

_____

5. List the conditions that will cause the F$_I$O$_2$ display in the monitored-data section of the e500 to show "- -".

_____

_____

_____

_____

_____

6. Describe the function of the PRESET VENT SETTINGS control on the e500.

6A. How does the operator gain access to the USER SET UP routine when the ventilator is powered on?

_____

_____

_____

_____

6B. How does the operator enter normal ventilating conditions after accessing the USER SET UP?

_____

_____

_____

_____

6C. What is the PRESET VENT SETTINGS function used for during ventilation?

_____

_____

_____

_____

6D. Describe how the PRESET VENT SETTINGS function is used as a safety measure for the patient.

_____

_____

_____

_____

7. Review the adjustable and nonadjustable alarms and messages available on the Newport e500.

7A. Where are most of the alarm controls and indicators located?

_____

_____

7B. Where is the tachypnea alarm located?

_____

_____

7C. How are the low and high minute volume alarms set?

_____

_____

_____

_____

_____

_____

_____

_____

_____

_____

7D. How does the e500 communicate the violation of either of the minute volume alarms?

_____

_____

7E. How are the low and high airway pressure alarms set?

_____

_____

_____

_____

_____

_____

_____

_____

7F. What is the time interval on the apnea alarm?

_____

7G. The high and low alarm thresholds for the F_IO_2 alarm are:

_____

_____.

7H. If the set baseline pressure is 10 cm H_2O, at what pressures will the high and low baseline pressure alarms be violated?

_____

_____

_____

7I. The ALARM MESSAGE display window shows "Prox Line Disconnect." To what condition is this referring?

_____

_____

7J. What are the conditions that cause the SUSTAINED HIGH BASELINE message to be displayed?

_____

_____

_____

_____

7K. What are the alarm limits for inspiratory time and I:E ratio?

_____

_____

_____

_____

_____

_____

8. Explain the corrective actions needed to remedy situations that can result in ventilator messages and alarms.

8A. Which alarm(s) will become active if the patient bites the endotracheal tube and does not let go?

_____

_____

_____

_____

8B. A patient is being ventilated with an e500 during transport to undergo computed tomography. During in-hospital transport, the DEVICE ALERT begins to blink while the ventilator is operational. What is the most likely cause, and how can this be corrected?

_____

_____

_____

_____

8C. During a patient ventilator system check, the respiratory therapist notices that the exhaled flow differs from the set values. What corrective action should the respiratory therapist take?

_____

_____

_____

_____

8D. During an attempt to make ventilator parameter changes, the I:E RATIO INVERSE VIOLATION alarm occurs. What should be done to correct this condition?

_____

_____

_____

_____

Think About This

What are the medical concerns for a ventilated patient who is traveling by airplane?

Helpful Web Site

- Newport Medical Instruments, Newport e500 Ventilator — http://www.ventilators.com/e500US.asp

NBRC-TYPE QUESTIONS NEWPORT E500

1. During a check of the patient and ventilator system, the respiratory therapist notices that the F_IO_2 data display shows "- -". Which of the following action(s) is (are) the most appropriate action?
   I. Calibrate the oxygen sensor.
   II. Check the oxygen high-pressure hose.
   III. Check the oxygen supply pressure.
   IV. Press and hold the F_IO_2 knob.
      A. II and IV only
      B. I and III only
      C. I, II, and III only
      D. IV only

2. Which of the following statements is true about the e500 ventilator?
   A. The internal battery can run the ventilator for 60 minutes when fully charged.
   B. Automatic leak compensation helps to minimize the chance of auto triggering.
   C. Compliance compensation will automatically adjust for leaks in the circuit.
   D. Biphasic pressure-release ventilation can be activated in both PC and VC ventilation.

3. How often should the compliance compensation calculation be run?
   A. Every 24 hours
   B. Every 48 hours
   C. After each patient
   D. Between circuit changes

4. The respiratory therapist answers a call to the ICU for a patient receiving mechanical ventilation with an e500. The nurse tells the respiratory therapist that the ventilator has been beeping approximately every 5 minutes. Which of the following is the most-appropriate action for the respiratory therapist to take?
   A. Calibrate the oxygen sensor.
   B. Plug the ventilator into an AC power source.
   C. Check the air and oxygen high-pressure hoses.
   D. Replace the ventilator, because it is malfunctioning.

5. During a check of the patient and ventilator system, the respiratory therapist notices that the exhaled flow differs from the set values on the e500. What action(s) should the respiratory therapist take to correct this situation?
   I. Check for circuit leaks.
   II. Clean the flow sensor screen.
   III. Initiate a compliance calculation.
   IV. Check for an exhalation valve malfunction.
      A. I and II only
      B. II and III only
      C. I, III, and IV only
      D. IV only

6. A decrease in the volume delivered during volume-targeted PC breaths might be caused by which of the following?
   A. Bronchospasm
   B. Proximal-line disconnect
   C. Decreased airway resistance
   D. Increased static compliance

SECTION VI: PURITAN BENNETT VENTILATORS

Puritan Bennett 840
Puritan Bennett 740
Puritan Bennett 760
Puritan Bennett 7200

"Things do not happen. Things are made to happen."
John F. Kennedy

KEY TERMS CROSSWORD PUZZLE

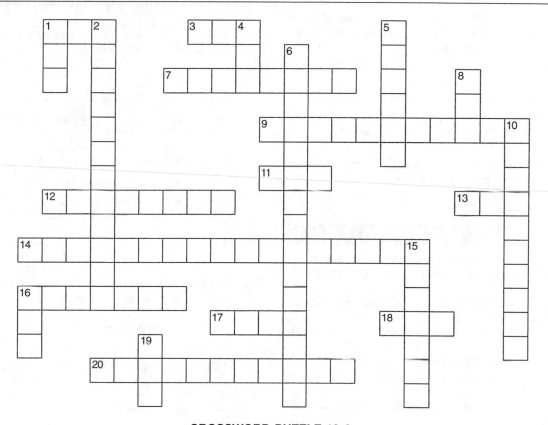

CROSSWORD PUZZLE 12-6

Use the clues to complete the crossword puzzle.

Across

1. This occurs when the ventilator is inoperative (*abbreviation*).
3. A method of breath delivery on the PB840 that targets a pressure based on the selected percentage of support set by the operator and the flow and volume readings from the patient (*abbreviation*).
7. The type of oxygen sensor used on the PB740.
9. The type of piston used in the PB740 and PB760 (*two words*).
11. This mode of ventilation becomes operational when **17 across** fails (*abbreviation*).

12. A factor that represents the amount of time it takes for inspiratory pressure to rise from 0% to 95% of the set pressure during PCV (*two words*).
13. The function that provides data reports that include data logs, chart summary reports, ventilator status reports, and host reports on the PB7200 (*abbreviation*).
14. A PB840 mode that is similar to PRVC (*three words*).
16. The type of ventilation that is similar to APRV.
17. This test runs automatically when the ventilator is powered on (*abbreviation*).

Chapter **12** Mechanical Ventilators: General-Use Devices

18. A PB840 unit that controls ventilation and connects to the patient circuit (*abbreviation*).

20. The type of pause used to measure lung compliance.

Down

1. This test should be run when a new circuit or humidifier is added (*abbreviation*).
2. On the PB7200, **1 across** acts as this type of relief valve, which opens at 140 cm H_2O.
4. Volume-targeted A/C breaths on the PB740 and PB760 (*abbreviation*).
5. A type of waveform available in VC ventilation.
6. On the PB7200, **1 across** acts as this type of valve, which opens during the start-up self-test and if pneumatic or electric power is lost.
8. Manages the controls and alarms on the PB840 (*abbreviation*).
10. The type of pause used to measure auto-PEEP.
15. The place on the PB840 where changes can be made without them becoming active (*two words*).
16. PB840 battery (*abbreviation*).
19. An extensive test that is generally run by a qualified service technician (*abbreviation*).

Puritan Bennett 840

LEARNING OBJECTIVES

Upon completion of this section, you will be able to:
1. Explain the three primary functions of the expiratory filter.
2. Identify a situation in which the battery has become operational in the back-up power source.
3. Describe how a short self-test (SST) is run by the operator.
4. List the tests performed during an SST.
5. Analyze a problem in ventilator cycling during PSV.
6. Provide a definition of the parameter settings in the lower screen.
7. List the information contained in the upper screen.
8. Describe the indicator lights on the STATUS INDICATOR PANEL and the BREATH DELIVERY UNIT.
9. Compare the vertical and horizontal adjustments on the available waveforms and loops.
10. Identify the potential causes of problems during the measurement of respiratory mechanics.
11. Explain the function of rise-time percent and expiratory sensitivity.
12. Define the modes of ventilation available, including their trigger, limit, and cycle parameters.
13. Contrast the function of the expiratory valve during PC and VC ventilation.
14. Define *PAV+*.
15. Explain the set-up and operation of PAV+.

16. Describe volume runaway during PAV+.
17. Compare apnea ventilation to safety ventilation.

ACHIEVING THE OBJECTIVES

1. Explain the three primary functions of the expiratory filter.

_____

_____

2. Identify a situation in which the battery has become operational in the back-up power source.

2A. Where is the indicator for the battery or *back-up power source* (BPS) located?

_____

_____

2B. What functions does the internal battery power in the case of an emergency?

_____

_____

2C. What does a green light in the upper right-hand portion of the front panel indicate?

_____

_____

2D. What does a yellow light in the upper right-hand portion of the front panel indicate?

_____

_____

2E. How can the operator tell whether the BPS is fully charged?

_____

_____

2F. What indicates that the BPS is still charging?

_____

_____

3. Describe how an SST is run by the operator.

3A. How long does it take to perform an SST?

_____

3B. How often should an SST be run?

_____

_____

3C. What is the first thing the respiratory therapist must do before initiating the SST?

_____

_____

3D. What selections must be made before the beginning of the SST?

_____

_____

_____

_____

3E. During the SST, what actions must the operator take?

_____

_____

_____

_____

4. List the tests performed during an SST.

_____

_____

_____

_____

5. Analyze a problem in ventilator cycling during PSV.

5A. What is the cycle variable in PSV?

_____

5B. What parameter on the PB840 enables adjustment of this cycle variable?

_____

5C. What adjustment should be made to the PSV cycle variable if air-trapping is noted?

_____

_____

_____

_____

_____

5D. The PSV cycle variable is set at 5%, and a spontaneous tidal volume is acceptable. However, there is patient-ventilator dysynchrony. What adjustment needs to be made to improve patient ventilator synchrony? Why?

_____

_____

_____

_____

_____

6. Provide a definition of the parameter settings in the lower screen.

6A. List the five areas of the lower screen.

_____

_____

_____

_____

6B. Where do the current set parameters appear on the lower screen?

_____

_____

6C. What parameter settings might appear on the lower screen?

_____

_____

_____

_____

_____

6D. What does pushing the VENT SETUP button allow the operator to do?

_____

_____

6E. How are parameter changes activated?

_____

_____

6F. What does the APNEA SETUP button allow the operator to do?

_____

_____

_____

_____

6G. Describe three additional screens that can be accessed through the OTHER SCREENS function key on the lower screen.

_____

_____

_____

_____

_____

7. List the information contained in the upper screen.

7A. What are the four areas contained in the upper screen?

_____

_____

7B. Give an example of patient information that is displayed at the very top of the screen.

_____

_____

7C. How can the operator define unfamiliar abbreviations used in the upper screen?

_____

_____

_____

_____

7D. Where do the alarm messages appear, and how are they grouped?

_____

_____

_____

_____

7E. How many high-priority alarms can be listed at any time?

_____

7F. What other information can be displayed on the upper screen?

_____

_____

_____

_____

_____

_____

7G. Explain the other information that can be displayed on the upper screen (from Question 7F).

_____

_____

_____

_____

_____

_____

_____

_____

_____

_____

_____

_____

_____

_____

_____

_____

_____

_____

8. Describe the indicator lights on the STATUS INDICATOR PANEL and the BREATH DELIVERY UNIT.

8A. Where is the STATUS INDICATOR PANEL located?

_____

_____

8B. The separate STATUS INDICATOR PANEL provides information about which ventilator functions?

_____

_____

_____

_____

8C. How are the different alarm priority levels displayed?

_____

_____

_____

_____

_____

_____

_____

_____

8D. What does the VENT INOP. message mean?

_____

_____

8E. What action must be taken when there is a VENT INOP. indication?

_____

_____

8F. What does *SVO* mean?

_____

_____

8G. What indicators are on the front of the breath-delivery unit?

_____

_____

_____

_____

9. Compare the vertical and horizontal adjustments on the available waveforms and loops.

9A. Where are the vertical and horizontal adjustments located on the PB840?

_____

_____

9B. How much of a waveform does the FREEZE function capture? _____

9C. Which adjustment controls time, and which controls size?

_____

_____

9D. Which adjustment can show an entire 48-second scalar?

_____

_____

10. Identify the potential causes of problems during the measurement of respiratory mechanics.

10A. What respiratory mechanic measurements can the PB840 perform?

_____

_____

10B. During which maneuvers are these measurements made?

_____

_____

_____

_____

_____

10C. Name three conditions that will result in error messages during measurements of respiratory mechanics.

_____

_____

_____

_____

11. Explain the function of rise-time percent and expiratory sensitivity.

11A. Define *inspiratory rise time*.

_____

_____

11B. How does rise-time percent work?

_____

_____

_____

_____

_____

_____

11C. What is the difference between a low rise-time percent setting and a high rise-time percent setting in terms of the way the ventilator operates?

_____

_____

_____

_____

11D. Name one advantage and disadvantage of using a low rise-time percent setting?

_____

_____

_____

_____

11E. Name one advantage and disadvantage of using a high rise-time percent setting?

_____

_____

_____

_____

_____

11F. During which modes is rise time percent available?

_____

11G. What does the expiratory sensitivity set on the PB840?

_____

_____

11H. During what mode is expiratory sensitivity active?

_____

11I. What is the relationship between expiratory sensitivity and inspiratory time?

_____

_____

_____

_____

12. Define the modes of ventilation available, including their trigger, limit, and cycle parameters.

	Mode/breath type	Trigger	Limit	Cycle
12A.	ACVC			
12B.	VC+			
12C.	PC			
12D.	SIMV-VC			
12E.	SIMV-PC			
12F.	PS			
12G.	VS			
12H.	BiLevel			
12I.	PAV+			

13. Contrast the function of the expiratory valve during PC and VC ventilation.

13A. How does the expiratory valve operate during VC breaths?

_____

_____

13B. How does the expiratory valve operate during PC breaths?

_____

_____

_____

_____

_____

13C. How does the expiratory valve operate during BiLevel? _____

_____

14. Define PAV+.

14A. PAV+ estimates what values in order to function?

_____

_____

14B. What equation is the basis for PAV+?

_____

_____

14C. How does PAV+ operate?

_____

_____

_____

_____

14D. How often are measurements of flow and volume made during the inspiratory phase?

_____

14E. What is the trigger for PAV+?

_____

_____

14F. What is the difference between exhalation sensitivity (E_{SENS}) during PAV+ and E_{SENS} during PSV?

_____

_____

_____

_____

_____

_____

15. Explain the set-up and operation of PAV+.

15A. What type of circuit is required for PAV+?

_____

15B. What steps must be followed to set up a new patient with PAV+?

_____

_____

_____

_____

_____

_____

_____

15C. What is the range for the % SUPPORT setting?

_____

15D. How is the WOB split between patient and ventilator when the % SUPPORT setting is 65%?

_____

15E. How does the WOB bar act as a guide for setting the % SUPPORT?

_____

_____

_____

_____

15F. How does the ventilator make the initial determination of the patient's compliance and resistance?

_____

_____

_____

_____

_____

_____

_____

_____

15G. How often does the ventilator recalculate the compliance and resistance after the initial calculation?

_____

15H. What will happen if a valid estimation of resistance and compliance is not made?

_____

_____

_____

_____

_____

15I. What monitored values are displayed during PAV+?

_____

_____

_____

_____

15J. Describe the condition that would cause inspiration to terminate early.

_____

_____

_____

16. Describe volume runaway during PAV+.
16A. What does the term *runaway* mean?

_____

_____

_____

_____

16B. What condition will cause volume runaway during PAV+?

_____

_____

_____

_____

16C. What safeguards are used to reduce the risk of overventilation?

_____

_____

_____

17. Compare apnea ventilation to safety ventilation.
17A. What initiates apnea ventilation (AV)?

_____

17B. What parameters are used for AV?

_____

_____

_____

17C. How is AV deactivated?

_____

_____

_____

_____

17D. What initiates SAFETY VENTILATION?

_____

_____

_____

_____

17E. What parameters are used for SAFETY VENTILATION?

_____

_____

_____

_____

Think About This

How is cruise control on an automobile similar to PAV+ on the PB840?

Helpful Web Site

■ Puritan Bennett, PB840 Ventilator — http://www. puritanbennett.com

NBRC-TYPE QUESTIONS PB840

1. A green light in the battery-status indicator section of a Puritan Bennett 840 indicates which of the following?
   A. The BPS is operational.
   B. The BPS is currently charging.
   C. Two hours of battery time are available.
   D. The battery has at least 2 minutes of charge available.

2. Which of the following describes the function of the expiratory filter?
   I. It humidifies the gas.
   II. It warms the exhaled gas.
   III. It protects the ventilator from microorganisms.
   IV. It captures condensation from exhaled gas.
      A. III only
      B. II and III only
      C. I and IV only
      D. I, II, III, and IV

3. The "idle" mode on the Puritan Bennett 840 does which of the following?
   A. Allows the BPS to charge.
   B. Reduces the flow to zero during disconnection.
   C. Helps prevent a spray of aerosol particles into the room.
   D. Occurs when the graphics interface is nonoperational.

4. A high-priority alarm is represented by which of the following?
   A. A "!!" in red that is steady and emits two tones.
   B. A "!!!" in red that blinks rapidly and emits a tone.
   C. A "!!!" in red that emits three beeps and blinks slowly if active.
   D. A "!" in red that blinks rapidly and beeps three times every 10 seconds.

5. Calculate the expiratory time for the ACVC mode when the wave pattern is square; $f = 14$ breaths/min; flow = 25 L/min; and $V_T = 450$ mL.
   A. 1.07 second
   B. 2.68 seconds
   C. 3.22 seconds
   D. 3.45 seconds

6. In Figure 12-12, which PB840 mode is shown?

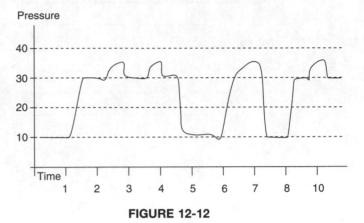

FIGURE 12-12

   A. PCV
   B. PAV+
   C. BiLevel
   D. ACVC

7. Overinflation of the lungs during PAV+ can be caused by which of the following?
   I. Underestimating patient compliance
   II. Overestimating patient compliance
   III. Underestimating airway resistance
   IV. Overestimating airway resistance
      A. I and III
      B. I and IV
      C. II and III
      D. II and IV

8. In what area of the PB840 are the current set parameters displayed?
   A. The Sandbox
   B. The Prompt area
   C. The top of the lower screen
   D. The top of the upper screen

9. Calculate the T_E during pressure ventilation when the T_I is locked at 0.85 second and the rate is set at 13 breaths/min.
   A. 1.07 second
   B. 3.76 seconds
   C. 3.98 seconds
   D. 4.19 seconds

10. VS on the PB 840 is the same as which of the following?
   A. APRV with a volume target
   B. CPAP with a volume target
   C. VC with a pressure target
   D. PSV with a volume target

Puritan Bennett 740

Upon completion of this section, you will be able to:

1. Name the power source requirements of the Puritan Bennett 740.
2. Describe the internal mechanisms involved in breath delivery.
3. Explain how to establish ventilator and alarm settings.
4. Assess an alarm situation, and identify the probable cause.
5. Identify messages that appear in the message window.
6. Compare the power-on self-test (POST) with the SST.
7. Define the functions of the various keys in the ventilator settings and patient status sections.
8. Compare flashing and constantly lit indicators in the ventilator status section.
9. Explain the functions of all modes of ventilation available on the PB740, including AV.
10. Identify functions that can be accessed through the menu key.
11. Describe the appropriate corrective action(s) to take when the VENT. INOP. alarm is activated.

ACHIEVING THE OBJECTIVES

1. Name the power source requirements of the Puritan Bennett 740.

1A. What pneumatic power requirements does the PB740 have?

_____

_____

_____

_____

1B. What are the electrical power requirements of the PB740?

_____

_____

2. Describe the internal mechanisms involved in breath delivery.

2A. Where is the information from the control panel processed and stored?

_____

_____

2B. How is breath delivery controlled on the PB740?

_____

_____

_____

_____

2C. What mechanism is responsible for providing gas flow to the patient?

_____

_____

2D. Within a PB740, trace gas from the ventilator inlet to the patient circuit.

_____

_____

_____

_____

3. Explain how to establish ventilator and alarm settings.

3A. Name the three sections of the front panel on the PB740.

_____

_____

_____

_____

_____

_____

_____

3B. What three steps must be followed to set new ventilator parameters or alarms?

_____

_____

_____

3C. The operator realizes that the wrong value for a new setting was dialed in, but it has not yet been accepted. How can the operator change it to the correct value?

_____

_____

3D. The operator changed the volume setting, but the value in the volume window did not change. What is the problem?

_____

_____

4. Assess an alarm situation, and identify the probable cause.

4A. What are the audible and visual differences between a high-priority alarm and a medium-priority alarm on the PB740?

_____

_____

_____

_____

_____

4B. The low exhaled tidal volume, low exhaled minute volume, low inspiratory pressure, and the disconnect alarms are all active at the same time. What is the probable cause of this situation?

_____

_____

4C. A patient is using the PSV mode in the PB740, which is indicating an active high exhaled tidal volume alarm. What are two probable causes for this situation?

_____

_____

4D. The high respiratory rate and low exhaled tidal volume alarms are active on a PB740 ventilating a patient with PSV. What is the most likely cause for this situation?

_____

_____

4E. List four causes for an occlusion alarm or partial-occlusion alarm on the PB740.

_____

_____

_____

_____

4F. During the ventilation of a patient who is using SIMV, the PB740 initiates AV. List two possible causes of this problem.

_____

_____

5. Identify messages that appear in the message window.

Match the message with its meaning.

5A. ___	DELIV GAS HI TEMP	1.	Internal power supply temperature high
5B. ___	FAN FAILED ALERT	2.	Missing air intake filter
5C. ___	HI BBU TEMP ALERT	3.	Room air temperature high
5D. ___	AIR INTAKE BLOCKED	4.	Internal temperature of ventilator high
5E. ___	LOSS OF POWER	5.	AC power disconnect
5F. ___	HI SYS TEMP ALERT	6.	High resistance on air intake filter
5G. ___	AIR INTAKE ABSENT	7.	AC power is lost, and batteries are low
5H. ___	LOSS OF AC POWER	8.	Fan is not operational, or fan filter is blocked

6. Compare the POST with the SST.

6A. Compare the initiation of the POST and the SST.

_____

6B. What does the POST check?

_____

6C. What does the SST check?

_____

_____

7. Define the functions of the various keys in the ventilator settings and patient status sections.

7A. List the pressures, rates, and volumes, with their ranges, displayed in the patient data area.

_____

_____

_____

_____

_____

7B. The alarms set in the patient data area and their ranges are:

_____

_____

_____

_____

_____.

7C. What mode and breath selection keys are included in the ventilator settings section on the front panel of the PB740?

_____

_____

7D. Name the parameters that are set in the ventilator settings section on the front panel of the PB 740.

_____

_____

_____

_____

7E. What do the four active keys located just below the message window on the front panel control?

_____

_____

_____

_____

_____

_____

_____

7F. What do the three additional function keys at the very bottom center of the ventilator settings section control?

_____

_____

_____

_____

_____

7G. What is the function of the SUPPORT PRESSURE control?

_____

_____

_____

8. Compare flashing and constantly lit indicators in the ventilator status section.

_____

_____

_____

_____

_____

_____

9. Explain the functions of all modes of ventilation available on the PB740, including AV.

9A. Which VC modes are available on the PB740?

_____

9B. Which spontaneous modes does the PB740 have?

_____

9C. What is the trigger variable for the VC modes?

_____

9D. What is the trigger variable for the spontaneous modes? _____

9E. How does the trigger variable for both the VC and spontaneous modes on the PB740 differ from that on other ventilators?

_____

_____

_____

_____

_____

269

9F. When should the apnea parameters be set for a new patient?

_____

_____

_____

9G. Under what circumstances can AV be triggered?

_____

_____

_____

_____

9H. What mode is used for AV on the PB740?

_____

10. Identify functions that can be accessed through the menu key.

10A. Which function, available through the menu key, provides additional pressure and flow to the patient who is receiving PSV to compensate for the work imposed by the resistance of the endotracheal tube?

_____

_____

10B. Which function corrects calculations for spirometric values when the SST is run?

_____

_____

10C. What is the range for the apnea interval?

_____

10D. Explain the VC ventilation flow-pattern selection.

_____

_____

_____

_____

11. Describe the appropriate corrective action(s) to take when the VENT. INOP. alarm is activated.

_____

_____

_____

_____

Think About This

What types of machines use pistons to operate?

Helpful Web Sites

- Puritan Bennett, PB740 Ventilator System — http://www.puritanbennett.com/_Catalog/PDF
- Puritan Bennett, Product Manuals — http://www.puritanbennett.com/Serv/manuals.aspx?ID=225

Name _____

Date _____

NBRC-TYPE QUESTIONS PB740

1. What type of internal mechanism does the PB740 have?
   A. Rotary piston
   B. Linear piston
   C. Flow-control valves
   D. Electromagnetic poppet valves

2. The operator can make the flow sensors on the PB740 respond with greater precision by doing which of the following?
   A. Running the ventilator as much as possible.
   B. Having preventative maintenance performed more frequently.
   C. Keeping the ventilator plugged in when not in use.
   D. Letting the ventilator run 10 minutes before patient connection.

3. In the PSV mode on the PB 740, the patient's peak flow is measured at 56 L/min. Inspiration will end when the flow tapers to which of the following?
   A. 10 L/min
   B. 14 L/min
   C. 17 L/min
   D. Cannot be determined

4. A patient with a tracheostomy who is being ventilated with the PB740 will be receiving a Passy-Muir valve. What ventilator adjustment does the respiratory therapist need to make?
   A. None
   B. Change the mode to PSV.
   C. Reduce exhaled volume alarm.
   D. Turn on the SPEAKING VALVE feature.

5. Which of the following is true concerning the PB740 ventilator?
   A. When not in use, the PB740 must be turned on to charge its internal battery.
   B. The PB740 is shielded from transmitting devices such as cellular phones and pagers.
   C. The low-pressure alarm cannot be used in the SPEAKING VALVE mode.
   D. ABV does not operate during VC ventilation.

271

Puritan Bennett 760

Upon completion of this section, you will be able to:
1. List the options and breath types that are available on the PB760 but not on the PB740.
2. Calculate T_I, T_E, and the I:E ratio when these variables are selected in PCV.
3. Explain the settings and functions of exhalation sensitivity, rise-time factor, and inspiratory and expiratory pause.
4. Identify the presence of auto-PEEP by using the end-expiratory flow valve in the message window.

ACHIEVING THE OBJECTIVES

1. List the options and breath types that are available on the PB760 but not on the PB740.

1A. What additional breath types are available for the modes on the 760?

_____

_____

1B. List the parameters that are available on the PB760 but not on the PB740.

_____

_____

_____

_____

_____

1C. Name the two features in the PB760 menu under USER SETTINGS that are not in the PB740.

_____

_____

_____

_____

1D. What features are different on the front-panel patient data section of the PB760?

_____

_____

_____

_____

_____

_____

_____

_____

2. Calculate T_I, T_E, and the I:E ratio when these variables are selected in PCV.

2A. Calculate the T_I and T_E with PCV settings as follows: an I:E ratio of 1:3 and a rate of 12 breaths/min.

_____

_____

_____

_____

2B. Calculate the I:E ratio with PCV settings as follows: a T_I of 0.95 s and a rate of 16 breaths/min.

_____

_____

_____

_____

2C. Calculate T_I and T_E with PCV settings as follows: an I:E ratio of 1:2 and a rate of 20 breaths/min.

_____

_____

_____

2D. Calculate the rate that should be set for PCV when the T_I is set to 1.2 s and the I:E ratio needs to be maintained at approximately 1:2.

_____

_____

_____

_____

_____

3. Explain the settings and functions of exhalation sensitivity, rise-time factor, and inspiratory and expiratory pause.

3A. What does the exhalation sensitivity adjust?

_____

_____

3B. What is the difference between exhalation sensitivity on the PB740 and that on the PB760?

_____

_____

_____

3C. Exhalation sensitivity is set at 50%, and the measured peak flow is 60 L/min. At what flow rate will inspiration end?

_____

_____

_____

3D. What changes should be made to exhalation sensitivity to decrease T_I?

_____

_____

_____

_____

_____

3E. Define the term *rise time*.

_____

_____

_____

3F. What is the range for adjusting rise time?

_____

3G. Explain the difference between a high rise-time setting (e.g., 100%) and a low rise-time setting (e.g., 5%).

_____

_____

_____

_____

_____

_____

3H. What is the purpose of an inspiratory pause?

_____

_____

3I. Explain the two ways to execute an inspiratory pause.

_____

_____

_____

_____

_____

_____

3J. How does the ventilator hold inspiration?

_____

_____

3K. What is the purpose of an expiratory pause?

_____

_____

3L. How is the time for an expiratory pause determined?

_____

_____

3M. List five factors that can end the expiratory pause measurement.

_____

_____

_____

_____

4. Identify the presence of auto-PEEP by using the end-expiratory flow value in the message window.

4A. What does the message window normally display?

_____

_____

4B. What effect does active breathing by the patient have on the auto-PEEP reading?

_____

_____

4C. What measurement will be shown in the message window after a successful expiratory pause?

_____

_____

_____

_____

4D. How long will the measurements be displayed in the message window?

_____

_____

Think About This

Why are computerized ventilators easy to upgrade?

Helpful Web Site

■ Puritan Bennett, PB760 Ventilator System — http://www.puritanbennett.com/prod/

Name _____

Date _____

NBRC-TYPE QUESTIONS PB740

1. Which of the following is the parameter that determines inspiratory time during PSV?
   A. I:E ratio
   B. Rise time
   C. Expiratory pause
   D. Exhalation sensitivity

2. Which of the following is the parameter that determines the length of time for the set pressure during PCV to be reached?
   A. Rise time
   B. Inspiratory time
   C. PCV timing variable
   D. Exhalation sensitivity

3. Calculate the I:E ratio in the PCV mode when the T_I is set to 0.75 second and the respiratory rate is set at 25 breaths/min.
   A. 0.45:1
   B. 1:2.2
   C. 1:2.6
   D. 1:3.2

4. Which of the following statements is false concerning the PB760?
   A. The expiratory pause can be held for 30 s.
   B. In AV the rise-time factor is fixed at 50%.
   C. In PCV the operator can set either T_I or the I:E ratio as the constant.
   D. Inspiratory pause ends automatically at the end of 2 s.

5. An expiratory pause maneuver will end when which of the following occurs?
   I. An alarm is initiated.
   II. The patient initiates a breath.
   III. The ventilator detects a leak.
   IV. The operator releases the key.
   A. IV only
   B. II only
   C. I and III only
   D. I, II, III, and IV

275

Copyright © 2010 by Mosby Inc., an affiliate of Elsevier Inc.

Chapter **12** **Mechanical Ventilators: General-Use Devices**

Puritan Bennett 7200

Upon completion of this section, you will be able to:

1. Explain the procedure for setting a mode and its parameters.
2. Adjust ventilator settings appropriately when the DECR RESP RATE FIRST message appears.
3. Identify conditions that activate emergency modes of ventilation.
4. Recognize breath delay when switching from CMV to SIMV, and provide an appropriate solution.
5. Describe the available flow waveforms and their effects on breath delivery, inspiratory time, and peak flow.
6. Recommend appropriate corrections to alarm situations.
7. List the weaning measurements available under the respiratory mechanics option.
8. Calculate the I:E ratio, inspiratory and expiratory time, and total cycle time during PCV.
9. Recommend an appropriate flow-trigger and base flow setting for a patient.
10. Compare the functions of the 1.0 version of flowby to those of the 2.0 version on the PB7200.

ACHIEVING THE OBJECTIVES

1. Explain the procedure for setting a mode and its parameters.

1A. What message is displayed in the window after initial start-up?

1B. If new parameters are not specified after initial start-up, how will the ventilator operate?

1C. List the three primary modes of ventilation on the PB7200.

1D. List the two available optional modes on the PB7200.

1E. What steps must be taken to set the primary modes of ventilation on the PB7200?

1F. How does the operator set the parameters for the primary modes of ventilation?

1G. What steps must be taken to activate the PC mode?

1H. How does setting the PC mode or the PC apnea ventilation mode differ from setting the other modes of ventilation?

1I. How is the PS mode accessed?

_____

_____

_____

_____

_____

_____

_____

2. Adjust ventilator settings appropriately when the DECR RESP RATE FIRST message appears.

2A. A change in which four parameters can cause the DECR RESP RATE FIRST message?

_____

_____

2B. What does a change in any one of the aforementioned four parameters do to cause this message to appear?

_____

_____

_____

_____

2C. How does decreasing the respiratory rate alleviate the problem?

_____

_____

_____

3. Identify conditions that activate emergency modes of ventilation.

3A. What causes AV to be initiated?

_____

_____

3B. What activates back-up ventilation?

_____

_____

_____

_____

3C. What are the parameters for back-up ventilation?

_____

_____

_____

_____

_____

3D. What activates the disconnect-ventilation mode?

_____

_____

_____

_____

_____

3E. What are the parameters for disconnect ventilation?

_____

_____

_____

4. Recognize breath delay when switching from CMV to SIMV, and provide an appropriate solution.

4A. What should be done to prevent the delay that might occur when switching from CMV to SIMV?

_____

_____

_____

5. Describe the available flow waveforms and their effects on breath delivery, inspiratory time, and peak flow.

5A. What dictates the amount of flow delivered during each waveform?

_____

_____

5B. How is the flow delivered during the rectangular waveform?

_____

_____

5C. How is the flow delivered during the descending-ramp waveform?

_____

_____

5D. How is the flow delivered during the sine curve?

_____

_____

5E. What effect does changing waveforms from constant to descending have on the T_I?

_____

_____

5F. What effect does changing waveforms from constant to sine have on the T_I?

_____

_____

_____

_____

_____

_____

6. Recommend appropriate corrections to alarm situations.

6A. A PB7200 in use on a patient initiates back-up ventilation. What action should the respiratory therapist take?

_____

_____

6B. A respiratory therapist responds to a stat call for a patient being volume-ventilated by a 7200. When the respiratory therapist enters the patient's room, he notices that the high-pressure limit light, the low exhaled tidal volume light, and the low exhaled minute volume light are lit continuously and the yellow caution light is on. What action should be taken?

_____

_____

_____

_____

_____

_____

6C. During PCV use the 7200 the high-pressure limit alarm is active. What action should the respiratory therapist take?

_____

_____

_____

_____

_____

_____

6D. While on rounds in the ICU, the respiratory therapist is told by a nurse that the apnea time interval and AV for a patient receiving PSV has initiated and been reset several times during the last hour. What actions should the respiratory therapist take?

_____

_____

_____

_____

_____

_____

7. List the weaning measurements available under the respiratory mechanics option.

_____

_____

_____

_____

8. Calculate the I:E ratio, inspiratory and expiratory time, and total cycle time during PCV.

8A. Calculate the I:E ratio for an apneic patient receiving PCV with the following settings: pressure of 25 cm H_2O; a T_I set at 1.2 second; a rate of 12 breaths/min; and a PEEP of +3 cm H_2O.

_____

_____

_____

8B. Calculate the T_I and T_E for the following settings: PCV; rate, 10 breaths/min; I:E ratio, 1:3; pressure, 20 cm H_2O; PEEP, +5 cm H_2O.

_____

_____

_____

8C. Calculate the T_E and I:E ratio for PCV at a rate of 16 breaths/min and a T_I of 1.5 s.

_____

_____

_____

_____

9. Recommend an appropriate flow-trigger and base flow setting for a patient.

9A. What is the appropriate flow-trigger and base flow setting for an adult 108 lb female?

_____

_____

9B. What is the appropriate flow-trigger and base flow setting for a 44-lb toddler?

_____

_____

9C. What is the appropriate flow-trigger and base flow setting for a 75-kg male?

_____

_____

10. Compare the functions of the 1.0 version of flowby to those of the 2.0 version on the PB 7200.

10A. What was the original intent of the flowby function (i.e., version 1.0)?

_____

_____

_____

_____

_____

10B. Flowby version 1.0 was active in which modes?

_____

_____

10C. What unintentional benefit did flowby version 1.0 have?

_____

_____

_____

_____

10D. Flowby version 2.0 is available during which modes?

_____

_____

10E. What is the flow sensitivity range for version 1.0?

_____

10F. What is the flow sensitivity range for version 2.0?

_____

10G. What is the base flow range for both versions?

_____

10H. How does nebulizer use affect the use of flowby in version 1.0?

_____

_____

_____

_____

10I. How does nebulizer use affect the use of flowby in version 2.0?

_____

_____

_____

_____

Think About This

What type of computer were you using in 1983?

Helpful Web Sites

■ Puritan Bennett, PB7200 Series Ventilator —http://www.puritanbennett.com/Serv/manuals.aspx?ID=22

■ http://www.puritanbennett.com

NBRC-TYPE QUESTIONS PB7200

1. Back-up ventilation on the PB7200 will occur when which of the following occur?
   I. Power failure
   II. Failure of the POST
   III. Three system errors within 24 hours
   IV. More than a 10% drop in AC voltage
   A. I and IV only
   B. II and III only
   C. I, II, and III only
   D. II, III, and IV only

2. On the PB7200, when the selected flow rate is unable to deliver the set volume within a time that provides an acceptable I:E ratio, which two of the following corrective actions can eliminate this problem?
   I. Increase the respiratory rate.
   II. Decrease the respiratory rate.
   III. Increase the inspiratory flow rate.
   IV. Decrease the inspiratory flow rate.
   A. I and II
   B. I and IV
   C. II and III
   D. III and IV

3. If both gas supplies to the PB7200 are lost, which of the following is initiated?
   A. Extended self-test
   B. Opening of safety valve
   C. Backup ventilation
   D. Disconnect ventilation

4. What causes autotriggering on a PB7200 set to PSV?
   A. PS level is set too low.
   B. PS level is set too high.
   C. Trigger sensitivity is set too low.
   D. Trigger sensitivity is set too high.

5. The peak flow setting during VC-CMV is 45 L/min with a rectangular flow waveform. The respiratory therapist wishes to change to the descending waveform. Which of the following is the flow rate setting that will maintain the current I:E ratio?
   A. 45 L/min
   B. 67.5 L/min
   C. 80 L/min
   D. 90 L/min

SECTION VII: RESPIRONICS

Respironics Esprit

"Morale is the state of mind. It is steadfastness and courage and hope. It is confidence and zeal and loyalty. It is élan, esprit de corps and determination."
General George Catlett Marshall

KEY TERMS CROSSWORD PUZZLE

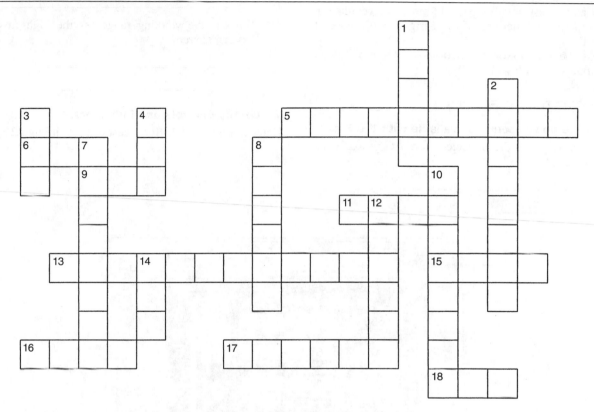

CROSSWORD PUZZLE 12-7

Use the clues to complete the crossword puzzle.

Across

5. Flashes red when 5 minutes or less is left (*two words*).
6. Volume-targeted ventilation (*abbreviation*).
9. A long self-test (*abbreviation*).
11. The first test the ventilator initiates (*abbreviation*).
13. Very important alarm (*two words*).
15. A setting in (*abbreviation*).
16. Not invasive positive pressure ventilation (*abbreviation*).
17. User interface.
18. A change in blower sound results from a change in this (*abbreviation*).

Down

1. A time interval set by the operator.
2. This helps eliminate breath-stacking (*hyphenated*).
3. Opened exhalation valve with closed air and oxygen valves (*abbreviation*).
4. A test to run after each patient (*abbreviation*).
7. This is illuminated when the ventilator malfunctions (*abbreviation*).
8. The color of the battery indicator.
10. Name for flow-cycle adjustment (*abbreviation*).
12. Gas source for the Esprit.
14. Maximum pressure alarm (*abbreviation*).

Chapter **12** **Mechanical Ventilators: General-Use Devices**

Upon completion of this section, you will be able to:

1. List the power sources available with the Esprit.
2. Identify controls and indicators.
3. Describe alarm functions.
4. Verify ventilator preparedness with the SST and the extended self-test (EST).
5. Set AV parameters.
6. Set and adjust breath types and modes of ventilation.
7. Compare the functions of the I-trigger with those of the E-trigger.
8. Describe the optional functions of O_2 monitoring, graphics, and Flow-Trak™.

ACHIEVING THE OBJECTIVES

1. List the power sources available with the Esprit.

1A. If the Esprit is disconnected from AC power, what happens?

_____

_____

1B. What types of battery back-ups does the Esprit have?

_____

_____

1C. What should be done to maintain the expected life of the lead-acid battery?

_____

_____

1D. What is the working range for the high-pressure oxygen source?

_____

_____

2. Identify controls and indicators.

Refer to Figure 12-13 for Questions 2A through 2G.

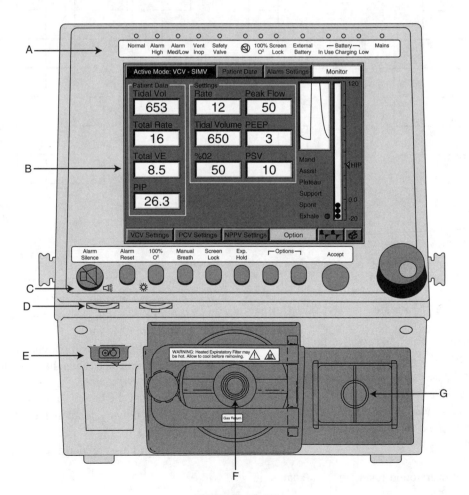

FIGURE 12-13

2A. What happens when the first button on the left in the row marked *C* is pressed?

_____

_____

2B. What happens when the third button from the left in the row marked *C* is pressed?

_____

_____

2C. What is the location of the button that will determine whether auto-PEEP is present?

_____

_____

2D. Which button helps to prevent accidental or inadvertent changes in the screen function?

_____

_____

2E. Where is the SAFETY VALVE OPEN alert located?

_____

_____

2F. Locate the audible alarm volume and display brightness controls.

_____

_____

2G. What elements that are common to all ventilator screens are located in the touch-screen area *B*?

_____

_____

_____

_____

_____

_____

3. Describe alarm functions.

3A. How are all alarm settings accessed?

_____

3B. What is different about accessing the high-pressure alarm?

_____

_____

_____

_____

3C. Name the priority alarm conditions and their audible and visual cues.

_____

_____

_____

_____

_____

_____

_____

_____

_____

_____

_____

3D. Give the names of two alarms that cannot be silenced.

_____

_____

3E. Give the names of four alarms that cannot be manually reset.

_____

_____

_____

_____

3F. Name the three situations that can cause the safety valve to open during ventilator operation.

_____

_____

_____

_____

_____

4. Verify ventilator preparedness with the SST and the EST.

4A. When should the SST be run?

_____

_____

4B. What does the SST verify?

_____

_____

_____

_____

_____

_____

_____

4C. What should be done if a ventilator does not pass an SST?

_____

_____

_____

_____

4D. When should the EST be run?

_____

_____

_____

_____

4E. How are the SST and EST accessed?

_____

_____

5. Set AV parameters.

5A. The apnea time interval range is:

_____

5B. What mode will AV use to ventilate the patient?

_____

_____

5C. What is the lowest breath rate that can be set for AV?

_____

_____

_____

5D. What parameters will be used for AV?

_____

_____

6. Set and adjust breath types and modes of ventilation.

6A. What should be selected before selecting the mode of ventilation?

_____

_____

6B. What are the available breath types on the Esprit ventilator?

_____

_____

6C. How is a breath type selected?

_____

_____

_____

_____

_____

6D. What are the available modes on the Esprit?

_____

_____

6E. List the parameters for VC ventilation (VCV)–A/C and VCV-SIMV modes.

_____

_____

_____

_____

6F. List the parameters for PCV-A/C and PCV-SIMV modes.

_____

_____

_____

_____

7. Compare the functions of the I-trigger with those of the E-trigger.

7A. Define *I-trigger*.

_____

_____

7B. How is the I-trigger set?

_____

_____

7C. What I-trigger variables are available for PCV, VCV, and noninvasive positive-pressure ventilation (NPPV)?

_____

_____

7D. What are the suggested initial settings for the I-trigger variables?

_____

_____

_____

7E. Define *E-trigger*.

_____

_____

7F. What is the range for the E-trigger setting?

_____

7G. Explain what an E-trigger setting of 30% means.

_____

_____

_____

8. Describe the optional functions of O_2 monitoring, graphics, and Flow-Trak™.

8A. When is the calibration for the optional O_2 sensor performed?

_____

_____

8B. What is the location of the O_2 sensor?

_____

_____

8C. List all the types of scalars and loops that are available when the graphics option is included.

_____

_____

8D. Name one use for the overlay image option.

_____

_____

8E. How does Flow-Trak™ function when used with volume-targeted breaths?

_____

_____

8F. How does Flow-Trak™ function if the patient has spontaneous efforts during volume ventilation?

_____

_____

_____

_____

Think About This

Who wrote the first account of mechanical ventilation use?

Helpful Web Site

■ Respironics, Esprit Ventilator Information — http://esprit.respironics.com

NBRC-TYPE QUESTIONS RESPIRONICS ESPRIT

1. On the Esprit, the EXP HOLD key is used to do which of the following?
   A. Measure auto-PEEP
   B. Measure expiratory resistance
   C. Calculate static lung compliance
   D. Administer a metered-dose inhaler

2. Pressing the alarm reset button on the Esprit will do all **EXCEPT** which of the following?
   A. Terminate the alarm silence.
   B. End the Occlusion-SVO alarm.
   C. Clear all visual alarm indicators.
   D. Reset AV to normal ventilation.

3. Which of the following is the alarm subscreen that can be activated while the VCV screen or the PCV screen is visible on the Esprit?
   A. Low tidal volume
   B. Low minute volume
   C. High respiratory rate
   D. High inspiratory pressure

4. The E-trigger on the Esprit is set at 2 L/min. The bias flow setting will be which of the following?
   A. Automatically 4 L/min
   B. Automatically 5 L/min
   C. Automatically 6 L/min
   D. Operator-selected

5. Where is the correct placement for the O_2 sensor in an Esprit patient circuit?
   A. The valve just after the humidifier
   B. Just before the exhalation valve
   C. Between the patient and the Y-connector
   D. Between the ventilator and the inspiratory bacteria filter

6. Which of the following are alarms that cannot be silenced on the Esprit?
   I. Low O_2 supply
   II. I-Time too long
   III. AV
   IV. Low back-up battery
   A. I and II only
   B. II and III only
   C. III and IV only
   D. I and IV only

7. Which of the following is the pressure support ventilation parameter change on the Esprit that will help reduce air-trapping on a ventilated patient with COPD?
   A. Increase I-trigger
   B. Increase E-trigger
   C. Decrease I-trigger
   D. Decrease E-trigger

8. Which of the following statements is not true regarding the Esprit?
   A. 100% O_2 increases the oxygen percentage to 100% for 2 minutes.
   B. The safety valve will open when the oxygen source is no longer operable.
   C. The alarm silence icon is yellow when the audible alarm has been disabled.
   D. The high-pressure limit in NPPV is automatically set at 10 cm H_2O above the inspiratory PAP setting.

Chapter **12** **Mechanical Ventilators: General-Use Devices**

Infant and Pediatric Ventilators

Upon completion of this chapter, you will be able to systematically review continuous positive airway pressure (CPAP) delivery devices and infant and pediatric ventilators by doing the following:

1. Naming the power sources required for each nasal CPAP device and each infant and pediatric ventilator.
2. Listing the modes of ventilatory support provided by each ventilator.
3. When given flow and inspiratory time (T_I), calculating the approximate tidal volume (V_T) delivered by a typical infant ventilator.
4. Describe noteworthy internal functions of each infant and pediatric ventilator.
5. Explain the location and function of the controls, monitors, alarm, and safety systems for each infant and pediatric ventilator.
6. Describe the precautions and key troubleshooting points for each nasal CPAP device or ventilator.

"There is always one moment in childhood when the door opens and lets the future in."
Deepak Chopra

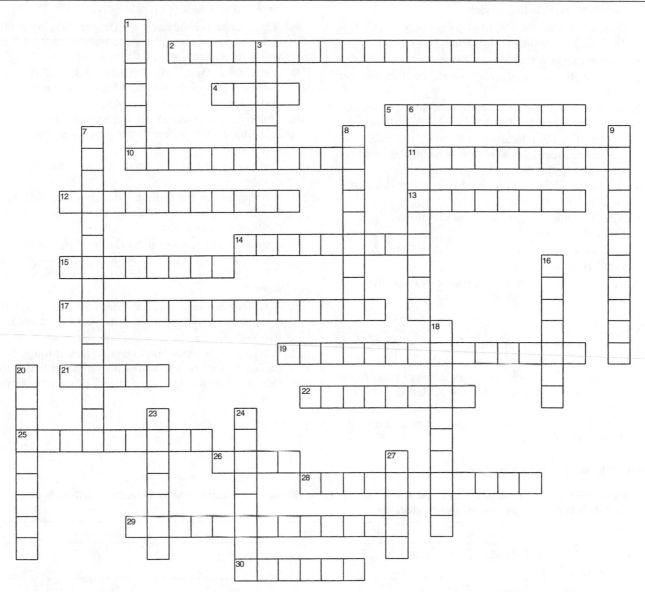

CROSSWORD PUZZLE 13-1
Created using Crossword Weaver, www.CrosswordWeaver.com.

Use the clues to complete the crossword puzzle.

Across

2. A special feature on the Cardinal Health V.I.P. Bird used to stabilize baseline pressure, prevent autocycling, and optimize assist sensitivity in the presence of leaks.

4. The type of flow set on the SensorMedics models.

5. Another name for *piston excursion* on the Sensor-Medics models.

10. This sensitivity control regulates the answer to **25 across.**

11. This driver powers the linear drive motor on the SensorMedics models (*two words*).

12. Reserves pressurized gas during the expiratory phase to meet flow demands up to 120 L/min on the Cardinal Health V.I.P. Bird.

13. A self-regulating mode of ventilation available on the Dräger EvitaXL.

14. Located on the rear panel on the Bunnell Life Pulse High-Frequency Jet Ventilator, this is a safety valve that releases internal pressure.

15. This type of voltage is applied to the electrical coil on the SensorMedics models.

17. The VarFlex on the Cardinal AVEA ventilator is this type of flow pneumotachometer (*two words*).

19. Another term for **18 down** (*two words*).

21. One of these equals 60 cycles, or breaths, per minute.

22. Another name for Airway Pressure Release Ventilation (APRV) on the Cardinal AVEA ventilator.

25. On the Cardinal Health V.I.P. Bird, the answer to **10 across** regulates the flow-termination point to provide expiratory _____.

26. A Bunnell Life Pulse is this type of ventilator (*abbreviation*).

28. The resistance to expiration at the airway produces this (*two words*).

29. An electromechanical-type valve located in the Cardinal Health V.I.P. Bird.

30. A type of flow system that provides inspiratory gas for spontaneous breaths.

Down

1. The type of triple-lumen tubes used with the Bunnell Life Pulse ventilator (*three words*).

3. The geometric design of the jet delivery ports of the Cardinal Health Infant Flow Nasal CPAP facilitates this effect.

6. A type of memory used to store alarm codes on the Dräger Babylog 8000.

7. A type of solenoid on the Bunnell Life Pulse Ventilator that activates the pinch valve.

8. A type of safety valve on the Dräger Babylog 8000 that directs excessive pressure build-up within the ventilator system through the exhalation valve.

9. Located on the Cardinal Health V.I.P. Bird, this control regulates the driving pressure to the exhalation valve jet venturi (*two words*).

16. This option is essential when the Dräger EvitaXL is being used with patients who weigh less than 6 kg (*two words*).

18. The subsystem at the heart of the SensorMedics models.

20. A dampener in the Cardinal Health V.I.P. Bird that stabilizes pressure and maintains driving pressure to the flow-control valve.

23. A type of flow sensor on the Cardinal Health AVEA ventilator that is compatible in applications with a maximum flow rate of less than 30 L/min (*two words*).

24. A type of sensor used on the SensorMedics models to track the movement of the piston between mechanical stops.

27. A type of valve that allows gas to flow through the patient box of the Bunnell Life Pulse ventilator to free the monitoring line of the hi-lo jet tube from moisture.

ACHIEVING THE OBJECTIVES

1. Name the power sources required for each nasal continuous positive airway pressure (nCPAP) device and each infant and pediatric ventilator.

	Device	Power sources
1A.	Cardinal Health Infant Flow Nasal CPAP System	
1B.	Cardinal Health AirLife™ nCPAP System Driver	
1C.	Cardinal Health Infant Flow SiPAP	
1D.	Fisher & Paykel Healthcare Bubble CPAP System	
1E.	Hamilton ARABELLA System	
1F.	Cardinal Health V.I.P. Bird Infant/Pediatric Ventilator	
1G.	Cardinal Health V.I.P. Sterling and Gold Infant/Pediatric Ventilators	
1H.	Dräger Babylog 8000 Infant Ventilator	
1I.	Dräger Babylog 8000 Plus Infant Ventilator	

Think About This

What are the differences between the United States and Europe in terms of electrical voltage?

Helpful Web Sites

- Fisher & Paykel, Bubble CPAP Patient Interface — http://www.fphcare.com
- Hamilton Medical, Inc, ARABELLA Infant Nasal CPAP System — http://www.hamilton-medical.com
- Cardinal Health, which owns VIASYS Healthcare, V.I.P. Bird Gold and Sterling Information — http://www.viasyshealthcare.com
- Dräger Medical AG & Co, Babylog 8000 Plus Information — http://www.draeger.com

2. List the modes of ventilatory support provided by each ventilator.

	Device	Modes of ventilation
2A.	Hamilton ARABELLA System	
2B.	Cardinal Health V.I.P. Bird Infant/ Pediatric Ventilator	
2C.	Cardinal Health V.I.P. Sterling and Gold Infant/Pediatric Ventilators	
2D.	Dräger Babylog 8000 Infant Ventilator	
2E.	Dräger Babylog 8000 Plus Infant Ventilator	
2F.	Cardinal AVEA Ventilator (for infant/ pediatric use)	
2G.	Dräger EvitaXL (for infant/pediatric use)	
2H.	Hamilton GALILEO Gold (for infant/ pediatric use)	
2I.	Maquet Servo^i Ventilator (for neonatal/pediatric use)	
2J.	Puritan Bennett 840™ (for infant/ pediatric use)	

Think About This

What are the advantages and disadvantages of having one type of ventilator that can be used with newborns, children, and adults?

Helpful Web Sites

- Hamilton Medical, Inc, GALILEO Product Documentation — http://www.hamilton-medical.com
- Dräger Medical UK Limited, Babylog 8000 Plus Technical Specifications — http://www.draeger.com
- Auckland District Health Board, Neonatal Ventilation — http://www.adhb.govt.nz
- Dräger Medical AG & Co, Information Booklets — http://www.draeger.com
- Cardinal Health, which owns VIASYS Healthcare, Archived Product Videos — http://www.viasyshealthcare.com

3. When given flow and inspiratory time (T$_I$), calculate the approximate tidal volume (V$_T$) delivered by a typical infant ventilator.

Fill in the blanks in the following table:

	T$_I$ (s)	Flow (L/min)	V$_T$ (mL)	Calculations
3A.	0.4	12		
3B.	0.5	10		
3C.	0.6	8		
3D.	0.75	15		
3E.		10	25	
3F.		8	10	
3G.	0.45		8	

Think About This

Which is more accurate: calculating the V$_T$ or measuring the volume with a pneumotachometer?

Helpful Web Site

- University of Washington Academic Medical Center, NICU-Web Home — http://depts.washington.edu

4. Describe noteworthy internal functions of each infant and pediatric ventilator.

4A. Cardinal Health V.I.P. Bird:

(1.) What is the maximum flow capability of the accumulator? _____

(2.) What device is used to stabilize pressure and maintain driving pressure to the flow-control valve?

_____

(3.) Which type of flow-control valve does the Cardinal Health V.I.P. Bird use?

_____

(4.) What device does the Cardinal Health V.I.P. Bird use to prevent automatic positive end-expiratory pressure (auto-PEEP) caused by continuous flow during time-cycled, pressure-limited ventilation?

_____

(5.) What occurs when there is a pressure decrease of greater than 0.25 cm H$_2$O below baseline pressure?

_____

_____

4B. Cardinal Health V.I.P. Sterling and Gold Infant/Pediatric Ventilators:

(1.) The dual-control mode of ventilation that is incorporated into the Cardinal Health V.I.P. Gold Infant/Pediatric Ventilator is:

_____.

(2.) Explain the function of both the Infant and Pediatric "Smart" Flow Sensors incorporated into the Cardinal Health V.I.P. Sterling and Gold Infant/Pediatric Ventilators.

_____

_____

_____

_____

(3.) Where are the "Smart" Flow Sensors placed in the ventilator circuit when used?

_____

_____

(4.) What is the difference in bias flow when setting up this ventilator for infant and pediatric use?

_____

_____

_____

_____

4C. Dräger Babylog 8000 Infant Ventilator:
(1.) How does this ventilator respond to a gas supply failure or electrical failure?

_____

_____

(2.) What happens if excessive pressure builds up within this ventilator?

_____

_____

4D. Dräger Babylog 8000 Plus Infant Ventilator:
(1.) What monitoring upgrades to the Babylog 8000 are incorporated into this ventilator?

_____

_____

_____

_____

(2.) What additional ventilator modes have been added to this ventilator?

_____

_____

4E. Bunnell Life Pulse High-Frequency Jet Ventilator:
(1.) Describe the features of the endotracheal tube that must be used with this ventilator.

_____

_____

_____

(2.) What is the function of each lumen of this endotracheal tube?

_____

_____

_____

_____

_____

(3.) A patient intubated with a standard endotracheal tube requires jet ventilation; how can this be accomplished?

_____

_____

_____

4F. SensorMedics 3100 and 3100A:
(1.) What type of drive mechanism does this ventilator use?

_____

(2.) Which control dictates the movement of this drive mechanism?

_____

(3.) What is the purpose of the Venturi-type air amplifier?

_____

_____

4G. SensorMedics 3100B High-Frequency Oscillatory Ventilator:
(1.) What is the difference between the drive mechanism of this ventilator and that of the 3100; between the mechanism of this ventilator and that of the 3100A?

_____

_____

(2.) What control is used to prevent inadvertent increases in mean airway pressure?

_____

(3.) What is the bias flow capability of this ventilator?

_____

(4.) What is the difference between the "Set Max Paw" alarm on this ventilator and that on the 3100; between the alarm on this ventilator and that on the 3100A?

_____

_____

4H. Cardinal Health AVEA Ventilator for infant/pediatric use:

(1.) What type of flow sensors are used on the three available models of this ventilator?

_____

_____

_____

_____

(2.) Which type of flow sensor accommodates heliox delivery on this ventilator?

_____

_____

_____

_____

_____

4I. Dräger EvitaXL Ventilator for infant/pediatric use:

(1.) What flow sensor must be used with this ventilator for patients who weigh less than 6 kg?

_____

_____

(2.) Describe the placement of this flow sensor.

_____

_____

(3.) What are the flow sensor's specifications?

_____

_____

_____

_____

(4.) Describe how aerosolized medication should be delivered when this ventilator is being used for an infant or pediatric patient.

_____

_____

_____

_____

_____

_____

_____

4J. Hamilton GALILEO Gold for infant and pediatric use:

(1.) What types of flow sensors are used on this ventilator for pediatric and infant patients?

_____

_____

(2.) When can the integrated nebulizer be used to deliver aerosolized medications in the infant application?

_____

_____

4K. Maquet Servo^i Ventilator for neonatal and pediatric use:

(1.) What type of flow sensor is used with this ventilator for infant patients?

_____

_____

(2.) What are the flow sensor's specifications?

_____

_____

_____

_____

4L. Puritan Bennett 840™ Ventilator for infant/pediatric use:

(1.) What option makes this ventilator compatible with neonate use?

_____

_____

(2.) What are the specifications of this option?

_____

_____

_____

_____

(3.) What else must be added to the ventilator to make it compatible with infant use?

_____

_____

Think About This

How are changes to mechanical ventilator design initiated?

Helpful Web Sites

- Bunnell Incorporated, Life Pulse High-Frequency Jet Ventilator — http://www.bunl.com

- Dräger Medical AG & Co, Babylog 8000 plus — http://www.draeger.com
- Maquet, Servo[i] Infant Ventilator — http://www.maquet.com
- Puritan Bennett, 840™ with NeoMode Software — http://www.puritanbennett.com
- SensorMedics, 3100B Operator's Manual — http://www.fda.gov

- Cardinal Health, which owns VIASYS Healthcare, AVEA and V.I.P. Bird Gold Videos — http://www.viasyshealthcare.com
- Cardinal Health, which owns VIASYS Healthcare/SensorMedics, 3100A High-frequency Oscillatory ventilator — http://www.viasyshealthcare.com
- Cardinal Health, which owns VIASYS Healthcare/SensorMedics, 3100B High-frequency Oscillatory Ventilator — http://www.viasyshealthcare.com

5. Explain the location and function of the controls, monitors, alarm, and safety systems for each infant and pediatric ventilator.

5A. Cardinal Health V.I.P. Bird — see Figure 13-1:

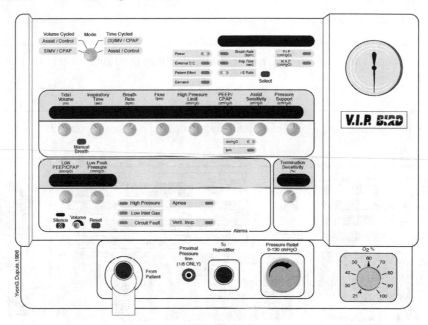

FIGURE 13-1
(Courtesy Yvon Dupuis.)

(1.) What is the location of the mode selector, and how are the modes grouped?

_____

(2.) What alarms are included in the alarm section on this ventilator's front panel?

_____

_____

(3.) What additional safety feature is incorporated into this ventilator, and where is its control located?

_____

_____

(4.) Explain the function of termination sensitivity.

_____

_____

(5.) What happens to the breath when the inspiratory flow fails to decrease to the termination sensitivity set percent?

_____

(6.) Which control knob on this ventilator will set flow sensitivity?

_____

(7.) When and how does leak compensation operate on this ventilator?

_____

_____

_____

(8.) What variables does the Bird Partner IIi Volume Monitor measure and display?

_____

_____

_____

(9.) How can a continuous artificial airway leak be detected within the circuit of this ventilator?

_____

_____

5B. Cardinal Health V.I.P. Sterling and Gold Infant/Pediatric Ventilators — see Figure 13-2:

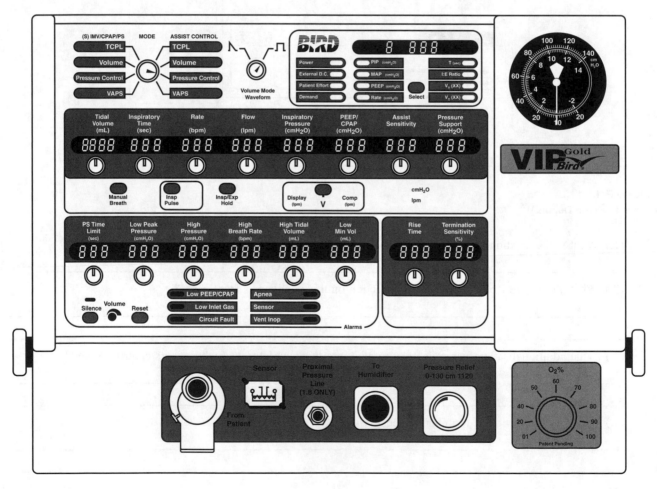

FIGURE 13-2
(Courtesy VIASYS Healthcare, Critical Care Division, Palm Springs, Calif.)

(1.) What is the location of the mode select switch, and how are the modes grouped?

_____

(2.) Which flow waveforms are available during volume-controlled breaths?

_____

(3.) How is the apnea interval determined and set?

_____

_____

_____

_____

_____

(4.) What is rise time and where is the control located on the Gold model?

_____

_____

_____

(5.) What is the difference between assist sensitivity and termination sensitivity on this ventilator?

_____

_____

_____

(6.) How is the bias flow adjusted on this ventilator?

_____

_____

_____

5C. Dräger Babylog 8000 Infant Ventilator — see Figure 13-3:

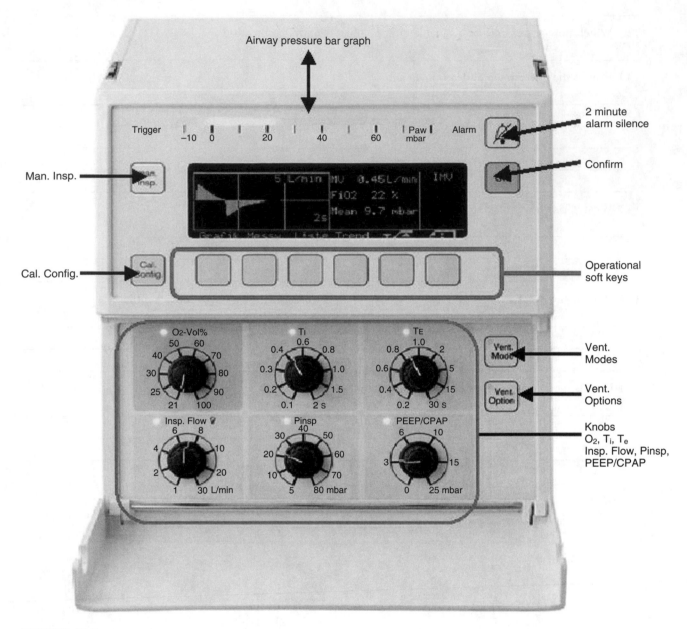

FIGURE 13-3
(Courtesy Dräger Medical AG & Co, Lübeck, Germany.)

(1.) What controls does the rotary dial panel contain?

_____

_____

(2.) What is the function of the soft keys?

_____

(3.) How are alarms silenced and reset on this ventilator?

_____

_____

(4.) Which alarms are set automatically by the ventilator, and what are their settings?

_____

_____

(5.) How are the alarms grouped on this ventilator?

_____

_____

_____

5D. Dräger Babylog 8000 Plus Infant Ventilator — see Figure 13-3:
   (1.) How are the monitoring parameters accessed on this ventilator?

_____

   (2.) How are the pressure-support ventilation and volume guarantee modes accessed on this ventilator?

_____

5E. Bunnell Life Pulse High-Frequency Jet Ventilator — see Figure 13-4.

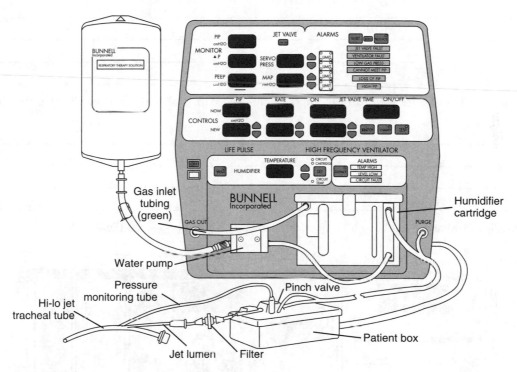

FIGURE 13-4
(Courtesy Bunnell Incorporated, Salt Lake City, Utah.)

(1.) What parameters can be adjusted in the controls area on the front panel?

_____

(2.) What does the jet valve time on/off button represent?

_____

(3.) What three buttons are located on the lower-right portion of the controls area, and what are their functions?

_____

_____

_____

Chapter **13** **Infant and Pediatric Ventilators**

(4.) List and explain the five parameters that are displayed in the monitor area.

_____

_____

_____

_____

_____

_____

(5.) List and explain the alarms located in the alarms area.

_____

_____

_____

_____

_____

_____

_____

(6.) What three buttons are located in the upper right-hand corner of the alarms area? What functions do they serve?

_____

_____

_____

_____

5F. SensorMedics 3100 and 3100A High-Frequency Oscillatory Ventilators — see Figure 13-5:

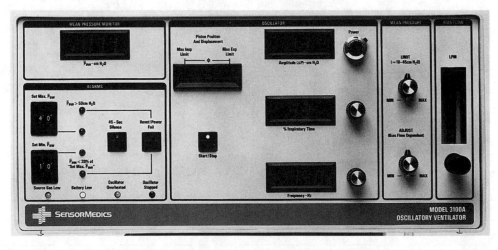

FIGURE 13-5
(Courtesy VIASYS Healthcare, Critical Care Division, Palm Springs, Calif.)

(1.) Describe the function of the flowmeter located to the right on the front panel.

_____

_____

(2.) What are the functions of the mean airway adjust and limit controls?

_____

_____

_____

_____

_____

(3.) Where is the mean airway pressure displayed?

_____

_____

(4.) Describe the function of each control and display in the oscillator section.

_____

_____

_____

_____

_____

_____

_____

_____

_____

_____

(5.) Where is the on/off switch located?

_____

_____

(6.) Describe the two switches in the alarms area.

_____

_____

_____

_____

_____

(7.) What is the difference among the following alarms: "Set Max $\bar{P}$aw", "Set Min $\bar{P}$aw," "$\bar{P}$aw > 50 cm H_2O," "$\bar{P}$aw < 20% of Set Max $\bar{P}$aw"?

_____

_____

_____

_____

_____

_____

_____

_____

_____

_____

_____

_____

_____

_____

_____

_____

_____

_____

_____

(8.) What happens to the ventilator if electrical power is interrupted and then restored?

_____

_____

_____

_____

(9.) If gas pressure fell to below 30 pound-force per square inch gauge (psig), which alarm would become visible?

_____

_____

(10.) At what temperature will the yellow "oscillator overheated" light-emitting diode (LED) become visible?

_____

_____

(11.) What is the function of the yellow "battery low" LED?

_____

_____

5G. SensorMedics 3100B High-frequency Oscillatory Ventilator — see Figure 13-5.

(1.) What controls on the 3100A have been eliminated from the 3100B?

_____

_____

(2.) What are the differences in the alarm limits and function of the 3100B in comparison with those of the 3100A?

_____

_____

_____

_____

(3.) How does the bias flow control differ on the 3100B?

_____

_____

Think About This

What types of ventilators are used with very small animals?

Helpful Web Sites

- Bunnell Incorporated, Life Pulse High-Frequency Jet Ventilator — http://www.bunl.com/jet.html
- Dräger Medical AG & Co, Babylog 8000 plus — http://www.draeger.com
- Mequet, Servo^i Infant Ventilator — http://www.maquet.com
- Puritan Bennett, 840$_{TM}$ with NeoMode Software — http://www.puritanbennett.com
- SensorMedics, 3100B Operator's Manual — http://www.fda.gov
- Cardinal Health, which owns VIASYS Healthcare, AVEA and V.I.P. Bird Gold videos — http://www.viasyshealthcare.com
- Cardinal Health, which owns VIASYS Healthcare/SensorMedics, 3100A High-Frequency Oscillatory Ventilator — http://www.viasyshealthcare.com
- Cardinal Health, which owns VIASYS Healthcare/SensorMedics, 3100B High-Frequency Oscillatory Ventilator — http://www.viasyshealthcare.com

6. Describe the precautions and key troubleshooting points for each nasal CPAP device or ventilator.

6A. Cardinal Infant Flow Nasal CPAP System, AirLife™ nCPAP System Driver, Infant Flow SiPAP, and Fisher & Paykel Bubble CPAP System:

(1.) What are the most likely causes of leaks in any CPAP system?

_____

_____

(2.) What may cause skin irritation and patient discomfort?

_____

_____

(3.) If the rims of a patient's nostrils are blanched, the cause is most likely:

_____.

(4.) What can be done to restore CPAP if the CPAP system is not maintaining the set pressure because the infant's mouth is open?

_____

_____

6B. Cardinal Health V.I.P. Bird Infant/Pediatric Ventilator:

(1.) In the assist/control time-cycled mode, the ventilator's "termination %" setting is flashing. What does this indicate, and what could be its cause?

_____

_____

_____

_____

(2.) What can be done to stop self-triggering when the ventilator is in the volume-cycled synchronized intermittent mandatory ventilation mode?

_____

_____

_____

_____

6C. Cardinal Health V.I.P. Bird Sterling and Gold Infant/ Pediatric Ventilators:

(1.) How can a patient being ventilated with a V.I.P. Bird Gold Ventilator be checked with regard to the presence of auto-PEEP?

_____

_____

_____

_____

_____

6D. Dräger Babylog 8000 and 8000 Plus Infant Ventilators:

(1.) What precautions should be taken when the volume guarantee mode is used on the 8000 Plus Ventilator?

_____

_____

_____

(2.) Name two reasons that the peak pressure, in the volume guarantee mode, might be less than the set Pinsp with no pressure plateau.

_____

_____

_____

_____

6E. Bunnell Life Pulse High-Frequency Jet Ventilator:

(1.) List four possible causes of a decrease in servo pressure.

_____

_____

(2.) List four possible causes of the "cannot meet PIP" (peak inspiratory pressure) alarm.

_____

_____

_____

(3.) _____

_____

(4.) _____

_____

6F. SensorMedics 3100/3100A High-Frequency Oscillatory Ventilators:

(1.) List two alarm situations that would cause the oscillator to stop.

_____

_____

(2.) What immediate action should be taken if the oscillator stops?

_____

_____

(3.) During operation the piston position is noted to have moved toward the maximum inspiratory limit. What action should be taken?

_____

_____

(4.) What could be the cause of the "Set Min Paw" alarm?

_____

_____

6G. SensorMedics 3100B High-Frequency Oscillatory Ventilator:

(1.) List three possible causes for "$\overline{P}aw$ > Set Max Alarm" condition?

_____

_____

_____

(2.) What procedure should be followed after a temporary disconnection, such as for routine suctioning?

_____

_____

_____

_____

_____

_____

6H. Cardinal Health AVEA Ventilator for infant/pediatric use:

(1.) Volumes that are consistently lower than set are being delivered to a pediatric patient, and there is no significant leakage around the endotracheal tube. What is the possible cause of this problem?

_____

_____

6I. Dräger EvitaXL Ventilator for infant/pediatric use:
(1.) Before placing the NeoFlow™ sensor into the circuit, what needs to be done to the sensor?

_____

_____

(2.) What happens to the ventilator if the neonatal flow sensor becomes partially occluded with water or secretions?

_____

_____

_____

_____

_____

_____

6J. Hamilton GALILEO Gold for infant and pediatric use:
(1.) What is the most likely cause of autocycling (self-triggering) during infant use?

_____

_____

(2.) Before beginning ventilation of an infant the "Check Flow Sensor Type" alarm becomes active. What will cause this situation? What action is necessary?

_____

_____

_____

_____

_____

6K. Maquet Servo^i Ventilator for neonatal and pediatric use:
(1.) What action should be taken when there is an audible and visual high-priority alarm with the message "Ventilating in Back-up Mode"?

_____

_____

_____

_____

_____

(2.) What could cause the ventilator to automatically increase the set flow rate during the use of nasal CPAP?

_____

_____

_____

6L. Puritan Bennett 840™ Ventilator for infant/pediatric use:
(1.) Why are low-compliance humidifiers most suitable for pediatric/neonatal use?

_____

_____

(2.) Why is it necessary to run a short self-test when resetting the ventilator for neonatal use?

_____

_____

_____

_____

Think About This

What are your thoughts on the advantages and disadvantages of a respiratory care department having separate infant ventilators versus having general-use ventilators with infant/pediatric capabilities?

Helpful Web Sites

- Bunnell Incorporated, Life Pulse High-Frequency Jet Ventilator — http://www.bunl.com/jet.html
- Dräger Medical AG & Co, Babylog 8000 plus — http://www.draeger.com
- Mequet, Servo^i Infant Ventilator — http://www.maquet.com
- Puritan Bennett, 840$_{TM}$ with NeoMode Software — http://www.puritanbennett.com
- SensorMedics, 3100B Operator's Manual — http://www.fda.gov
- Cardinal Health, which owns VIASYS Healthcare, AVEA and V.I.P. Bird Gold videos — http://www.viasyshealthcare.com
- Cardinal Health, which owns VIASYS Healthcare/SensorMedics, 3100A High-Frequency Oscillatory Ventilator — http://www.viasyshealthcare.com
- Cardinal Health, which owns VIASYS Healthcare/SensorMedics, 3100B High-Frequency Oscillatory Ventilator — http://www.viasyshealthcare.com

NATIONAL BOARD FOR RESPIRATORY CARE (NBRC)—TYPE QUESTIONS

1. The SensorMedics 3100A and 3100B High-Frequency Oscillatory Ventilator has what type of internal mechanism?
   A. Pinch valves
   B. Rotary drive piston
   C. Linear drive piston
   D. Proportional solenoid valves

2. Lowering the frequency setting on the Sensor Medics 3100A or 3100B High-Frequency Oscillatory Ventilator will cause which of the following?
   A. Increased volume
   B. Decrease volume
   C. Decreased piston travel time
   D. Changed percent inspiratory time

3. Which of the following infant ventilators requires a triple-lumen, uncuffed endotracheal tube?
   A. Cardinal Health V.I.P. Bird
   B. Dräger Babylog 8000 Plus
   C. Bunnell Life Pulse High-Frequency Jet Ventilator
   D. SensorMedics 3100A High-Frequency Oscillatory Ventilator

4. During a time-cycled, pressure-limited breath with the Cardinal Health V.I.P. Bird Gold model, a minimum tidal volume may be guaranteed by an automatic increase in which of the following?
   A. Rise time
   B. Flow rate
   C. Inspiratory phase
   D. Inspiratory pressure

5. A neonate requiring mechanical ventilation is being set up on a Dräger Babylog 8000 in the intermittent mandatory ventilation mode. Which combination of inspiratory time and expiratory time will provide a mandatory rate of 45 breaths/min with a ratio of inspiratory time to expiratory time of 1:3?
   A. 0.18 second, 0.55 second
   B. 0.33 second, 1.00 second
   C. 0.50 second, 1.50 second
   D. 0.75 second, 2.25 seconds

6. The continuous positive airway pressure (CPAP) device that can provide bi-level airway pressure for small infants is which of the following?
   A. Hamilton ARABELLA System
   B. Cardinal Health Infant Flow SiPAP™
   C. Cardinal AirLife™ nCPAP (nasal CPAP) System Driver
   D. Fisher & Paykel Healthcare Bubble CPAP System

7. Calculate the maximum available tidal volume for time-triggered, pressure-limited, time-cycled ventilation when inspiratory time is 0.5 second and the flow is set at 7 L/min.
   A. 35 mL
   B. 42 mL
   C. 58 mL
   D. 210 mL

8. Calculate the flow rate to deliver 4 mL/kg volume to a 1250-gram neonate with a 0.75-second inspiratory time.
   A. 0.003 L/min
   B. 0.4 L/min
   C. 3 L/min
   D. 4 L/min

9. Which mode on the Dräger Babylog 8000 Plus should **NOT** be used when there is a significant positional endotracheal tube leak?
   A. CPAP
   B. Pressure-limited SiPAP
   C. Synchronized intermittent mandatory ventilation (SIMV) + volume guarantee
   D. Pressure-limited SIMV

10. Heliox delivery is available through which of the following ventilators?
    A. Dräger Babylog 8000 Plus
    B. Cardinal Health V.I.P. Bird Gold
    C. Cardinal Health AVEA
    D. Maquet Servo[i]

LEARNING OBJECTIVES

Upon completion of this chapter you will be able to:

1. Give the value in liters/minute of the logic flow for the patient-disconnect feature of the Airon pNeuton model A ventilator.
2. Calculate the length of time between a low-battery event and a ventilator-inoperative event with the Bio-Med Crossvent ventilator when there is a power loss.
3. State the value for the gas supply pressure that will result in a low source pressure alarm with the Crossvent 3.
4. Describe the operating features, alarms, and ventilator parameter ranges of the following ventilators: Bio-Med MVP-10, Impact Uni-Vent 750, Pulmonetic Systems LTV 1200, Puritan Bennett LP10, Newport Medical Instruments HT50, and Pulmonetic Systems LTV 950.
5. Compare the alarm functions on the Dräger Oxylog 2000 to those on the Oxylog 3000.
6. Describe the affect of oxygen flow on oxygen delivery in the Dräger Oxylog 3000.
7. Explain the function of the apnea alarm on the Uni-Vent 750.
8. Provide the value for logic gas consumption on the Uni-Vent Eagle™ 754.
9. State the liter flow required to operate the internal logic of the Percussionaire Bronchotron TXP.
10. Review the function of the Smiths Medical Pneupac™ ventiPAC low-pressure "eyeball" alarm.
11. State the method of delivery (i.e., invasive or noninvasive) available with the Dräger Carina™*home* Ventilator.
12. Give the value for the maximum oxygen bleed-in with the Dräger Carina™*home* Ventilator.
13. Discuss the ability of the Newport HT50 to provide enriched oxygen delivery.
14. Describe the adjustment of the positive end-expiratory pressure/continuous positive airway pressure (PEEP/CPAP) control on the HT50 ventilator.
15. Tell how long the internal ventilator battery will operate on the Pulmonetic Systems LTV 800.
16. Name the two operator-adjustable alarms on the Respironics BiPAP Focus™.
17. Explain the possible cause of a discrepancy between the set fractional inspired oxygen (F_IO_2) and the delivered F_IO_2 for the Respironics BiPAP (bilevel positive airway pressure) Vision.
18. Give the patient size limit for the Respironics BiPAP Synchrony ventilator.
19. List the alarms available on the Puritan Bennett GoodKnight 425.

"Life's a voyage that's homeward bound."
Herman Melville

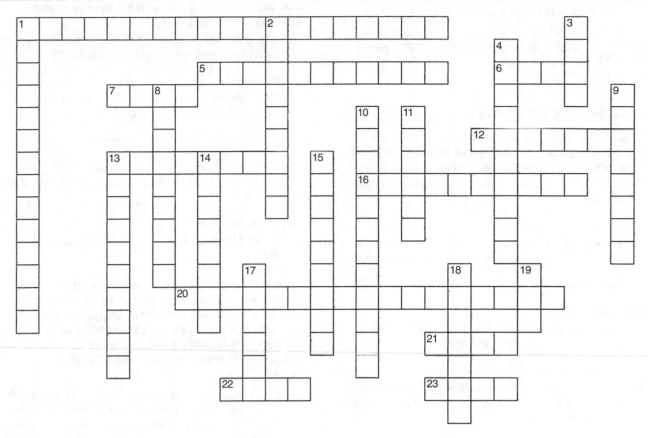

CROSSWORD PUZZLE 14-1
Created using Crossword Weaver, www.CrosswordWeaver.com.

Use the clues to complete the crossword puzzle.

Across

1. When oxygen enters the Pulmonetic Systems LTV 1000, it blends with air in this chamber. (*two words*).
5. A high-frequency flow interruptor ventilator.
6. The peak pressure setting for bilevel ventilation.
7. Positive end-expiratory pressure (PEEP) on a home care ventilator (*abbreviation*).
12. **9 down** needs to be attached to this ventilator
13. Not distal.
16. A type of expiration valve.
20. That which adjusts the incoming gas pressure on the Impact Uni-Vent 750. (*two words*).
21. On the Bio-Med Crossvent, this type of breath is 1.5 times the normal.
22. A mode of ventilation available on the Smiths Medical Pneupac TM VentiPAC transport ventilator. (*abbreviation*).
23. A level 3 alarm.

Down

1. The Crossvent can use this module instead of a blender (*two words*)
2. With the Carina*home* this type of trigger level is recommended for patients with obstructive or restrictive lung disease
3. An alternative to traditional invasive ventilation (*abbreviation*)
4. A _____ leakage valve is used to bleed in oxygen on the Carina*home* ventilator
8. A digital trigger sensitivity system used by the (*two words*)
9. Not an internal PEEP valve.
10. A portable body respirator (*two words*)
11. This ventilator has an oxygen-conserving device called an ir/mix injector.
13. A noninvasive respiratory support device (*two words*

14. A tank respirator (*two words*)
15. A type of patient interface for **3 down** (*two words*)
17. A level 2 alarm
18. This system consumes 4 L/min of extra gas in the MVP-10
19. A level 1 alarm

ACHIEVING THE OBJECTIVES

1. Give the value in liters/minute of the logic flow for the patient-disconnect feature with the Airon pNeuton model A ventilator.

1A. Why does the disconnect alarm require 1 L/min to operate?

_____

1B. How much gas does the pNeuton model A ventilator use for its pneumatically operated control system?

_____

Think About This

Why can a pneumatically operated ventilator be used during magnetic resonance imaging?

Helpful Web Site

- Airon Corporation, pNeuton Models A and S Operating Guides and Model A Training Video — http://www.pneuton.com

2. Calculate the length of time between a low-battery event and a ventilator-inoperative event with the Bio-Med Crossvent Ventilator when there is a power loss.

2A. What is the operational time of a fully charged direct current (DC) battery for the Crossvent?

_____

2B. How much remaining time does the DC battery have when the "Low Battery, Connect External Power" message is displayed on the liquid-crystal graph screen?

_____

Think About This

Why should most ventilators be plugged in even if they are not being used?

Helpful Web Site

- Bio-Med Devices, Inc, homepage — http://www.biomeddevices.com/index.html?intro2.html&3

3. State the value for the gas supply pressure that will result in a low source pressure alarm with the Crossvent 3.

3A. The Crossvent requires how much gas pressure to ensure adequate gas flow to the patient?

_____

3B. What source gas pressure will activate a low source pressure alarm?

_____

Think About This

What sizes of oxygen cylinders are used during flight transports?

Helpful Web Site

- Bio-Med Devices Homepage — www.biomeddevices.com

4. Describe the operating features, alarms, and ventilator parameter ranges of the following ventilators: Bio-Med MVP-10, Impact Uni-Vent 750, Pulmonetic Systems LTV 1200, Puritan Bennett LP10, Newport Medical Instruments HT50, and Pulmonetic Systems LTV 950.

4A. MVP-10:

(1.) List the operating features (i.e., target population, designation, power source, internal gas consumption, battery duration, and modes of ventilation):

_____

_____

_____

_____

_____

_____

(2.) List the alarms:

_____

_____

_____

_____

_____

_____

_____

(3.) List the ventilator parameter ranges:

_____
_____
_____
_____
_____

4B. Uni-Vent 750:
(1.) List the operating features:

_____
_____
_____
_____
_____
_____

(2.) List the alarms:

_____
_____
_____
_____
_____

(3.) List the ventilator parameter ranges:

_____
_____
_____
_____
_____

4C. Pulmonetic Systems LTV 1200:
(1.) List the operating features:

_____
_____
_____
_____
_____

(2.) List the alarms:

_____
_____
_____
_____
_____

(3.) List the ventilator parameter ranges:

_____
_____
_____
_____
_____

4D. LP10:
(1.) List the operating features:

_____
_____
_____
_____
_____

(2.) List the alarms:

_____
_____
_____
_____

(3.) List the ventilator parameter ranges:

_____
_____
_____
_____
_____
_____

4E. HT50:

(1.) List the operating features:

_____

_____

_____

_____

_____

_____

(2.) List the alarms:

_____

_____

_____

_____

_____

_____

(3.) List the ventilator parameter ranges:

_____

_____

_____

_____

_____

_____

4F. LTV 950:

(1.) List the operating features:

_____

_____

_____

_____

_____

_____

(2.) List the alarms:

_____

_____

_____

_____

_____

_____

(3.) List the ventilator parameter ranges:

_____

_____

_____

_____

_____

Think About This

Which of these ventilators is best-suited for a patient with a wheelchair?

Helpful Web Sites

- Bio-Med Devices, Inc, MVP-10 Ventilator Information — http://www.biomeddevices.com
- Pulmonetic Systems, Inc, LTV 1200 Ventilator Information — http://www.pulmoneticsystems.com
- Newport Medical Instruments, HT50 Ventilator Information — http://www.newportnmi.com
- Pulmonetic Systems, Inc, LTV 950 Ventilator Information — http://www.pulmoneticsystems.com
- International Ventilator Users Network, Home Ventilator Guide — http://www.ventusers.org

5. Compare the alarm functions on the Dräger Oxylog 2000 with those on the Oxylog 3000.

_____

_____

_____

_____

_____

_____

_____

_____

_____

_____

_____

_____

_____

_____

_____

_____

Think About This

If a practitioner is with a patient during transport, why should transport ventilators have alarms?

Helpful Web Sites

- Dräger Medical AG & Co, Oxylog 2000 — http://www.draeger.com
- Dräger Medical AG & Co, Oxylog 3000 — http://www.draeger.com

6. Describe the affect of the oxygen flow on oxygen delivery in the Oxylog 3000.

_____

_____

_____

_____

_____

_____

_____

_____

Think About This

How can the Oxylog 3000 deliver fractional inspired oxygen (F_IO_2) between 21% and 40%?

Helpful Web Site

- Dräger Oxylog 3000 — http://www.draeger.com/

7. Explain the function of the apnea alarm on the Uni-Vent 750.

7A. Explain the function of the apnea alarm on the Uni-Vent 750.

_____

_____

_____

_____

_____

_____

Think About This

What are the advantages and disadvantages of automatic apnea alarm settings?

Helpful Web Site

- Impact Instrumentation, Inc, Uni-Vent series information — http://www.impactinstrumentation.com/portable_ventilators.htm

8. Provide the value for logic gas consumption on the Uni-Vent Eagle™ 754.

_____

_____

_____

_____

_____

Think About This

What are the criteria to be included in the Strategic National Stockpile?

Helpful Web Site

- Impact Instrumentation Inc, Uni-Vent series information — http://www.impactinstrumentation.com/portable_ventilators.htm

9. State the liter flow required to operate the internal logic of the Percussionaire Bronchotron TXP.

_____

_____

_____

_____

_____

Think About This

What types of patients would benefit from high-frequency ventilation during transport?

Helpful Web Sites

- Percussionaire Corporation — http://www14.inetba.com/percussionaire/

10. Review the function of the Smiths Medical Pneupac™ ventiPAC low-pressure "eyeball" alarm.

_____

_____

_____

_____

_____

Think About This
How much gas supply should be available during a transport?

Helpful Web Site
■ Smiths Medical, Pneupac™ ventiPAC Ventilator — http://www.smiths-medical.com

11. State the method of delivery (i.e., invasive or noninvasive) available with the Dräger Carina™*home* ventilator.

11A. What types of interfaces can be used with this unit?

_____

_____

11B. What modes of ventilation does this unit offer?

_____

_____

Think About This
What is meant by a seamless transition from hospital to home?

Helpful Web Site
■ Dräger Medical AG & Co, Carina™*home* ventilator — http://www.draeger.com

12. Give the value for the maximum oxygen bleed-in with the Dräger Carina™*home* ventilator.

12A. How can this unit be modified to increase F_IO_2?

_____

_____

_____

12B. How can the F_IO_2 be determined?

_____

_____

_____

_____

_____

Think About This
Which method of supplemental oxygen delivery is appropriate for hospital use of the Carina™*home* ventilator?

Helpful Web Site
■ Dräger Carina™ *home* — www.draeger.com

13. Discuss the ability of the Newport HT50 to provide enriched oxygen delivery.

13A. Describe the function of the air-oxygen entrainment mixer.

_____

_____

_____

_____

13B. How does the oxygen-blending bag kit operate?

_____

_____

_____

_____

_____

Think About This
Which oxygen-delivery system is most appropriate for the hospital and which for the home?

Helpful Web Site
■ Newport Medical Instruments, HT50 ventilator information — http://www.newportnmi.com

14. Describe the adjustment of the positive end-expiratory pressure/continuous positive airway pressure (PEEP/CPAP) control on the HT50 ventilator.

14A. What happens to the sensitivity setting when PEEP is initiated?

_____

_____

14B. What is the range of PEEP available on the HT50?

_____

14C. During pressure-control ventilation with PEEP, what is the maximum amount of PEEP that can be set?

_____

Think About This

Can auto-PEEP occur during home ventilation?

Helpful Web Site

■ Newport Medical — www.newportnmi.com

15. Tell how long the internal ventilator battery will operate on the Pulmonetic Systems LTV 800.

_____

_____

Think About This

Which transport or home care ventilator has the battery with the longest operation time?

Helpful Web Site

■ Cardinal Health, Pulmonetic Systems LTV 800 — http://www.viasyshealthcare.com

16. Name the two operator-adjustable alarms on the Respironics BiPAP (bilevel positive airway pressure) Focus™.

_____

_____

_____

_____

Think About This

It's estimated that more than 12 million American adults have sleep apnea (National Heart, Lung, and Blood Institute).

Helpful Web Site

■ BiPAP Focus™ — http://bipapfocus.respironics.com

17. Explain the possible cause of a discrepancy between the set F_IO_2 and the delivered F_IO_2 for the Respironics BiPAP Vision.

_____

_____

_____

_____

_____

_____

_____

_____

Think About This

Other than those with sleep apnea, what other patients could benefit from BiPAP?

Helpful Web Site

■ BiPAP Vision — http://bipapvision.respironics.com

18. Give the patient size limit for the Respironics Synchrony ventilator.

_____

_____

Think About This

Is it age or weight that dictates whether a person is considered a pediatric patient or an adult patient?

Helpful Web Site

■ BiPAP Synchrony — http://bipapsynchrony. respironics.com

19. List the alarms available on the GoodKnight 425.

_____

_____

Think About This

Getting used to BiPAP or CPAP is like training for an athletic event: the patient needs to work up to it.

Helpful Web Site

■ Puritan Bennett GoodKnight 425 — http://www. puritanbennett.com

1. Transport ventilators' capabilities should include all **EXCEPT** which of the following?
   A. Ability to operate in extreme temperatures
   B. Easily recognizable controls
   C. A full range of modes from which to choose
   D. Sufficient shielding

2. The transport ventilator that can operate up to an altitude of 15,000 feet is:
   A. Airon pNeuton
   B. Bio-Med Crossvent
   C. Dräger Oxylog 3000
   D. Smiths Medical Pneupac™ ventiPAC

3. A 2-kg premature newborn requires transport to a level 3 neonatal unit. The ventilator that needs to be used for this transport is which of the following?
   A. Bio-Med MVP-10
   B. Dräger Oxylog 2000
   C. Impact Uni-Vent 750
   D. Impact Uni-Vent Eagle™ 754

4. During a transport in which the patient is using a ventiPAC ventilator, the respiratory therapist notices the eyeball indicator turning red. The most appropriate action to take at this time is which of the following?
   A. Suction the patient's airway immediately.
   B. Change out the gas supply to the ventilator.
   C. Analyze the oxygen concentration being delivered.
   D. Remove the patient from the ventilator and manually ventilate.

5. The ventilators that can be used invasively or noninvasively in the home are which of the following?
   I. Puritan Bennett LP10
   II. Pulmonetic Systems LTV 800
   III. Dräger Carina™ *home*
   IV. Puritan Bennett GoodKnight 425
   A. I and II only
   B. II and III only
   C. III and IV only
   D. I and IV only

6. A mechanically ventilated home care patient using an LP10 needs an increase in her fractional inspired oxygen (F_IO_2) from 21% to 30%. This can be accomplished by which of the following methods?
   A. Attaching an external blender.
   B. Pulling out the air/mix selector.
   C. Delivering oxygen via the oxygen-enrichment adapter.
   D. Delivering oxygen directly into the rear-panel air-inlet port.

7. The transport ventilator that can deliver respiratory rates up 700 breaths/min is which of the following?
   A. pNeuton
   B. Crossvent
   C. Pneupac™ ventiPAC
   D. Percussionaire Bronchotron TXP

8. An MVP-10 is set to deliver 3 L/min of desired F_IO_2 to a mechanically ventilated patient. Estimate how many minutes an "E" size cylinder with 1900 psi will last.
   A. 34 minutes
   B. 68 minutes
   C. 119 minutes
   D. 159 minutes

9. During a patient transport with the Crossvent, the alarm menu begins to flash "Low Battery, Connect External Power" on the liquid-crystal graph screen. How much internal battery time is left?
   A. 5 minutes
   B. 10 minutes
   C. 15 minutes
   D. 20 minutes

10. The F_IO_2 delivery of the Oxylog 2000 is dependent on which of the following?
    I. Air/mix switch setting
    II. The gas source being used
    III. Attachment of the blending bag kit
    IV. Flow rate of the oxygen bleed into the system
    A. I and II only
    B. II and III only
    C. III and IV only
    D. I and IV only

15 Sleep Diagnostics

Upon completion of this chapter, you will be able to:

1. Describe the various stages of sleep in adults and children.
2. Discuss the physiologic effects of sleep on cardiopulmonary function in healthy individuals.
3. List the measurements most commonly recorded during polysomnography.
4. Summarize the clinical and laboratory criteria used to diagnose obstructive, central, and mixed apnea.
5. Describe various strategies that can be used to monitor arterial oxygen saturation, nasal-oral airflow, and the respiratory effort of patients with obstructive sleep apnea syndrome.
6. Explain the physiologic consequences of obstructive sleep apnea.
7. Name several diseases commonly associated with central sleep apnea.

"People need dreams; there's as much nourishment in 'em as food."
Dorothy Gilman

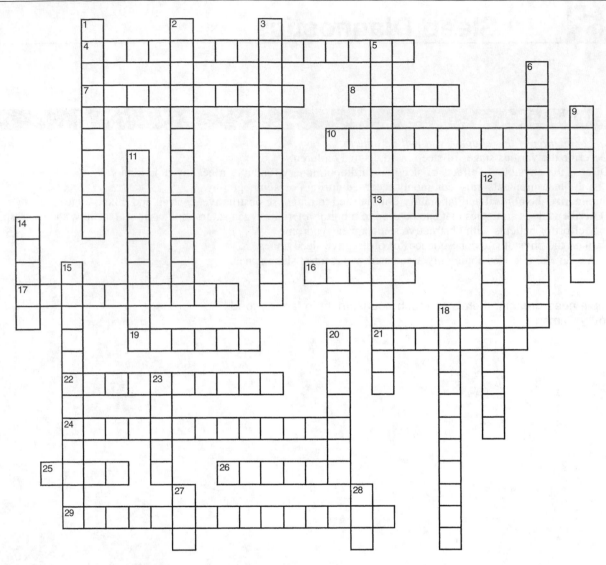

CROSSWORD PUZZLE 15-1
Created using Crossword Weaver, www.CrosswordWeaver.com.

Use the clues to complete the crossword puzzle.

Across

4. A pattern based on a 24-hour cycle (*two words*).

7. The type of apnea characterized by the answer to **13 across** and **15 down** (*two words*).

8. These waveforms are present in stage 1 sleep (*abbreviation*).

10. A device similar in function to the answer of **17 across**.

13. Lack of airflow resulting from occlusion of the upper airways despite continued respiratory efforts (*abbreviation*).

16. These waveforms are the "deep-sleep waves."

17. A device used to measure nasal-oral airflow.

19. The sleep that consists of four stages (*hyphenated*).

21. Spend as much as 75% of their sleep in the answer to **9 down**.

22. The number of periods of not breathing divided by the total number of hours of sleep (*two words*).

24. Waveforms with waxing and waning amplitude that occur at a frequency of 9 to 13 cycles per second (*two words*).

25. These waveforms are the "busy" waves of the brain.

26. A type of obesity characterized by a neck size of >17 inches for men and >16 inches for women.

29. The measurement and recording of variations in airflow, electroencephalograms, electro-oculograms, and arterial blood gases during sleep.

Down

1. Large vertical slow waves with amplitudes of at least 75 μV with an initial negative deflection.
2. This is reduced by approximately 10% during 9 down (*two words*).
3. _____ 10-20 electroencephalographic (EEG) system.
5. Making prolonged electrocardiographic recordings on a portable tape recorder while the patient conducts normal daily activities (*two words*).
6. Cardiac sequelae to a respiratory disorder (*two words*).
9. Sleep periods that last from a few minutes to half an hour; it is during these periods that dreaming occurs.
11. A solution used to secure electrodes to the scalp.
12. An abnormal, repeating pattern of breathing characterized by progressive hypopnea alternating with hyperpnea and ending in a brief apnea.
14. These waveforms are the "drowsy waves" that appear on electroencephalograms when the individual is awake but relaxed and sleepy.
15. The type of apnea characterized by the absence of airflow and respiratory efforts (*two words*).
18. The _____ pattern of breathing occurs when the abdomen and lower rib cage move in opposite directions.
20. A response to sensory stimulation to induce active wakefulness.
23. These waveforms are the "relaxed" waves of the brain.
27. Records eye movements (*abbreviation*).
28. The number of periods of not breathing and shallow breathing divided by the total number of hours of sleep (*abbreviation*).

ACHIEVING THE OBJECTIVES

1. Describe the various stages of sleep in adults and children.

1A. What are the two distinct states of sleep?

_____

1B. What are the electrographic and behavioral differences between these two states of sleep for individuals 12 months of age and older?

_____
_____
_____
_____
_____
_____
_____

1C. Which sleep stage is known as *quiet sleep*?

_____

1D. Which waveforms are present during wakefulness and during the onset of quiet sleep?

_____

1E. Describe the electroencephalographic and electro-oculographic findings during stage 1 of quiet sleep.

_____
_____
_____
_____
_____
_____

1F. How is the transition to stage 2 of quiet sleep identified?

_____
_____
_____
_____
_____

1G. What does the electro-oculogram show during stage 2?

_____

1H. What enables you to distinguish stages 3 and 4 from the other stages?

_____

_____

1I. How are stages 3 and 4 differentiated?

_____

_____

_____

_____

_____

1J. How long do stages 1 through 4 usually last?

_____

1K. Which stages of sleep are known as *slow-wave sleep*?

_____

1L. What type of waveform is present during rapid eye movement (REM) sleep?

_____

_____

_____

_____

1M. Dreams that are remembered occur during which state of sleep?

_____

1N. What is the sleep-stage distribution in normal, healthy adults?

_____

_____

_____

_____

1O. How long does REM sleep usually last during a typical 8-hour period of sleep for a healthy adult?

_____

_____

Think About This

Why do infants spend most of their sleep in REM?

Helpful Web Sites

■ eMedicine from WebMD, "Sleep Stage Scoring," Michael B. Russo — http://www.emedicine.com

■ Missouri University of Science and Technology, Psychology World, "Stages of Sleep" — http://web.mst.edu

2. Discuss the physiologic effects of sleep on cardiopulmonary function in healthy individuals.

2A. During which stages of sleep is a person predisposed to apneic periods?

_____

_____

_____

_____

_____

_____

_____

2B. How does minute ventilation change during non-REM slow-wave sleep?

_____

_____

2C. What happens to the partial pressure of arterial oxygen (PaO_2) and the partial pressure of arterial carbon dioxide ($PaCO_2$) during non-REM slow-wave sleep?

_____

_____

_____

2D. During which sleep stage is there an increase in upper airway resistance?

_____

2E. What effect does sleep have on heart rate and blood pressure?

_____

_____

_____

_____

_____

_____

_____

_____

2F. During which stage of sleep is cardiac output reduction pronounced?

_____

_____

2G. What effect does sleep have on blood vessels?

_____

_____

_____

_____

Think About This
Can sleep disturbances cause permanent cardiovascular problems?

Helpful Web Site
■ *Cardiovascular Research* Journal, "An Update on: Cardiovascular and Respiratory Changes During Sleep in Normal and Hypertensive Subjects," Federico Lombardi and Gianfranco Parati — http://cardiovascres.oxfordjournals.org

3. List the measurements most commonly recorded during polysomnography.

3A. How is cardiac function measured during polysomnography? _____

3B. How are the stages of sleep identified?

_____

3C. What three physiologic parameters of breathing are measured?

_____

_____

3D. What are the most common ways of measuring the parameters answered in Question 3C?

_____

_____

_____

_____

_____

_____

_____

_____

_____

3E. How are arousal responses and movements monitored during polysomnography?

_____

_____

_____

3F. What measurement is used to assess eye movement during polysomnography?

_____

_____

_____

_____

_____

_____

_____

Think About This
Why is continuous video monitoring important during polysomnography?

Helpful Web Sites
■ eMedicine from WebMD, "Polysomnography: Overview and Clinical Application," Carmel Armon et al — http://www.emedicine.com
■ American Association for Respiratory Care, *Respiratory Care* Journal, "AARC Clinical Practice Guideline: Polysomnography" — http://www.rcjournal.com

4. Summarize the clinical and laboratory criteria used to diagnose obstructive, central, and mixed apnea.

4A. What does a patient with obstructive sleep apnea (OSA) typically report?

_____

_____

_____

4B. What are the criteria for the diagnosis of OSA?

_____

_____

_____

_____

_____

_____

319

4C. How can OSA be differentiated from central sleep apnea (CSA)?

_____

_____

_____

_____

4D. How can mixed sleep apnea be differentiated from OSA and CSA?

_____

_____

4E. Identify the type of sleep apnea shown in Figure 15-1.

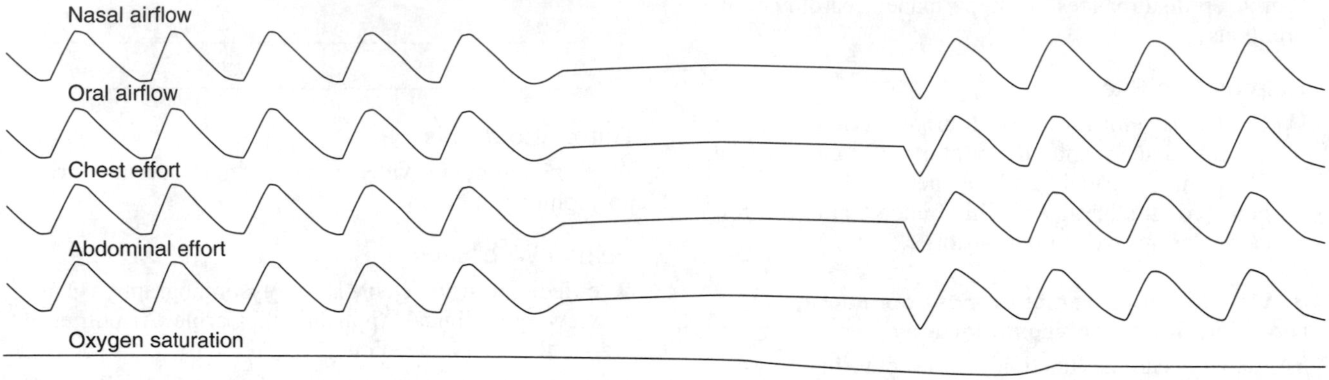

_____

FIGURE 15-1
(Redrawn from Sheldon SH, Spire JP, Levy HB: *Pediatric sleep medicine*, Philadelphia, 1992, WB Saunders.)

4F. What type of individual has the greatest risk for developing OSA?

_____

_____

4G. What other factors increase an individual's risk for OSA?

_____

_____

4H. What factors may augment the symptoms of patients with mild OSA?

_____

_____

Think About This

How is neonatal apnea diagnosed?

Helpful Web Sites

- *Chest* Journal, "Adult Obstructive Sleep Apnea: Pathophysiology and Diagnosis," Susheel P. Patil et al — http://www.chestjournal.org
- eMedicine from WebMD, "Sleep Apnea," M Steffan — http://www.emedicine.com

5. Describe various strategies that can be used to monitor arterial oxygen saturation, nasal-oral airflow, and the respiratory effort of patients with OSA syndrome.

5A. What are the advantages and disadvantages of the three methods that may be used to monitor arterial oxygen saturation during polysomnography, as expressed in the following table?

Method	Advantages	Disadvantages

5B. How is nasal-oral airflow monitored during a sleep study?

_____

_____

_____

5C. What is the most common problem that can occur while nasal-oral airflow is being monitored?

_____

_____

_____

_____

5D. How can respiratory effort be measured during a sleep study?

_____

_____

_____

_____

_____

5E. What equipment can be used to monitor respiratory effort?

_____

_____

_____

_____

_____

_____

_____

Think About This

What role do home sleep studies play in the diagnosis of sleep apnea?

Helpful Web Site

■ WebSciences International, "Value of Monitoring Esophageal Pressure During Polysomnography," R.D. Chervin et al — http://www.websciences.org

6. Explain the physiologic consequences of OSA.

6A. What physiologic consequence of sleep apnea causes "unexplained" nocturnal death?

_____

_____

_____

_____

6B. How do pulmonary hypertension and right-sided heart failure develop from sleep apnea?

_____

_____

_____

_____

6C. Systemic vasoconstriction caused by sleep apnea will cause what clinical feature of sleep apnea?

_____

6D. What are the physiologic causes of excessive daytime sleepiness, personality changes, intellectual deterioration, and behavioral disorders commonly seen in patients with sleep apnea?

_____

_____

_____

_____

6E. Restless sleep in sleep apnea is due to what physiologic consequence?

_____

Think About This
What effect does OSA have on diabetes?

Helpful Web Sites
■ *Journal of Applied Physiology*, "Physiological and Genomic Consequences of Intermittent Hypoxia," Eugene C. Fletcher — http://jap.physiology.org

■ Duval County Medical Society, "Sleep Related Respiratory Disorders: A Review For The Primary Care Physician," Mitchell S. Rothstein — http://www.dcmsonline.org

7. Name several diseases commonly associated with CSA.

7A. What three mechanisms have been suggested as accountable for the cessation of respiratory drive associated with CSA?

_____

_____

_____

_____

7B. Name two neuromuscular diseases that involve respiratory muscles and that are associated with CSA.

_____

_____

7C. What other types of problems are thought to cause CSA?

_____

_____

_____

_____

Think About This
How does sleeping at a high altitude cause CSA?

Helpful Web Sites
■ University of Pennsylvania Health System, *Health Encyclopedia*, Central Sleep Apnea [entry] — http://www.pennhealth.com

■ eMedicine from WebMD, "Central Sleep Apnea," Rahul K. Kakkar — http://www.emedicine.com

NATIONAL BOARD FOR RESPIRATORY CARE (NBRC)–TYPE QUESTIONS

1. The appearance of sleep spindles and K-complexes on a sleeper's electroencephalogram indicates what non–rapid eye movement (REM) sleep stage?
   A. Stage 1
   B. Stage 2
   C. Stage 3
   D. Stage 4

2. The type of electroencephalographic waveform that is indicative of REM sleep is which of the following?
   A. Alpha waves
   B. Beta waves
   C. Delta waves
   D. Theta waves

3. The key to recognizing obstructive sleep apnea when the results of a sleep study are analyzed is which of the following?
   A. No airflow and no respiratory effort
   B. No airflow with increasing respiratory effort
   C. Reduced airflow with minimal respiratory effort
   D. No airflow with no or minimal respiratory effort

4. The physiologic consequences of obstructive sleep apnea include all of the following **EXCEPT**:
   A. Pulmonary edema
   B. Acute hypercapnia
   C. Cardiac arrhythmias
   D. Systemic hypertension

5. For a patient to be diagnosed with sleep apnea, the minimum number of apneic events that have to occur per hour is:
   A. 3
   B. 5
   C. 7
   D. 9

6. During which stage of sleep is the threshold for arousability to respiratory stimuli low?
   A. Non-REM stage 2
   B. Non-REM stage 3
   C. Non-REM stage 4
   D. REM sleep

7. High-voltage, slow-wave electroencephalographic activity, absence of eye movements, and tonic electromyographic activity are present during which of the following sleep stages?
   A. Non-REM stage 2
   B. Non-REM stage 3
   C. Non-REM stage 4
   D. REM sleep

8. During which stage of sleep does breathing normally become irregular?
   A. Non-REM stage 2
   B. Non-REM stage 3
   C. Non-REM stage 4
   D. REM sleep

9. The variables that are measured during a sleep screening are which of the following?
   I. Pulse oximetry oxygen saturation (SpO_2)
   II. Tibialis electromyogram results
   III. Diaphragm electromyogram results
   IV. The results of a Holter monitoring electrocardiogram
   A. I and IV only
   B. I, II, and IV only
   C. II, III, and IV only
   D. II and IV only

10. Which of the following could be a cause of central sleep apnea?
    A. Nuchal obesity
    B. Nasopharyngeal narrowing
    C. Myasthenia gravis
    D. Cor pulmonale